Recurrent Pregnancy Loss

Asher Bashiri • Avi Harlev
Ashok Agarwal
Editors

Recurrent Pregnancy Loss

Evidence-Based Evaluation, Diagnosis and Treatment

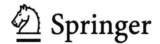

Editors
Asher Bashiri
Director Maternity C and Recurrent
  Pregnancy Loss Clinic
Department of Obstetrics and
  Gynecology
Soroka University Medical Center
Faculty of Health Sciences
Ben-Gurion University of the Negev
Be'er Sheva, Israel

Avi Harlev
Recurrent Pregnancy Loss Clinic
Fertility and IVF Unit
Department of Obstetrics and
  Gynecology
Soroka University Medical Center
Ben Gurion University of the Negev
Be'er Sheva, Israel

Ashok Agarwal
American Center for Reproductive
  Medicine
Cleveland Clinic
Cleveland, OH, USA

ISBN 978-3-319-27450-8   ISBN 978-3-319-27452-2   (eBook)
DOI 10.1007/978-3-319-27452-2

Library of Congress Control Number: 2015960757

Springer Cham Heidelberg New York Dordrecht London
© Springer International Publishing Switzerland 2016

Printed on acid-free paper

Springer International Publishing AG Switzerland is part of Springer Science+Business Media (www.springer.com)

To my father who supported me
To my mother who gave me the spirit
To my children who gave me the power
To my wife who showed me the way
To all my brothers and sisters who were there for me
And to all my mentors who helped me to treat the patients.

-Prof. Asher Bashiri

We dedicate this book to our patients for the privilege of trying our best to learn, diagnose, and treat RPL—a complex medical disorder.

-Asher Bashiri, MD
-Avi Harlev, MD
-Ashok Agarwal, PhD

Foreword

Recurrent pregnancy loss, depending on the definition, affects 2–3 % of all women attempting to get a child, and there are indications that the incidence may be increasing. It spite of its high incidence and the anger and grief that are suffered by the affected couples, the research activity on the topic as measured by the number of publications and presentations at scientific congresses is low compared with the activity in other areas of involuntary childlessness. The result of this relative inactivity is that our knowledge about causes and treatments of recurrent pregnancy loss is limited. Still approximately 1/3 of all patients with recurrent pregnancy loss 5 years after getting the diagnosis have not got the desired child in spite of all what can be offered to them.

It is often stated that in 50 % of couples with recurrent pregnancy loss a cause can be found; however, more correctly I think that in 50 % of couples a risk factor can be found, which is not the same as finding a cause. With all what is known today very few cases of recurrent pregnancy loss are caused by a single pathogenic factor; the vast majority may have a multifactorial background involving the interaction of multiple genetic and environmental risk factors. This complexity renders the research in recurrent pregnancy loss very difficult because you need very large patient and control populations to be able to detect causal factors, the importance of which can be confirmed in other studies, and you need large populations of patients to test therapeutic interventions to be able to detect any effect. Since very few dedicated recurrent pregnancy loss clinics exist, it is difficult to collect the large populations of patients needed for good studies.

Several books about recurrent pregnancy loss have been published in the recent years, and some would pose the question: why publish a new book? Reading a book reviewing a particular disease area has advantages compared with reading the original articles in the area. Because much research in recurrent pregnancy loss is based on small and few studies, there are large "white" areas on the map, and where there is knowledge there is in most cases substantial controversy. A book provides an easily accessible overview on a large research area, and the contributions from various authors can highlight the areas of agreement and areas of controversy.

The book by Bashiri, Harlev, and Agarwal provides an extensive overview of all relevant aspects of recurrent pregnancy loss seen from both the health-care giver's and patient's perspectives. Contributions from prominent researches in the field will focus on both well-known risk factors for recurrent pregnancy loss such as uterine, endocrine, and chromosomal abnormalities but much focus will also be on the fields of genetic and immunological factors associated with recurrent pregnancy loss, since in these areas diagnostic techniques are developing rapidly and new knowledge relating to recurrent pregnancy loss is accordingly accumulating fast. More "soft" topics that have previously often been ignored such as the relevance of lifestyle factors in recurrent pregnancy loss and the importance of understanding and coping with the emotions of the couples suffering from the problem will be extensively dealt with.

The book will be an interesting read for all people meeting and taking care of couples with recurrent pregnancy loss: scientists, physicians, nurses, and midwifes. I hope it will stimulate more high-quality research in the area and improve healthcare givers' skills in managing these often deeply stressed and depressed patients.

Copenhagen, Denmark   Ole B. Christiansen, DMSc
Aalborg, Denmark

Preface

Most current guidelines define recurrent pregnancy loss (RPL) as two or more consecutive pregnancy losses before 20–22 weeks of gestation. Initially, RPL was defined as three consecutive pregnancy losses; however, significant developments in medicine, such as the introduction of low molecular weight heparin, advanced laboratory tests like antiphospholipid antibodies, and advanced imaging modalities including 3D ultrasound, contributed significantly to this change. Thus, we should reconsider the relevant medical developments that influence the definition of RPL, evaluation, and treatment of this specific condition.

Despite the research and the above-mentioned developments, we are still far from understanding the total picture of RPL. More than 50 % of RPL cases are considered unexplained even after a thorough RPL etiology workup. This means that research must be expanded and consist mainly of multicenter trials. This approach will help overcome the methodologic weaknesses of the current studies, which are mostly small study groups that make it difficult to draw valid conclusions.

As a consequence, patients suffering from RPL can be very frustrated, and the inaccessible nature of professional evaluation and treatment due to the very few specialized RPL clinics serves to increase their frustration. This means that most patients will see their general gynecologist, who is not well equipped with all the needs of those patients and unfortunately will not have the chance to refer to clinics that have such knowledge and resources.

The reason for writing the book is to put RPL on the front line of OB-GYN research. Our book consists of the most updated literature on RPL, with chapters written by leading international experts in the field. The primary intended audience is OB-GYN specialists, who can get the best overview on this topic and have all the information necessary to evaluate and treat the patients. Other specialists who could benefit include hematologists, rheumatologists, endocrinologists, immunologists, radiologists, psychiatrists, psychologists, and social workers. The fact that we still have several approaches to some topics means that we still don't have the best answers in all situations, but this book will help to increase awareness of RPL for all specialists in the field, even if they don't treat these patients directly.

We want to thank all the people who contributed to this important book, especially the authors who wrote excellent chapters, the excellent and continuous support from the Springer Editorial team of Michael D. Sova and Kristopher Springer, and lastly the support of our family members.

Beer-Sheva, Israel   Asher Bashiri, MD
Beer-Sheva, Israel   Avi Harlev, MD
Cleveland, OH, USA   Ashok Agarwal, PhD

Contents

Contributors

Ashok Agarwal, PhD Cleveland Clinic, Case Western Reserve University, Cleveland, OH, USA

Asher Bashiri, MD Director Maternity C and Recurrent Pregnancy Loss Clinic, Department of Obstetrics and Gynecology, Soroka University Medical Center, Faculty of Health Sciences, Ben-Gurion University of the Negev, Be'er Sheva, Israel

Neta Benshalom-Tirosh, MD Department of Obstetrics and Gynecology, Faculty of Health Sciences, Soroka University Medical Center, Ben-Gurion University of the Negev, Be're Sheva, Israel

Jamie L. Borick, MD International program, Faculty of Health Sciences, Ben Gurion University of the Negev, Be're Sheva, Israel

David Chitayat, MD, FABMG, FACMG, FCCMG, FRCPC Department of Obstetrics and Gynecology, The Prenatal Diagnosis and Medical Genetics Program, Mount Sinai Hospital, Toronto, ON, Canada

Ole Bjarne Christiansen, PhD, DMSc Fertility Clinic 4071, Rigshospitalet, Copenhagen University Hospital, Copenhagen, Denmark

Department of Obstetrics and Gynecology, Aalborg University Hospital, Aalborg, Denmark

Tullio Ghi, PhD Department of Obstetrics and Gynecology, University of Parma, Parma, Italy

David Gilad, MMedSc Department of Physiology and cell Biology, Joyce and Irwing Goldman Medical school, Ben-Gurion University, Be'er Sheva, Israel

Avi Harlev, MD Recurrent Pregnancy Loss Clinic, Fertility and IVF Unit, Department of Obstetrics and Gynecology, Soroka University Medical Center, Ben Gurion University of the Negev, Be'er Sheva, Israel

Gershon Holcberg, MD, PhD Placental Research Laboratory, Maternity-C Department and High Risk Pregnancy, Faculty of Health Sciences, Soroka University Medical Center, Ben Gurion University of the Negev, Be'er Sheva, Israel

Maor Kabessa Faculty of Health Sciences, Ben Gurion University of Negrev, Be'er Sheva, Israel

Kinue Katano, MD, PhD Department of Obstetrics and Gynecology, Graduate School of Medical Sciences, Nagoya City University, Nagoya, Japan

Tamao Kitaori, MD, PhD Department of Obstetrics and Gynecology, Graduate School of Medical Sciences, Nagoya City University, Nagoya, Japan

Arie Koifman, MD Institute of human genetics, Department of Obstetrics and Gynecology, Soroka University Medical Center, Faculty of Health Sciences, Ben-Gurion University of the Negev, Be'er Sheva, Israel

Astrid Marie Kolte, MD Recurrent Pregnancy Loss Unit, Fertility Clinic 4071, University Hospital Copenhagen, Rigshospitalet, Copenhagen, Denmark

Deepak Kumar Cleveland Clinic, Center for Reproductive Medicine, Cleveland, OH, USA

William H. Kutteh, MD, PhD, HCLD Department of Obstetrics and Gynecology, Vanderbilt University, Memphis, TN, USA

Elisabeth Clare Larsen, MD, PhD Fertility Clinic, Rigshospitalet, Copenhagen University Hospital, Copenhagen, Denmark

Gayatri Mohanty, MPhil Redox Biology Laboratory, Department of Zoology, Ravenshaw University, College Square, Cuttack, India

Henriette Svarre Nielsen, MD, DMSci Fertility Clinic, Rigshospitalet, Copenhagen University Hospital, Copenhagen, Denmark

Yasuhiko Ozaki, MD, PhD Department of Obstetrics and Gynecology, Graduate School of Medical Sciences, Nagoya City University, Nagoya, Japan

Angel Porgador, PhD National Institute for Biotechnology in the Negev, Ben Gurion University of the Negev, Be'er Sheva, Israel

Iris Raz, CNM, MHA Department of Obstetrics and Gynecology, Faculty of Health Sciences, Soroka University Medical Center, Ben-Gurion University of the Negev, Be'er Sheva, Israel

Luna Samanta, PhD Redbox Biology Laboratory, Department of Zoology, Ravenshaw University, Cuttack, Odisha, India

David Segal, MD Division of Obstetrics and Gynecology, Faculty of Health Science, Soroka University Medical Center, Ben-Gurion University of the Negev, Be'er Sheva, Israel

Avishai Shemesh The Shraga Segal Department of Microbiology, Immunology and Genetics, Ben Gurion University of the Negev, Be're Sheva, Israel

Naama Steiner, MD Recurrent Pregnancy Loss Clinic, Department of Obstetrics and Gynecology, Soroka Medical Center, Be're Sheva, Israel

Mayumi Sugiura-Ogasawara, MD, PhD Department of Obstetrics and Gynecology, Graduate School of Medical Sciences, Nagoya City University, Nagoya, Japan

Dan Tirosh, MD Department of Obstetrics and Gynecology, Faculty of Health Sciences, Soroka University Medical Center, Ben-Gurion University of the Negev, Be're Sheva, Israel

Hildee Weiss Beachwood, OH, USA

David Yohai, MD Department of Obstetrics and Gynecology, Soroka Medical Center, Ben Gurion University of the Negev, Be're Sheva, Israel

Hanna Ziedenberg, PhD Nursing Department, Faculty of Health Sciences, Recanati School for Community Health Professions, Ben-Gurion University of the Negev, Kibutz Beet Kama, Israel

Part I

Introduction to Recurrent Pregnancy Loss

Recurrent Pregnancy Loss: Definitions, Epidemiology, and Prognosis

Asher Bashiri and Jamie L. Borick

Introduction

Originally, RPL was termed habitual abortion and was defined as three or more consecutive miscarriages before 20 weeks gestation [1]. Due to an increasing number of childless couples, the improved availability of diagnostic tests, and most importantly the minimal difference in the prognostic value between two and three losses, the ASRM updated the definition of RPL to 2 or more clinical pregnancies losses documented by either ultrasonography or approved in a histopathologic examination [2].

Approximately 15 % of all clinically recognized pregnancies in women less than 35 years old result in spontaneous miscarriage [3]. If RPL is due to chance alone, then it would occur in 2.25 % of couples with two losses, or in 0.34 % of couples with three losses. Yet, it is seen in 5 % of couples with two or more losses and in 1–2 %

of those with three or more losses. These findings suggest that most RPL is not due to chance alone and should be investigated clinically [4, 5].

The prognosis for couples with RPL is not determined by a single parameter, but by the specific characteristics and risk factors of each couple. The circumstances of previous losses, past medical history, maternal age, as well as emotional factors affecting the couple. These and other details are particularly important for the clinician's construct of both the investigative plan and the treatment approach. In the following chapter, we aim to review the factors contributing to RPL prognosis in order to develop a multifaceted approach to tailor an individual approach for patients.

Misleading Numbers and Inconclusive Studies: Epidemiological Issues

Different definitions of recurrent pregnancy loss, or recurrent miscarriage, are currently employed by various societies on reproduction around the world. The Royal College of Obstetricians and Gynaecologists (RCOG) and the European Society of Human Reproduction and Embryology (ESHRE) define recurrent miscarriage as three or more consecutive losses before 24 weeks gestation [1, 6], while ASRM defines RPL as two previous losses [2]. These differences affect the incidence and prevalence of RPL in countries using different guidelines and lead to a different

A. Bashiri, MD
Director Maternity C and Recurrent Pregnancy Loss Clinic, Department of Obstetrics and Gynecology, Soroka Medical Center, Faculty of Health Science, Ben Gurion University of the Negev, 84101 Be'er Sheva, Israel
e-mail: abashiri@bgu.ac.il

J.L. Borick, MD (✉)
International program, Faculty of Health Sciences, Ben Gurion University of the Negev, Be're Sheva, Israel
e-mail: borickj@post.bgu.ac.il

© Springer International Publishing Switzerland 2016
A. Bashiri et al. (eds.), *Recurrent Pregnancy Loss*, DOI 10.1007/978-3-319-27452-2_1

approach to the subgroup of couples with two previous losses. Although the ASRM defines recurrent pregnancy loss as two losses before 20 weeks gestation, they suggest using this definition to initiate primary investigation of couples while including only couples with three or more previous losses in clinical studies [2]. This, however, has not been followed universally.

Recently, the validity of RPL as a clinical entity has been questioned. High success rates of subsequent pregnancies, high percentages of unexplained etiology, and a general lack of causation due to the difficulty in conducting proper studies are the major role players weighing into this discussion [7]. These factors may be attributed to trouble obtaining correct epidemiological values and inconsistencies in measurements across studies. For example, the estimated prevalence of RPL in the general population varies. This is often due to inconsistencies in determining the populations that belong in the numerator and denominator. The numerator may include women with two or more or three or more miscarriages. This number is affected by the gestational age in which a pregnancy is diagnosed, since the earlier the pregnancy is diagnosed the more miscarriage will be diagnosed as well [8]. Furthermore, the denominator is often framed in different terms. It can include the number of women at a specific time point who may be at risk of RPL, all women of childbearing age, or all women regardless of age [5]. These different options of defining the denominator have implications in determining the incidence and prevalence of RPL and may account for the variations observed in the literature.

The various definitions of pregnancy diagnosis also leave room for epidemiological inconsistencies. Biochemical pregnancy is defined as a pregnancy with documented elevation of HCG levels that has not been visualized by ultrasonography [9]. However, the ASRM officially requires the pregnancy to be diagnosed and documented either by ultrasound or histology [2]. Therefore, biochemical pregnancy losses are not included as previous pregnancy failures in the couple's history. Since biochemical pregnancy losses were reported to occur in up to 60 % of cases, by

chance alone, 20 % of women with biochemical pregnancies will have three losses [8]. Additionally, it has been suggested that women with RPL tend to check and diagnose their pregnancies earlier, leading to higher rates of recognized loss in this group compared to the general population [10]. As a result, biochemical pregnancies are not counted as pregnancy losses. Conversely, recent studies emphasize the prognostic value of a couple with a history of biochemical pregnancies and pregnancies of unknown location (also termed non-visualized pregnancies) [11, 12]. Moreover, non-visualized pregnancy loss in a woman with two or more clinically diagnosed miscarriages decreases the relative risk of having a live birth by 10 % [1].

Maternal Age and Its Link to Aneuploidy

Age is the most significant factor determining prognosis for live birth [13]. As a woman ages, the cellular mechanisms that govern the meiotic spindle formation and function have a higher rate of error. It is estimated that 30 % of embryos are aneuploid in 40-year-old women. This increases to 50 % at the age of 43, and approaches 100 % after 45 years of age [14]. Anderson et al. [15] reported that the risk of a spontaneous abortion increases from 8.9 % at the ages of 20–24 to 74.7 % after the age of 44, and that the risk rose most significantly at the age of 35. The study also found that the risk for spontaneous abortion was associated with the number of previous miscarriages, but maternal age was found to be an independent risk factor [15]. It should be noted that although the risk rises more steeply starting at 35 years, significant effects of age were observed only after 40 years of age [16]. Indeed, RPL occurs by chance alone one hundred times more frequently in women aged 40–44 compared to the 20–24 year olds [10]. Clearly seen in Fig. 1.1, women with RPL have a poorer prognosis as age increases.

Some studies suggest that poorer prognosis for live birth after the age of 35 is directly linked to diminished ovarian reserve (DOR). In a study

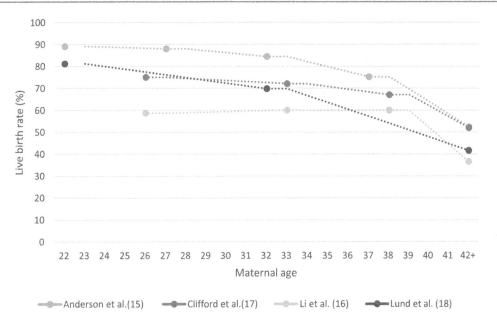

Fig. 1.1 Trend lines demonstrate that as maternal age increases, live birth rate decreases, with a sharp decline at ~40 years. Ages are medians of ranges given in the literature

of patients with DOR undergoing IVF, Levi et al. [19] not only found higher rates of RPL in older patients (>40 compared to 35–40 and <35) but also found higher rates of recurrent miscarriage in patients with elevated FSH levels reflecting DOR in each of the age groups. They further reported that higher rates of aneuploidy were found in embryos of patients with RPL compared with those who did not have RPL [19]. This is consistent with other studies indicating that abnormal FSH and estradiol levels are associated with RPL and aneuploidy [20, 21]. Furthermore, infertility or subfertility could also play a role in the high rates of miscarriage at increased ages, but this will be discussed in more detail further on [22].

Aneuploidy is a significant cause of fetal loss and is directly linked to advanced maternal age (AMA). It accounts for approximately 50 % of first trimester abortions, 30 % of second trimester abortions, and 3 % of stillborn births [14]. Trisomy is the most common cause of aneuploidy by far, followed by other polysomies and structural anomalies inherited from parental anomalies.

The rate of aneuploidy in the products of conception from couples with RPL compared to the general population is debatable. Table 1.1 summarizes previous studies reports. Generally, we can conclude that fetal aneuploidy is positively associated with AMA [25, 26] and unexplained RPL [15], while it is negatively associated with the number of previous miscarriages [24, 27, 28].

Poor placentation and implantation failure are also associated with AMA. Higher rates of perinatal complications including preterm birth, stillbirth, and infertility as well as increased comorbidities including diabetes, obesity, and hypertension have been reported [29]. The increased complication rates of AMA could potentially lead to RPL in women who postpone their reproductive lives.

Karyotyping the Products of Conception

Karyotyping the products of conception (POC) after the second miscarriage may provide reassurance to the couple as unknown etiologies tend to provoke more stress. Suigura-Ogasawara et al. [30] found that of the 70 % of couples with unexplained RPL, 41 % had abnormal karyotype in

Table 1.1 The rate of aneuploidy in RPL patients compared to the general population

	Type of study	Number of cases	% aneuploidy in RPL	Rate of aneuploidy compared to the general population	Caveats
Carp et al. [20]	Retrospective analysis	126	29 %	Lower	Only used in patients with three or more miscarriages
Li et al. [16]	Retrospective, observational analysis	105	32.4 %	Similar	
Ogasawara et al. [24]	Retrospective analysis	234	51.3 %	Similar	Abnormal karyotypes were less common as number of miscarriages increased
Marquard et al. [25]	Retrospective cohort study	50	78 % (>35 years old)	Higher	Patients with AMA were used
Stephenson et al. [26]	Prospective cohort study	197	40 % (>35 years old), 64 % (<35 years old)	Similar	
Stern et al. [27]	Retrospective analysis	94	57 %	Similar	Abnormal karyotypes were less common as number of miscarriages increased
Sullivan et al. [28]	Retrospective analysis	122	25.4 %	Lower	

their subsequent pregnancy (see Fig. 11.1 in Chap. 11). This not only gives couples a reason for their miscarriage but it also increases the probability that their recurrent loss was due to chance alone, providing them reassurance to a live birth in their future pregnancy. Additionally, it may be more cost effective, with an average savings of $524 per couple, to analyze the POC before performing a standard work-up after two losses, especially in women >35 years old [31].

The Numbers Matter

The number of previous miscarriages is an important prognostic factor. Demonstrated in Fig. 1.2, as the number of miscarriages increases, the prognosis worsens [16–18, 30]. Li et al. [16] found that live birth rate was 64 % in couples with two miscarriages, but as low as 43.2 % in women with six or more miscarriages. Additionally, Lund et al. [18] found a 71.9 % success rate after 5 years in women with three previous

losses versus 50.2 % success after six or more losses. Using a 5-year follow-up instead of risk per pregnancy is a beneficial estimate of success for patients because it approximates the overall outcome of having a child [18].

Maternal age must also be taken into account when developing a prognosis based on the number of previous miscarriages. The prospect for a live birth is dually affected as the quantity of miscarriages increases in couples with RPL because subsequent pregnancies occur at a later maternal age. Brigham et al. found that in 20-year-old women, the live birth rate after two miscarriages was 92 %, and 85 % after 5 miscarriages. These figures decreased to 77 % in 35-year-old women with two previous losses, and 62 % after five losses. At age 45, the numbers were much lower with a 60 % success rate after two losses, and 42 % after 5 losses [13].

Although the prognosis decreases as the number of miscarriages increases, it is important to reiterate that even women in their early forties with 5 or more losses still achieve a live birth rate

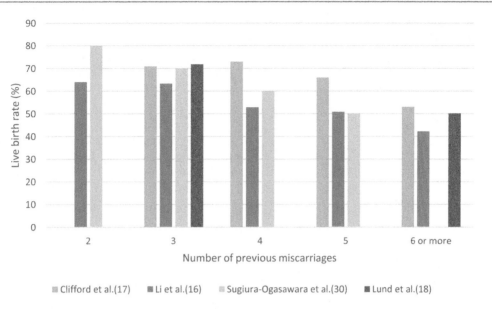

Fig. 1.2 Our figure shows that across studies, the live birth rate decreases as the number of previous miscarriages decreases

of anywhere from 42 to 53 % [13]. Besides advising them about their worse prognosis, couples with five or more losses may warrant a different evaluation. As of now, all couples are evaluated in the RPL clinic equally, whether they are after two miscarriages or six. There is no literature that addresses this issue, but we suggest that further studies are needed for this subgroup to determine the most effective diagnostic evaluation and treatment available.

Two vs. Three

There are few implications in changing the definition of RPL from three or more to two or more losses. A small difference (30 vs. 33 %) in the index pregnancy of two as opposed to three pregnancy losses strongly supports the evaluation after two losses in order to provide the best outcome to couples [32].

Jaslow et al. [33] found no statistically significant differences in diagnostic factors identified in 1020 women with two losses versus three or more. Additionally, according to Bashiri et al. [4], there are no statistically significant differences in outcome for patients with primary RPL who had

two versus three pregnancy losses. The study found there were higher levels of TSH in women with three versus two pregnancy losses (16.3 vs. 2.6 %, $p=0.033$), and subsequent spontaneous pregnancy occurred more frequently in women with three pregnancy losses (91.7 vs. 77.4 %, $p=0.011$). Low molecular weight heparin (LMWH) therapy was also used more in women with three or more losses (40.3 vs. 18.6 %, $p=0.016$), and there were higher rates of chronic disease, unemployment, and consanguinity. Brigham et al. [13] also found no statistical differences between couples with 2 or more or 3 or more idiopathic miscarriages. Furthermore, Bhattacharya et al. [34] found that there was no statistical difference between two, three, and even four losses in estimating future pregnancy outcome in 143,595 pregnancies adjusted for maternal age, year of pregnancy, and smoking history.

The change in definition of RPL has led to earlier evaluation of couples with RPL in order to seek out an etiology. This shift raises two important considerations. First, some reviews evaluating the epidemiology of RPL struggle with the inclusion of patients with two losses because of the higher likelihood that the RPL is due to chance.

As the number of miscarriages increases in a couple, the likelihood of the couple having an underlying cause increases and as a result, successful treatment reported in trials also increases. The second consideration involves a cost-benefit analysis, although this is beyond the scope of this review.

Primary vs. Secondary RPL

Primary RPL is defined as pregnancy loss with no previous live births, while secondary RPL refers to women with pregnancy loss and at least one live birth [35]. It has been suggested that secondary RPL couples make up 40–61 % of all people with RPL [35, 36]. Although some studies have found differences in couples with primary versus secondary RPL, the implications for the two groups remain to be seen.

Christiansen et al. [5] suggested that primary RPL may involve an innate immunological process after compiling data that found higher rates of thrombophilia, NK cell activity, and the effectiveness of allogenic lymphocyte immunization in primary RPL. Conversely, while secondary RPL may be linked more strongly to adaptive immunity, suggesting there are higher rates of antipaternal antibodies, HLA-DR3, and effectiveness of treatment with IVIg in secondary compared to primary RPL. The effectiveness of immunomodulating treatment will be discussed in a later chapter. However, these findings are currently more motivating for research opportunities.

Alternatively, Bashiri et al. [35] determined that there were no statistically significant prognostic differences in couples with primary versus secondary RPL in terms of live births (75.9 and 70.9 %, $p = 0.262$, respectively). However, higher pregnancy complications were observed in women with primary RPL such as preterm delivery, fetal growth restriction, and gestational diabetes mellitus after adjustment for age and gravidity. All diagnostic laboratory results were comparable in primary and secondary RPL patients, except for more cases of elevated prolactin in maternal blood. Most studies have agreed that there is no statistical difference [13,

16, 17, 37], and therefore, patients with primary and secondary RPL can be advised and evaluated in the same manner, although women with RPL should be monitored closely for obstetric complications.

While there is no difference in the evaluation of couples with primary versus secondary RPL, we often encounter unique circumstances in our clinic. In our area we have two special communities, the Ultra-Orthodox Jewish and the Bedouins. Both communities are characterized by families having 5–10 or more children. Couples are referred to the RPL clinic with secondary RPL after having 3, 4, and even 5 children. We desire to provide them with the counsel that they seek, but we struggle to prioritize these couples due to the limited time and resources in our publicly funded clinic, with a long queue of primary RPL couples. So far, our policy has been to perform a full patient history, discuss their prognosis, and advise them to continue to attempt to conceive. Then, if they insist on a further evaluation, we provide them the full evaluation. The logic behind this approach is that there is a possibility of acquiring pathology such as antiphospholipid syndrome, hypothyroidism, and uncontrolled diabetes.

Infertility and Superfertility

Infertility, defined as the inability to conceive after 1 year of regular intercourse without the use of contraceptives, has a negative impact on an RPL couple's prospects of having a live birth [38]. Li et al. [16] found that those with RPL and a history of infertility had a lower live birth rate than those without (50.6 and 61.3 %). Additionally, women with infertility have reported a higher rate of fetal loss, with an odds ratio of 3.92 [38]. Studies supporting these results suggest that many infertile women are unknowingly having repeated early miscarriages [39]. Infertile women also continue attempting conception at an older age, which may contribute to their increased risk [22].

On the other hand, superfertility has also been associated with RPL. It is described as a monthly fecundity rate of >60 % (normal: ~20 %) [40],

Fig. 1.3 Etiology of RPL

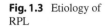 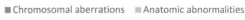

■ Unexplained   ■ Chromosomal aberrations   ■ Anatomic abnormalities
■ Endocrine   ■ Antiphospholipid syndrome

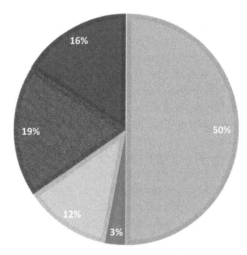

and the pathophysiology is attributed to dysregulation of the endometrium that allows implantation after the optimal window. Superfertile women conceive very easily but have complicated pregnancies and RPL [41] due to poorer placentation and more apparent pregnancy loss. Although it has not been described as a known etiology, superfertility is a new frontier of RPL that will be discussed later in this book.

Gestational Age

Gestational age is an important part of the couple's history, as timing of previous losses could point to different etiologies. The majority of pre-clinical miscarriages are due to aneuploidy (70 %) [42] while thrombophilia and cervical incompetence are more causes of second trimester loss [43]. Still, no etiology is restricted to a certain gestational age, and every couple with RPL deserves a complete work-up.

Additionally, knowledge of the gestational age in the current pregnancy will provide reassurance as it advances. Detection of the fetal heartbeat confers the most reassurance for a live

birth, since pregnancy loss occurs in only 2–6 % of women without RPL after fetal heartbeat detection [45]. This important finding should be visualized at 6 weeks gestation the latest [44]. It is thought that a couple with RPL has a three to five times higher chance of miscarriage after seeing a fetal heartbeat than the general population [14], as couples with RPL lose their pregnancy after a detected fetal heartbeat in 10.2–32 % of cases [45]. However, even if a fetal heartbeat is not determined around 6 weeks gestation, a repeat scan is indicated after 7 or more days before diagnosing an abortion [44].

RPL Etiology

Many entities have been examined to determine the source of RPL, but few have been significant enough to warrant investigation in all couples. Figure 1.3 demonstrates the proportions in which the etiologies contribute to RPL—parental chromosomal aberrations, uterine anomalies, endocrine abnormalities, autoimmune disorders, and thrombophilias. The next few sections discuss the known etiologies and the prognosis for patients who fall into these categories.

Parental Chromosomal Aberrations

Parental chromosomal anomalies account for 2–4 % of RPL in couples [32]. However, in unpublished data, Bashiri et al. have found a higher rate of chromosomal rearrangements at 11 % in an analysis of their patient database karyotyping approximately 500 couples. Translocations are the most common aberrations, followed by inversions, insertions, and mosaicism [32]. In light of its frequency and causality, the ASRM recommends chromosomal analysis of both partners during their initial evaluation [3]. Factors that have been associated with a higher likelihood of chromosomal aberrations include RPL in first-degree relatives and early age of onset of RPL [46]. The prognosis for couples with chromosomal abnormalities is difficult to express, with cumulative live birth rates ranging from 55 to 83 % for natural conception [3, 47, 48].

Couples with an abnormal karyotype can be advised to continue attempting pregnancy or they may be offered preimplantation genetic diagnosis (PGD). Continual attempts to conceive improve the chances of eventually having a child. Although the likelihood of miscarriage is higher for carriers, the prognosis for a live child is similar to those without aberrations [46].

Preimplantation genetic testing encompasses both screening and diagnostic measures and is currently the only intervention available to prevent pregnancy loss due to aneuploidy and chromosomal aberrations. PGD is a diagnostic tool for parents with known genetic anomalies. It has been found to reduce the rate of miscarriage in parents with structural chromosomal aberrations once they have become pregnant, but its ability to provide a better outcome for live birth compared to natural conception over time is controversial [49]. ESHRE determined that patients undergoing PGD for chromosomal abnormalities had the lowest pregnancy rate of all groups undergoing PGD, at less than 30 % per transfer. This was attributed to the concomitant infertility or subfertility in these patients [50] and the method used to detect healthy embryos. However, once pregnancy was achieved, women with chromosomal abnormalities had a live birth rate of 83 % in one clinical trial [51]. It is thought that a new method using microarray to determine healthy embryos will be more effective, but committees have not yet made recommendations [49]. Preimplantation genetic screening (PGS) is used largely for detecting aneuploidy and is reserved for patients with advanced maternal age, repeated implantation failure, and unexplained recurrent miscarriage. However, 11 studies have shown no benefit of PGS in terms of live birth. Moreover, PGS was suggested to negatively impact the pregnancy rate compared to natural conception in women with unexplained RPL [49, 50, 52]. Accordingly, a report by the American College of Obstetricians and Gynecologists (ACOG) concerning PGS does not support its use for AMA, recurrent unexplained miscarriage, or recurrent implantation failures [53].

Anatomic Abnormalities

Anatomic abnormalities cause 10–15 % of all RPL cases [32]. Septated uterus is the most common congenital abnormality, accounting for approximately 55–66 % of all uterine abnormalities in women with RPL [54]. Bicornuate and unicornuate make up the remaining 33 % of congenital anomalies. Acquired malformations that may contribute to RPL include polyps, fibroids, and intrauterine adhesions [54, 55]. The prevalence of uterine anomalies is approximately 3 times higher in those with RPL compared to the general population (12.6 and 4.3 %, respectively) [3]. Sugiura-Ogasawara et al. [56] found a live birth rate of untreated women with either a septated or bicornuate uterus of 59.5 %, with a cumulative birth rate of 78 %. These findings vary from others due to the fact that the septated and bicornuate uterus were combined in the study and usually treatment for a bicornuate uterus is not offered. For those with a septated uterus who wish to undergo treatment or continue to have pregnancy loss after diagnosis, hysteroscopic septectomy is offered although no randomized control trials have been performed to evaluate the effectiveness of treatment [57]. Nevertheless, Grimbizis et al. [58] performed a review of

9 retrospective and observational studies and found a cumulative live birth rate of 83.2 %, while another review of 18 retrospective trials have found an overall live birth rate of 45 % after hysteroscopic septectomy [59]. These two seemingly contradictory studies may represent the outcomes in different general groups of women. While Grimbizis et al. reviewed articles with some unspecified birth histories, Nouri et al. used articles that included women with complicated histories including infertility and RPL [58, 59]. Still, hysteroscopic septectomy should be discussed and offered to patients who have a history of RPL and a septate uterus due to its association with increased birth weight and decreased preterm delivery [60]. Unicornuate has the worst prognosis, with a live birth rate of 43.7 % with no available recommended surgical intervention [61].

Intrauterine adhesions (IUA) are also associated with RPL. Women with previous miscarriages have an increased risk of IUA, with a prevalence of 19–24 %, and an odds ratio of 1.99 in women with 2 or more miscarriages compared to one previous miscarriage [62, 63]. Although no previous studies have shown a poorer prognosis for women with RPL after repeated dilation and curettage, this may be a topic worth investigating due to its potential complications since a live birth rate of 71–88 % was found in women with IUA after treatment and a miscarriage rate of 26–30 % in untreated women [63, 64].

Lastly, it remains unclear if fibroids are associated with spontaneous miscarriage, although the size and location of the fibroids are important for prognosis determination [32]. Submucosal fibroids sized 5 cm or greater are more predictive of RPL and infertility, while intramural and subserosal remain to be associated with RPL [55, 65]. Saravelos et al. [66] found that women with RPL have a higher prevalence of fibroids than women with infertility. They suggest that women with repeated second trimester losses should be evaluated for fibroids and undergo myomectomy if present. It has been shown that myomectomy increases the chance of a successful pregnancy from 57 to 93 % [56], and should be considered in women with fibroids. See Chap. 7 for a further description of uterine anomalies.

Endocrine Abnormalities

Endocrine abnormalities affect both the implantation and maintenance of an embryo, and are the source of 17–20 % of all RPL [32]. Diabetes mellitus (DM) must be evaluated in patients with RPL using HbA1C, since uncontrolled DM increases the risk for fetal loss [3]. However, once controlled, DM is no longer a risk factor for RPL. Insulin resistance has been found at higher rates in women with RPL in the early stages of their pregnancy, with insulin resistance observed in 27 % of women with RPL compared to 9.5 % in the general population [67]. Zolghadri et al. [68] found that women with RPL had a higher prevalence of abnormal results in their glucose tolerance tests (17.6 % compared to 5.4 % of women without RPL). Furthermore, they found that those with abnormal glucose tolerance had better outcomes when taking metformin than those untreated, with an abortion rate of 15 and 55 % respectively. Therefore, these studies suggest insulin resistance is an important factor in RPL that warrants screening and treatment, although committee recommendations of this nature have not been made [67–69].

Overt hypothyroidism is seen in 0.2 % of pregnancies and subclinical hypothyroidism (SCH) is seen in 2–3 % [70]. All women with RPL should have their TSH levels monitored [3]. Although lowering the upper limit of a normal TSH level in pregnancy from 5.0 to 2.5 has been discussed, no conclusion in this matter has been made [71]. Pregnant women with known hypothyroidism must be monitored closely, as the rate of fetal loss is estimated to be 31 % in untreated women compared to 4 % in well-treated women [72]. Women with RPL have been found to have higher rates of hypothyroidism (10.5 %) and SCH (19 %) [73]. Furthermore, patients with SCH have been found to have higher rates of RPL [74]. A study by Benhadi et al. [75] of almost 2500 women showed that higher TSH levels were positively correlated with higher rates of pregnancy loss. Given the evidence that SCH may be associated with adverse outcomes, the Endocrine Society recommends that women with SCH are treated with T_4 regardless of their thyroid antibody titers [76].

Thyroid autoimmunity has been directly linked with RPL [77], and 22–37 % [76] of women with RPL have positive thyroid antibodies (Tg-Ab or TPOAb), with as many as 10 % being thyroid antibody positive despite euthyroidism [74]. Kaprara et al. [78] reviewed 14 studies which found higher rates of miscarriage groups with thyroid antibodies compared to those without, with statistical significance in 10 out of 14. Additionally, 9 studies detected higher rates of auto-antibodies in groups with RPL compared to those without RPL, with statistical significance in 6 out of 9 [78]. Interestingly, high titers have not been shown to correlate with worse outcome than lower titers [70]. Levothyroxine is given for the treatment of autoimmune hypothyroidism [75]. Treatment for euthyroid women with positive thyroid antibody titers is not recommended [76], although levothyroxine has been shown in three studies to decrease fetal loss in thyroid antibody positive women [79–81].

The actual prevalence of PCOS in patients with RPL is not known, although Hudecova et al. [82] found similar live birth and miscarriage rates in both groups in a long-term follow-up. There is no correlation between PCOS and a high aneuploidy rate [82], and ultrasonographic polycystic ovaries and abnormal luteinizing hormone levels were not predictive of future miscarriage [84]. Although PCOS is not directly linked to RPL, hyperandrogenism, obesity, and hyperinsulinism are common sequelae in PCOS and have also been found in higher rates in women with RPL [81, 82].

Luteal phase defects have been studied for RPL and their association with endometrial dysfunction. However the lack of diagnostic criteria made the effects of varying luteal phase hormones on pregnancy impossible to quantify [83]. Therefore, according to the 2012 ASRM guidelines [3], progesterone treatment for luteal phase defects is not recommended. However, a recent systematic review by Carp made a compelling argument for treatment with dydrogesterone, a progestogen, in a review of 13 studies demonstrating a 13 % absolute reduction in the miscarriage rate among the treated vs. the untreated group [85].

Hyperprolactinemia is associated with RPL, and it may be involved in the pathogenesis of reproductive failure in patients with APS, PCOS, and hypothyroidism [3, 79, 86]. Hirahura et al. [86] found that treatment with bromocriptine was very effective for women with elevated prolactin levels, leading to a live birth rate of 85.7 %. On the other side, Li et al. [87] found that women with prolactin concentrations in the lower end of the physiological range had an increased risk of miscarriage when adjusted for all other factors.

Thrombophilias

Hereditary thrombophilias (HT) elicit a prothrombotic state that has been associated with RPL. The most common HT is Factor V Leiden [88]. It is found in ~5 % of the general population of Caucasians, 1 % Africans, and is almost absent in Asians [88]. Other thrombophilias include prothrombin gene mutation, protein C deficiency, protein S deficiency, and antithrombin III deficiency. Certain thrombophilias produce a higher risk environment than others, and routine screening for HT is not mandatory in all patients with RPL. The association between Factor V Leiden mutation and pregnancy loss is thought to be as low as 4.2 % [89]. ACOG's most recent practice bulletin [90] divides HT into high-risk and low-risk groups, recommending prophylactic treatment based on the genetic mutation and history of venous thromboembolism (VTE). Histories of VTE or high-risk thrombophilia were considered as indications for prophylactic therapy with LMWH or unfractionated heparin [90]. In spite of this, it has been found that as many as 40 % of physicians screen patients without recommendations [91]. In clinical practice, HT is hard to ignore. Early studies have supported screening [91], and discounting a possible cause of RPL, however small it may be, in couples by foregoing a genetic test or prophylactic treatment is difficult to do when the stakes are so high. See chapter on hereditary thrombophilia for further discussion of therapeutic options.

Acquired thrombophilia, mostly attributed to antiphospholipid syndrome (APS), is seen in 5–20 % of patients with RPL [33]. Testing for

APS is indicated after 3 or more unexplained miscarriages before week 10, one unexplained miscarriage after 10 weeks gestation, or a history of preeclampsia or placental insufficiency that led to delivery before 34 weeks gestation. Anticardiolipin, lupus anticoagulant, anti-β2-glycoprotein I, and antiphosphatidylserine are the only tested antiphospholipid antibodies, and they must be found positive twice at a 12-week interval or greater [92]. The inclusion of other antiphospholipid antibodies has increased false positive results, leading to vastly greater percentages describing the incidence of APS in past studies [31].

Antiphospholipid antibodies induce thrombosis, inhibit differentiation of the trophoblast, and provoke dysregulation of the maternal immune system [3]. Inflammation may also participate in producing these effects on the trophoblast. Fetal loss rate, e.g., pregnancy loss after 20 weeks, was reported to be 50–90 % without treatment [93]. A Cochrane review of randomized control trials has shown that low-dose aspirin with heparin leads to a live birth rate of 70–80 % [94]. Although these results are encouraging, this subgroup is still at an increased risk for miscarriage. An observational study by Bouvier et al. [95] found that women with RPL and obstetric APS undergoing treatment continued to have increased rates of fetal loss as well as neonatal and obstetric complications, producing lower rates of live births compared to women without APS. Therefore, a desired successful and uncomplicated pregnancy after the diagnosis and treatment for APS is not always accomplished.

Lifestyle and Habits

Smoking, alcohol, and caffeine are three of the most discussed environmental factors associated with spontaneous single abortion. However, no direct correlation between these factors and RPL was reported. All three factors have been shown to be dose-dependent causes of single abortions, and obtaining a full patient history including questions about these factors may uncover a possible causation [3, 33].

Obesity

Obesity is defined as a BMI of ≥ 30 kg/m [96]. It has been a topic of discussion in the field of RPL due to its increasing prevalence and association with PCOS, type II diabetes mellitus, and hormone abnormalities. Differing results have been found concerning the association of obesity with RPL. Metwally et al. [97] found that while there was an association between obesity and miscarriage, the evidence was weak in 16 articles published including both spontaneous and assisted conception. They criticized the data for using varying definitions of obesity and advanced maternal age. Boots et al. [98] performed a similar review of the literature, including spontaneous conceptions only. They found stronger evidence of recurrent early miscarriage in obese patients with an odds ratio of 3.51. Furthermore, Lashen et al. [99] found an increased rate of recurrent miscarriage in women with high BMI compared to those without, with odds ratio of 4.68 in a study of 4932 women. Therefore, it is likely that obesity directly affects RPL, but more studies are needed to confirm these results.

Unexplained RPL

Although it is commonly recognized that unexplained RPL (URPL) occurs in about 50 % of all RPL [32], as seen in Fig. 11.1 in Chap. 11, Sugiura-Ogasawara et al. [30] found an abnormal karyotype in the POC of 41.1 % of URPL patients, and therefore suggest that true unexplained RPL may only be present in 24.5 % of the total RPL population. Saravelos et al. [10] has shown that women with URPL have a similar risk of miscarriage compared to the general population (14–26 and 15–25 %). However, they do not suggest that all URPL is due to chance alone, but that this group should be separated into two subgroups. Those who fall under type I have RPL that is actually due to chance alone, while those in type II have truly unexplained RPL. Younger women with higher incidence of clinically diagnosed pregnancy losses and normal karyotypes in the POC are classified as type II, while women who do not meet these criteria are type I [10]. This has interesting implications for counseling these two groups, but is still not widely accepted.

A variety of therapies have been attempted on women with URPL including immunotherapy, low-dose aspirin, and psychological support [32, 100]. Interestingly, psychological support alone has offered promising results. Clifford et al. [17] found better outcomes in couples with URPL who received supportive care during early pregnancy compared to those who did not (26 and 51 % respectively). Other studies have supported these results [13, 101]; however, additional studies should be conducted due to the lack of randomization. It has been shown that women with RPL experience increased levels of anxiety. In fact, Mevorach-Zussmanet et al. [102] found that variables which compose a woman's reproductive status are directly associated with her psychological health. They suggest that the anxiety is a long-term condition, often not resolved by TLC therapy, and may produce poor outcome in subsequent pregnancies. As was discussed earlier, PGS is not a standard of care, as the chance of having a live birth in URPL is good. It is typically only in cases in infertility, AMA, and primary RPL as a last resort.

When May I Get Pregnant Again, and Is It Ok to Try Now?

Many patients with RPL wish to know if it will be possible for them to achieve conception, and if they should wait a certain amount of time to decrease their risk of another miscarriage. Psychological stress can become an extremely important factor in counseling women who feel their "biological clock is ticking." Kaandorp et al. [103] found a median time to pregnancy of 21–23 weeks in women with unexplained RPL, which is comparable to the average time to pregnancy for women in the general population, and can be reassuring for patients who wish to become pregnant soon after their last miscarriage.

Additionally, inter-pregnancy intervals (IPIs) have been a source of speculation for prognosis. Questions have been raised over whether psychological stress and physical recovery should delay conception after a miscarriage. However, since the World Health Organization [104] suggested at least 6 months between miscarriage and conception, studies have shown that IPIs are equivalent in prognosis [105, 106]. Furthermore, some studies have suggested that a shorter IPI of less than 6 months carries a better prognosis [107]. Bentolila et al. [106] showed that shorter IPI (<6 months) was associated with a better pregnancy outcome, although the group with an IPI of more than 6 months had equivalent outcomes when adjusted for maternal age and fertility problems. Therefore, patients who desire to become pregnant soon after miscarriage may be reassured that they are not at an increased risk of adverse effects compared to those who delay conception.

Conclusion

Each couple with RPL has a different prognosis according to their individual history and the results of their diagnostic work-up. The prognosis can be dynamic from the first meeting until right before pregnancy. Therefore, although it is difficult to create an exact percentage for each couple's prognosis, advising them on their potential for a live birth can help make important therapeutic and reproductive decisions. Maternal age provides the best indication for prognosis, with the lowest rates of live birth seen in women over 40 years old. Higher incidence of previous miscarriages worsens prognosis and decreases the likelihood that the miscarriages are due to chance alone. While primary and secondary RPL have similar live birth rates, women with primary RPL should be monitored more closely for obstetric complications during the pregnancy. Concomitant infertility also contributes to a poor outcome. All of these factors affect the prognosis of the couple aside from etiology. Each etiology confers its own rate of live birth and varies based on whether it is treated or untreated. Some therapy—diabetes control for example—provides near normal live birth rates, while others, like PGD for parental chromosomal aberrations, are more controversial.

In conclusion, each couple should be carefully evaluated and advised with emotional support in order to provide the best possible outcome.

References

1. Jauniaux E, Farquharson RG, Christiansen OB, Exalto NE, (ESHRE). Evidence-based guidelines for the investigation and medical treatment of recurrent miscarriage. Hum Reprod. 2006;21:2216–22.
2. Practice Committee of the American Society for Reproductive Medicine. Definitions of infertility and recurrent pregnancy loss. Fertil Steril. 2013;99(1):63. doi:10.1016/j.fertnstert.2012.09.023. http://dx.doi.org.
3. Practice Committee of the American Society for Reproductive Medicine. Evaluation and treatment of recurrent pregnancy loss: a committee opinion. Fertil Steril. 2012;98(5):1103–11. doi:10.1016/j.fertnstert.2012.06.048. http://dx.doi.org.
4. Bashiri A, Ratzon R, Amar S, Serjienko R, Mazor M, Shoham-Vardi I. Two vs. three or more primary recurrent pregnancy losses- are there any differences in epidemiologic characteristics and index pregnancy outcome? J Perinat Med. 2012;40:365–71.
5. Christiansen OB. Epidemiology of recurrent pregnancy loss. In: Carp H, editor. Recurrent pregnancy loss: causes, controversies and treatment. 1st ed. UK: Informa healthcare; 2007. p. p1–14.
6. Royal College of Obstetricians and Gynaecologists (RCOG). The investigation and treatment of couples with recurrent first-trimester and second-trimester miscarriage. Green-top guideline; no. 17. London (UK): RCOG. 2011.
7. Christiansen OB. Recurrent miscarriage is a useful and valid clinical concept. Acta Obstet Gynecol Scand. 2014;93:852–7. doi:10.1111/aogs.12456.
8. Chard T. Frequency of implantation and early pregnancy loss in natural cycles. Baillieres Clin Obstet Gynaecol. 1991;5(1):179–89.
9. Farquharson RG, Jauniaux E, Exalto N. Updated and revised nomenclature for description of early pregnancy events. Hum Reprod. 2005;20(11):3008–11.
10. Saravelos S, Li T. Unexplained recurrent miscarriage: how can we explain it? Hum Reprod. 2012;27:1882–6.
11. Kolte A, van Oppenraaj R, Quenby S, Farquharson R, Stephenson M, Goddin M, Christiansen O. (ESHRE). Non-visualized pregnancy losses are prognostically important for unexplained recurrent miscarriage. Hum Reprod. 2014;29(5):931–7.
12. Zeadna A, et al. A comparison of biochemical pregnancy rates between women who underwent IVF and fertile controls who conceived spontaneously. Hum Reprod. 2015;30(4):783–8.
13. Brigham S, Colon C, Farquharson G. A longitudinal study of pregnancy outcome following idiopathic recurrent miscarriage. Hum Reprod. 1999;14:2868–71.
14. Fritz M. Recurrent early losses. In: Fritz M, Speroff L, editors. Clinical gynecologic endocrinology and infertility. 8th ed. Philadelphia, PA: Lippincott Williams & Wilkins; 2011. p. 1191–220.
15. Nybo Andersen A, Wohlfahrt J, Christens P, Olsen J, Melbye M. Maternal age and fetal loss: population based register linkage study. BMJ. 2000;320:1708–12.
16. Li TC, Iqbal T, Anstie B, Gillham J, Amer S, Wood K, Laird S. An analysis of the pattern of pregnancy loss in women with recurrent miscarriage. Fertil Steril. 2002;78(5):1100–6.
17. Clifford K, Rai R, Regan L. Future pregnancy outcome in unexplained recurrent first trimester miscarriage. Hum Reprod. 1997;12(2):387–9.
18. Lund M, Kamper-Jorgensen M, Nielson HS, Lidegaard O, Nybo Anderson A, Christiansen O. Prognosis for live birth in women with recurrent miscarriage: what is the best measure of success? Obstet Gynecol. 2012;119(1):37–43. doi:10.1097/AOG.0b013e31823c0413.
19. Levi A, Raynault M, Bergh P, Drews M, Miller B, Scott R. Reproductive outcome in patients with diminished ovarian reserve. Fertil Steril. 2001;76(4):666–9.
20. Hofmann GE, Khoury J, Thie J. Recurrent pregnancy loss and diminished ovarian reserve. Fertil Steril. 2000;74:1192–5.
21. Nasseri A, Mukherjee T, Grifo J, Noyes N, Krey L, Copperman A. Elevated day 3 follicle stimulating hormone and/or estradiol may predict fetal aneuploidy. Fertil Steril. 1999;71:715–8.
22. Cano F, Simon C, Remohi J, Pellicer A. Effect of ageing on the female reproductive system: evidence for a role of uterine senescence in the decline in female fecundity. Fertil Steril. 1995;64:584–9.
23. Carp H, Toder V, Aviram A, Daniely M, Mashiach S, Barkai G. Karyotype of the abortus in recurrent miscarriage. Fertil Steril. 2001;75(4):678–82.
24. Ogasawara M, Aoki K, Okada S, Suzumori K. Embryonic karyotype of abortuses in relation to the number of previous miscarriages. Fertil Steril. 2000;73:300–4.
25. Marquard K, Westphal L, Milki A, Lathi R. Etiology of recurrent pregnancy loss in women over the age of 35 years. Fertil Steril. 2010;94(4):1473–7. doi:10.1016/j.fertnstert.2009.06.041.
26. Stephenson MD. Frequency of factors associated with habitual abortion in 197 couples. Fertil Steril. 1996;66:24–9.
27. Stern J, Dorfman A, Gutierez-Najar M. Frequency of abnormal karyotype among abortuses from women with and without a history of recurrent spontaneous abortion. Fertil Steril. 1996;65:250–3.
28. Sullivan A, Silver R, LaCoursiere D, Porter T, Branch D. Recurrent fetal aneuploidy and recurrent miscarriage. Obstet Gynecol. 2004;104(4):784–8.
29. Nelson S, Telfer E, Anderson R. The ageing ovary and uterus: new biological insights. Hum Reprod Update. 2013;19(1):67–83. doi:10.1093/humupd/dms043.

30. Sugiura-Ogasawara M, Ozaki Y, Suzumori N. Management of recurrent miscarriage. J Obstet Gynaecol. 2014;40(5):1174–9. doi:10.1111/jog.12388.

31. Foyouzi N, Cedars M, Huddleston H. Cost-effectiveness of cytogenetic evaluation of products of conception in the patient with a second pregnancy loss. Fertil Steril. 2012;98(1):151–5. doi:10.1016/j.fertnstert.2012.04.007.

32. Ford H, Schust D. Recurrent pregnancy loss: etiology, diagnosis, and therapy. Rev Obstet Gynecol. 2009;2(2):76–83.

33. Jaslow CR, Carney JL, Kutteh WH. Diagnostic factors identified in 1020 women with two versus three or more recurrent pregnancy losses. Fertil Steril. 2010;93(4):1234–43.

34. Bhattacharya S. Townsend, Bhattacharya S. Recurrent miscarriage: are three miscarriages one too many? analysis of a Scottish population-based database of 151,021 pregnancies. Eur J Obstet Gynecol Reprod Biol. 2010;150(1):24–7. doi:10.1016/j.ejogrb.2010.02.015.

35. Bashiri A, Shapira E, Ratzon R, Shoham-Vardi I, Sejienko R, Mazor M. Primary vs. secondary recurrent pregnancy loss- epidemiological characteristics, etiology, and next pregnancy outcome. J Perinat Med. 2012;40(2012):389–96.

36. Jivraj S, Anstie B, Cheong YC, Fairlie FM, Laird SM, Li TC. Obstetric and neonatal outcome in women with a history of recurrent miscarriage: a cohort study. Hum Reprod. 2001;16:102–6.

37. Morikawa M, Yamada H, Kato EH, Shimada S, Sakuragi N, Fujimoto S, Minakami H. Live birth rate varies with gestational history and etiology in women experiencing recurrent spontaneous abortion. Eur J Obstet Gynecol Reprod Biol. 2003; 109(1):21–6.

38. Whitley E, Doyle P, Roman E, De Stavola B. The effect of reproductive history on future pregnancy outcomes. Hum Reprod. 1999;14(11):2863–7.

39. Hakim R, Gray R, Zacur H. Infertility and early pregnancy loss. Am J Obstet Gynecol. 1995;172:1510–7.

40. Teklenburg G, Salker M, Heijnen C, Macklon NS, Brosens JJ. The molecular basis of recurrent pregnancy loss: impaired natural embryo selection. Mol Hum Reprod. 2010;12:886–95. doi:10.1093/molehr/gaq079.

41. Wilcox A, Baird D, Weinberg C. Time of implantation of the conceptus and loss of pregnancy. N Engl J Med. 1999;340(23):1796–9.

42. Ohno M, Maeda T, Matsunobu A. A cytogenetic study of spontaneous abortions with direct analysis of chorionic villi. Obstet Gynecol. 1991;77(3):394–8.

43. Drakeley A, Quenby S, Farquharson R. Mid-trimester loss—appraisal of a screening protocol. Hum Reprod. 1998;13(7):1975–80.

44. Appiah A, Johns J. Endocrine and ultrasonic surveillance of pregnancies in patients with recurrent miscarriage. In: Christiansen O, editor. Recurrent pregnancy loss. 1st ed. Wiley-Blackwell: Hoboken, NJ; 2014. p. 103–14.

45. Li TC, Spring PG, Bygrave C, Laird SM, Serle E, Spuijbroek M, Adekanmi O. The value of biochemical and ultrasound measurements in predicting pregnancy outcome in women with a history of recurrent miscarriage. Hum Reprod. 1998;13(12):3525–9.

46. Franssen MT, Korevaar JC, van der Veen F, Leschot NJ, Bossuyt PM, Goddijn M. Reproductive outcome after chromosome analysis in couples with two or more miscarriages: index [corrected]-control study. BMJ. 2006;332(7544):759–63.

47. Sugiura-Ogasawara M, Ozaki Y, Sato T, Suzumori N, Suzumori K. Poor prognosis of recurrent aborters with either maternal or paternal reciprocal translocations. Fertil Steril. 2004;81:367–73.

48. Carp H, Guetta E, Dorf H, Soriano D, Barkai G, Schiff E. Embryonic karyotype in recurrent miscarriage with parental karyotypic aberrations. Fertil Steril. 2006;85(2):446–50.

49. Brezina P, Kutteh W. Clinical applications of preimplantation genetic testing. BMJ. 2015;350:g7611. doi:10.1136/bmj.g7611.

50. Harper J, Wilton L, Traeger-Synodinos J, Goossens V, Moutou C, SenGupta S, et al. The ESHRE PGD Consortium: 10 years of data collection. Hum Reprod Update. 2012;18:234–47.

51. Twisk M, Mastenbroek S, van Wely M, Heineman MJ, Van der Veen F, Repping S. Preimplantation genetic screening for abnormal number of chromosomes (aneuploidies) in in vitro fertilisation or intracytoplasmic sperm injection. Cochrane Database Syst Rev. 2006;1.

52. Rubio C, Simon C, Vidal F, Rodrigo L, Pehlivan T, Remohi J, et al. Chromosomal abnormalities and embryo development in recurrent miscarriage couples. Hum Reprod. 2003;18:182–8.

53. Preimplantation Genetic Screening for Aneuploidy. ACOG Committee Opinion No.430. American College of Obstetricians and Gynecologists. Obstet Gynecol. 2009;113:766–7.

54. Salim R, Regan L, Woelfer B, Backos M, Jurkovic D. A comparative study of the morphology of congenital uterine anomalies in women with and without a history of recurrent first trimester miscarriage. Hum Reprod. 2003;18(1):162–6.

55. Bajekal N, Li TC. Fibroids, infertility and pregnancy wastage. Hum Reprod Update. 2000;6(6):614–20.

56. Sugiura-Ogasawara M, Ozaki Y, Kitaori T, Kumagai K, Suzuki S. Midline uterine defect size is correlated with miscarriage of euploid embryos in recurrent cases. Fertil Steril. 2010;93(6):1983–8. doi:10.1016/j.fertnstert.2008.12.097.

57. Kowalik CR, Goddijn M, Emanuel MH, Bongers MY, Spinder T, de Kruif JH, Mol BW, Heineman MJ. Metroplasty versus expectant management for women with recurrent miscarriage and a septate uterus. Cochrane Database Syst Rev. 2011;6:CD008576. doi:10.1002/14651858.CD008576.pub3.

58. Grimbizis GF, Camus M, Tarlatzis BC, Bontis JN, Devroey P. Clinical implications of uterine malformations and hysteroscopic treatment results. Hum Reprod Update. 2001;7(2):161–74.
59. Nouri K, Ott J, Huber JC, Fischer EM, Stögbauer L, Tempfer CB. Reproductive outcome after hysteroscopic septoplasty in patients with septate uterus—a retrospective cohort study and systematic review of the literature. Reprod Biol Endocrinol. 2010;8:52. doi:10.1186/1477-7827-8-52.
60. Freud A, Harlev A, Weintraub AY, Ohana E, Sheiner E. Reproductive outcomes following uterine septum resection. J Matern Fetal Neonatal Med. 2014;1–4.
61. Raga F, Bauset C, Remohi J, Bonilla-Musoles F, Simón C, Pellicer A. Reproductive impact of congenital Müllerian anomalies. Hum Reprod. 1997;12(10):2277–81.
62. Yu D, Wong YM, Cheong Y, Xia E, Li TC. Asherman syndrome—one century later. Fertil Steril. 2008;89(4):759–79. doi:10.1016/j.fertnstert.2008.02.096.
63. Hooker A, Lemmers M, Thurkow A, Heymans M, Opmeer B, Brölmann H, Mol B, Huirne J. Systematic review and meta-analysis of intrauterine adhesions after miscarriage: prevalence, risk factors and long-term reproductive outcome. Hum Reprod Update. 2014;20(2):262–78. doi:10.1093/humupd/dmt045.
64. Pabuçcu R, Atay V, Orhon E, Urman B, Ergün A. Hysteroscopic treatment of intrauterine adhesions is safe and effective in the restoration of normal menstruation and fertility. Fertil Steril. 1997;68(6):1141–3.
65. Casini ML, Rossi F, Agostini R, Unfer V. Effects of the position of fibroids on fertility. Gynecol Endocrinol. 2006;22(2):106–9.
66. Saravelos S, Yan J, Rehmani H, Li TC. The prevalence and impact of fibroids and their treatment on the outcome of pregnancy in women with recurrent miscarriage. Hum Reprod. 2011;26(12):3274–9. doi:10.1093/humrep/der293.
67. Craig L, Ke R, Kutteh W. Increased prevalence of insulin resistance in women with a history of recurrent pregnancy loss. Fertil Steril. 2002;78(3):487–90.
68. Zolghadri J, Tavana Z, Kazerooni T, Soveid M, Taghieh M. Relationship between abnormal glucose tolerance test and history of previous recurrent miscarriages, and beneficial effect of metformin in these patients: a prospective clinical study. Fertil Steril. 2008;90(3):727–30.
69. Tian L, Shen H, Lu Q, Norman RJ, Wang J. Insulin resistance increases the risk of spontaneous abortion after assisted reproduction technology treatment. J Clin Endocrinol Metab. 2007;92(4):1430–3.
70. Casey B, Dashe J, Wells C, McIntire D, Byrd W, Leveno K, Cunningham F. Subclinical hypothyroidism and pregnancy outcomes. Obstet Gynecol. 2005;105:239–45.
71. Ke RW. Endocrine basis for recurrent pregnancy loss. Obstet Gynecol Clin North Am. 2014;41(1):103–12. doi:10.1016/j.ogc.2013.10.003.
72. Abalovich M, Gutierrez S, Alcaraz G, Maccallini G, Garcia A, Levalle O. Overt and subclinical hypothyroidism complicating pregnancy. Thyroid. 2002;12:63–8.
73. Bernardi L, Cohen R, Stephenson M. Impact of subclinical hypothyroidism in women with recurrent early pregnancy loss. Fertil Steril. 2013;100(5):1326–31. doi:10.1016/j.fertnstert.2013.07.1975.
74. Negro R, Mestman J. Thyroid disease in pregnancy. Best Pract Res Clin Endocrinol Metab. 2011;25(6):927–43. doi:10.1016/j.beem.2011.07.010.
75. Benhadi N, Wiersinga WM, Reitsma JB, et al. Higher maternal TSH levels in pregnancy are associated with increased risk for miscarriage, fetal or neonatal death. Eur J Endocrinol. 2009;160(6):985–91.
76. De Groot L, Abalovich M, Alexander EK, Amino N, Barbour L, Cobin RH, Eastman CJ, Lazarus JH, Luton D, Mandel SJ, Mestman J, Rovet J, Sullivan S. Management of thyroid dysfunction during pregnancy and postpartum: an Endocrine Society clinical practice guideline. J Clin Endocrinol Metab. 2012;97(8):2543–65. doi:10.1210/jc.2011-2803.
77. Abramson J, Stagnaro-Green A. Thyroid antibodies and fetal loss: an evolving story. Thyroid. 2001;11(1):57–63.
78. Kaprara A, Krassas GE. Thyroid autoimmunity and miscarriage. Hormones. 2008;7(4):294–302.
79. Negro R, Mangieri T, Coppola L, Presicce G, Casavola EC, Gismondi R, Locorotondo G, Caroli P, Pezzarossa A, Dazzi D, Hassan H. Levothyroxine treatment in thyroid peroxidase antibody-positive women undergoing assisted reproduction technologies: a prospective study. Hum Reprod. 2005;20(6):1529–33.
80. Negro R, Formoso G, Coppola L, Presicce G, Mangieri T, Pezzarossa A, Dazzi D. Euthyroid women with autoimmune disease undergoing assisted reproduction technologies: the role of autoimmunity and thyroid function. J Endocrinol Invest. 2007;30(1):3–8.
81. Lincoln SR, Ke RW, Kutteh WH. Screening for hypothyroidism in infertile women. J Reprod Med. 1999;44(5):455–7.
82. Hudecova M, Holte J, Olovsson M, Sundström PI. Long-term follow-up of patients with polycystic ovary syndrome: reproductive outcome and ovarian reserve. Hum Reprod. 2009;24(5):1176–83. doi:10.1093/humrep/den482.
83. Weghofer A, Munne S, Chen S, Barad D, Gleicher N. Lack of association between polycystic ovary syndrome and embryonic aneuploidy. Fertil Steril. 2007;88(4):900–5.
84. Cocksedge K, Li TC, Saravelos SH, Metwally M. A reappraisal of the role of polycystic ovary syndrome in recurrent miscarriage. Reprod Biomed Online. 2008;17(1):151–60.
85. Carp H. Gynecol Endocrinol. 2015;31(6):422–30.
86. Hirahara F, Andoh N, Sawai K, et al. Hyperprolactinemic recurrent miscarriage and results of

randomized bromocriptine treatment trials. Fertil Steril. 1998;70:246–52.

87. Li W, Ma N, Laird SM, Ledger WL, Li TC. The relationship between serum prolactin concentration and pregnancy outcome in women with unexplained recurrent miscarriage. J Obstet Gynaecol. 2013; 33(3):285–8. doi:10.3109/01443615.2012.759916.

88. De Stefano V, Chiusolo P, Paciaroni K, Leone G. Epidemiology of factor V Leiden: clinical implications. Semin Thromb Hemost. 1998;24(4):3 67–79.

89. Rodger MA, Betancourt MT, Clark P, et al. The association of factor V Leiden and prothrombin gene mutation and placenta-mediated pregnancy complications: a systematic review and meta-analysis of prospective cohort studies. PLoS Med. 2010;7(6), e1000292. doi:10.1371/journal.pmed.1000292.

90. James A. Practice bulletin no. 123: thromboembolism in pregnancy. Obstet Gynecol. 2011;118(3):718–29.

91. Davenport W, Kutteh W. Inherited thrombophilias and adverse pregnancy outcomes a review of screening patterns and recommendations. Obstet Gynecol Clin N Am. 2014;41:133–44. doi:10.1016/j.ogc. 2013.10.005. http://dx.doi.org.

92. Miyakis S, Lockship M, Atsumi T, Branch D, Brey R, Cervera R, Derksen R, De Groot P, Koike T, Meroni P, Reber G, Shoenfeld Y, Tincani A, Vlachoyiannopoulos P, Krilis S. International consensus statement on an update of the classification criteria for definite antiphospholipid syndrome (APS). J Thromb Haemost. 2006;4:295–306. doi:10.1111/j.1538-7836.2006.01753.x.

93. Kwak-Kim J, Agcaoili MSL, Aleta L, Liao A, Ota K, Dambaeva S, Beaman K, Kim JW, Gilman-Sachs A. Management of women with recurrent pregnancy losses and antiphospholipid antibody syndrome. Am J Reprod Immunol. 2013;69:596–607. doi:10.1111/aji.12114.

94. Empson M, Lassere M, Craig JC, Scott JR. Recurrent pregnancy loss with antiphospholipid antibody: a systematic review of therapeutic trials. Obstet Gynecol. 2002;99:135–44.

95. Bouvier S, Cochery-Nouvellon E, Lavigne-Lissaide G, Mercier E, Marchetti T, Balducchi JP, Mares P, Gris JC. Comparative incidence of pregnancy outcomes in treated obstetric antiphospholipid syndrome: the NOH_APS observational study. Blood. 2014;123(3):404–13.

96. World Health Organization. Obesity: preventing and managing the global epidemic. Report of a WHO consultation on obesity. Geneva, Switzerland: World Health Organization; 1999.

97. Metwally M, Ong K, Ledger W, Li TC. Does high body mass index increase the risk of miscarriage after spontaneous and assisted conception? A meta-analysis of the evidence. Fertil Steril. 2008;90(3): 714–26. doi:10.1016/j.fertnstert.2007.07.1290.

98. Boots C, Stephenson M. Does obesity increase the risk of miscarriage in spontaneous conception: a systematic review. Semin Reprod Med. 2011;29(6): 507–13. doi:10.1055/s-0031-1293204.

99. Lashen H, Fear K, Sturdee DW. Obesity is associated with increased risk of first trimester and recurrent miscarriage: matched case-control study. Hum Reprod. 2004;19:1644–6.

100. Stephenson M, Kutteh W. Evaluation and management of recurrent early pregnancy loss. Clin Obstet Gynecol. 2007;50(1):132–45.

101. Stray-Pederson B, Stray-Pederson S. Etiologic factors and subsequent reproductive performance in 195 couples with a prior history of habitual abortion. Am J Obstet Gynecol. 1984;148:140–6.

102. Mevorach-Zussman N, Bolotin A, Shalev H, Bilenko N, Mazor M, Bashiri A. Anxiety and deterioration of quality of life factors associated with recurrent miscarriage in an observational study. J Perinat Med. 2012;40(5):495–501.

103. Kaandrop S, van Mens T, Middeldorp S, Hutton BA, Hof M, van der Post J, van den Veen F, Goddijn H. Time to conception and time to live birth in women with unexplained recurrent miscarriage. Hum Reprod. 2014;29(6):1146–52.

104. World Health Organization. Report of a WHO technical consultation on birth spacing. 2005. www.who. int/making_pregnancy_safer/documents/birth_ spacing.pdf.

105. Sholapurkar SL. Is there an ideal interpregnancy interval after a live birth, miscarriage or other adverse pregnancy outcomes? J Obstet Gynaecol. 2010;30(2):107–10.

106. Bentolila Y, Ratzon R, Shoham-Vardi I, Serjienko R, Mazor M, Bashiri A. Effect of interpregnancy interval on outcomes of pregnancy after recurrent pregnancy loss. J Matern Fetal Neonatal Med. 2013;26(14):1459–64. doi:10.3109/14767058.2013.784264.

107. Love ER, Bhattacharya S, Smith NC, Bhattacharya S. Effect of interpregnancy interval on outcomes of pregnancy after miscarriage: retrospective analysis of hospital episode statistics in Scotland. BMJ. 2010;341:c3967.

Implantation, Physiology of Placentation

2

Gershon Holcberg, David Segal, and Asher Bashiri

Introduction

Human reproduction is a very inefficient process. The maximum probability of conception in any menstrual cycle is 30 %. Only 50–60 % of all conceptions advance beyond 20 weeks of gestation. Studies reveal that anywhere from 10 to 25 % of all clinically recognized pregnancies will end in miscarriage. *Chemical pregnancies* may account for 50–75 % of all miscarriages. Implantation, trophoblast development, and placentation are crucial in the establishment and development of normal pregnancy. Abnormalities

G. Holcberg, MD, PhD (✉)
Maternity-C department and High Risk Pregnancy, Placental Research Laboratory, Faculty of Health Sciences, Soroka University Medical Center, Ben-Gurion University of the Negev, Be'er Sheva, Israel
e-mail: holcberg@bgu.au.il

D. Segal, MD
Division of Obstetrics and Gynecology, Faculty of Health Science, Soroka University Medical Center, Ben-Gurion University of the Negev, Be'er Sheva, Israel
e-mail: Segald@bgu.ac.il

A. Bashiri, MD
Director Maternity C and Recurrent Pregnancy Loss Clinic, Department of Obstetrics and Gynecology, Soroka University Medical Center, Faculty of Health Sciences, Ben-Gurion University of the Negev, Be'er Sheva, Israel
e-mail: abashiri@bgu.ac.il

of these events can lead to pregnancy complications known as the great obstetrical syndromes: preeclampsia, intrauterine growth restriction, fetal demise, and recurrent pregnancy loss (Fig. 2.1). The definition of repeated pregnancy loss (RPL) varies; however, most include two or more failed clinical pregnancies as documented by ultrasonography or histopathologic examination [1].

In this chapter only a few pitfalls related to RPL will be discussed. However, these events play a significant role in the development of normal pregnancy. Pre-implantation, vascularization, invasion, and oxidative stress are the main players in the regulation and function of these events and are the leading elements in good pregnancy outcomes. It seems that the mechanisms of RPL are dependent more on the maternal genetic predisposition (activation or silencing of several genes) than on the fetal chromosomal count [2].

Preimplantation

Human reproduction is characterized by a high incidence of peri-implantation loss [3]. The highly dynamic nature of the human endometrium is well documented. In response to the rise and fall in ovarian hormones, it proliferates, differentiates, sheds, and regenerates approximately 400 times during reproductive years. This process of continuous reshaping and regeneration of the endometrium depends on the presence of adult stem

© Springer International Publishing Switzerland 2016
A. Bashiri et al. (eds.), *Recurrent Pregnancy Loss*, DOI 10.1007/978-3-319-27452-2_2

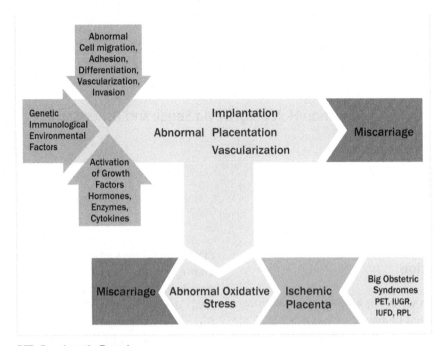

PET - Preeclamptic Toxemia
IUGR - Intra Uterine Growth Restriction
IUFD - Intra Uterine Fetal Death
RPL - Recurrent Pregnancy Loss

Fig. 2.1 Schematic depiction of the possible role of inter-action between several factors involved in the formation of the hypoxic placenta and its role in RPL. As shown, most complications are related to very early events in pregnancy. The abnormal genetic information influenced by environmental hazard and several immunological events lead to abnormal cross talking information during pre- and implantation period the Abnormal activation of placental biological molecules (growth factors/cytokines hormones and enzymes that lead to Abnormal activation of placental biological molecules growth factors cyto-kines, hormones, enzymes Elevatuon of d circulating bio-logical molecules Clinical manifestations of: Abortion, PET, IUFD, IUGR and RPL

cells, migratory resident cells, coordinated influx of specialized immune cells, controlled inflamma-tion, and angiogenesis [4]. Increasing evidence suggests that some women may experience RPL when a "super-receptive" endometrium allows embryos of low viability to implant, presenting as a clinical pregnancy before miscarrying [5–7].

The concept of super-receptivity is supported by the recent observation of a reduced interval between pregnancies in women with RPL com-pared to that reported by normally fertile women [8]. Further evidence comes from studies demon-strating lower levels of endometrial mucin-1, an anti-adhesion molecule that contributes to the barrier function of the epithelium in women with RPL [6]. Moreover, endometrial stromal cells (H-EnSCs) of women with RPL demonstrate

abnormal decidualization in vitro [7]. This phenotype may result in the window of implanta-tion being extended [7] (Fig. 2.2), while reducing the ability of the decidualized endometrium to be "selective" in response to embryo quality [9]. This concept is consistent with the previously reported association between implantation occur-ring later in the luteal phase and preclinical preg-nancy loss [10].

The preparatory process for pregnancy starts with the postovulatory surge in circulating pro-gesterone levels. This process inhibits estrogen-dependent proliferation of the uterine epithelium and induces secretory transformation of the uter-ine glands. Subsequently, the luminal epithelium expresses an evolutionarily conserved repertoire of molecules essential for stable interaction

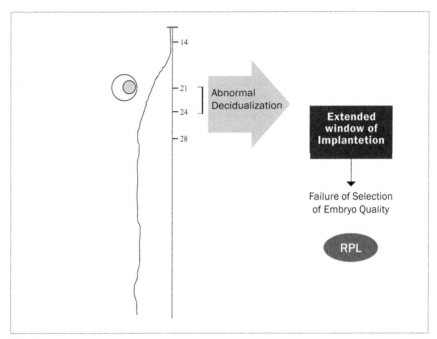

RPL - Recurrent Pregnancy Loss

Fig. 2.2 Receptivity window—defined as the stage of endometrial maturation when the blastocyst can become implanted. Must be synchronized with embryo development and defined as the human window of receptivity—days 20–24 of a 28-day cycle. An intimate cross-talk between the embryo and the uterus is needed for blastocyst implantation. This process, which consists of an interaction between trophoblast cells and endometrium, is initially dependent on the presence of estrogen and progesterone, although further morphological and biochemical changes are evoked within the uterine wall by signals from the embryo and invading trophoblast. MLCP, resulting in actomyosin contraction. Detachment of the rear end: focal contacts disassemble and integrins detach from the substrate. Invasion denotes cellular movement within tissues and requires degradation of

and adherence of a blastocyst, thus enabling implantation. The receptivity is a transient endometrial state, confined to only a few days in the mid-secretory phase of the cycle, and depends on paracrine signals from decidualizing endometrial stromal cells (ESCs) underlying the luminal epithelium [11]. This process is defined by mesenchymal-to-epithelial transformation of endometrial fibroblasts into secretory decidual cells [12]. Decidualization is indispensable for pregnancy as it confers immunotolerance to the fetal semi-allograft, controls trophoblast invasion, and both nourishes and protects the peri-implantation conceptus against a variety of physiological stressors associated with pregnancy [13]. The decidual ESCs operate as gatekeepers of different immune cells at the implantation site. The differentiating ESCs secrete interleukin-11 (IL-11) and IL-15, implicated in recruitment and differentiation of uterine natural killer (NK) cells, which in turn are a rich source of angiogenic factors [14–16]. In most species, the implanting embryo triggers the decidual process. In humans, however, decidualization is under maternal control and is initiated during the mid-secretory phase of each menstrual cycle in response to elevated progesterone and rising cellular cAMP levels [17]. ESCs first mount an acute auto-inflammatory response upon decidualization, which in turn triggers the expression of key receptivity genes in the overlying endometrial surface epithelium [18]. This pro-inflammatory phenotype is transient, determines the duration of the window of implantation, and is followed by an anti-inflammatory response essential for post-implantation embryo support and coordinated trophoblast invasion [18] (Fig. 2.2). In the absence of pregnancy, falling progesterone levels reactivate the expression of inflammatory mediators in decidualizing ESCs, triggering apoptosis, influx of immune cells, extracellular matrix (ECM) breakdown, and menstrual shedding [19, 20]. An inevitable consequence of menstruation is the need for cyclic regeneration and renewal of the endometrium. The regenerative capacity of the human endometrium is indeed remarkable. It is rich in mesenchymal stem-like cells (MSCs) residing predominantly around the vessels. They are recruited to the endometrium in response to hypoxic, proteolytic, and inflammatory stimuli associated with cyclic menstruation, pregnancy, and parturition. In fact, purified ESCs also express elevated levels of pluripotency factors, and are more agreeable to induced pluripotent stem cell reprogramming compared with conventional somatic cells. Molecular phenotyping indicates that ESCs are closely related to follicular dendritic cells (FDCs). The ESCs and FDCs both originate from perivascular platelet-derived growth factor receptor β-positive (PDGFRβ+) adult stem/precursor cells, differentiate in response to inflammatory signals, and are key to local and systemic maternal immunotolerance in pregnancy, respectively [21]. New data demonstrate that coordinated migration and invasiveness of decidualizing ESCs in response to embryonic and trophoblast signals are key to successful implantation. In addition, endometrial cells are capable of invading distant sites, leading to pelvic endometriosis or uterine adenomyosis [22, 23].

Migration and Invasion of Trophoblast

The migratory and invasive capacity of mature ESCs and progenitor cells is increasingly recognized to support the intense tissue remodeling associated with endometrial regeneration, decidualization, embryo implantation, and trophoblast invasion. The lack of fine-tuning of ESC migration and invasion and deregulation of these cell functions contributes to common reproductive disorders, such as implantation failure and recurrent pregnancy loss (RPL).

Cellular Movement

Cellular movement in response to a signal can be classified into two major types: chemokinesis and chemotaxis. Chemokinesis occurs when a factor stimulates cell motility without determining the direction of migration; chemotaxis takes place when cells migrate toward a chemoattractant in a concentration gradient [24]. Chemokinesis is a random and nondirected type of migration, whereas chemotaxis is directed locomotion in response to an external cue.

Implantation

Implantation, a critical step for the establishment of pregnancy, requires complex molecular and cellular events resulting in uterine growth and differentiation, blastocyst adhesion and invasion, and placental formation. Successful implantation necessitates a receptive endometrium, a normal and functional embryo at the blastocyst stage, and a synchronized dialogue between the mother and the developing embryo [25]. In addition to the well-characterized role of sex steroids, the complexity of blastocyst implantation and placentation is exemplified by the role played by a number of cytokines and growth factors in these processes. Indeed, the process of implantation is orchestrated by hormones such as sex steroids and hCG; growth factors such as TGF-B, HB-EGF, and IGF-1; cytokines such as Leukemia Inhibitory Factor, Interleukin-6, and Interleukin-11; adhesion molecules including L-selectin and E-cadherin; the extracellular matrix (ECM) proteins; and prostaglandins [25]. Embryonic implantation is initiated by the recognition and adhesion between the blastocyst surface and the uterine endometrial epithelium. Adhesion occurs when a free-floating blastocyst comes into contact with the endometrium during the "receptive window" during which it is able to respond to the signals from the blastocyst. This contact is then stabilized in a process known as *adhesion,* in which the trophoblast cells establish contact with the micro-protrusions present on the surface of the endometrium known as pinopodes [26].

The last step of implantation is the *invasion* process, which involves penetration of the embryo through the luminal epithelium into the endometrial stroma; this activity is mainly controlled by the trophoblast [27]. The trophoblast lineage is the first to differentiate during human development, at the transition between morula and blastocyst. Initially, at day 6–7 post-conception, a single layer of mononucleated trophoblast cells surrounds the blastocoel and the inner cell mass. At the site of attachment and direct contact to maternal tissues, trophoblast cells fuse to form a second layer of post-mitotic multinucleated syncytiotrophoblast [28]. Once formed, the syncytiotrophoblast grows by means of steady incorporation of new mononucleated trophoblast cells from a proximal subset of stem cells located at the cytotrophoblast layer [29]. Tongues of syncytiotrophoblast cells begin to penetrate the endometrial cells, and gradually the embryo is embedded into the stratum compactum of the endometrium. A plug of fibrin initially seals the defect in the uterine surface, but by days 10–12 the epithelium is restored [30]. Only at around the 14th day do mononucleated cytotrophoblasts break through the syncytiotrophoblast layer and begin to invade the uterine stroma at sites called trophoblastic cell columns. Such cells constitute the extravillous trophoblast and have at least two main subpopulations: interstitial trophoblast, comprising all those extravillous trophoblast cells that invade uterine tissues and that are not located inside vessel walls and lumina; and endovascular trophoblast, located inside the media or lining the spiral artery lumina and partly occluding them (sometimes this subtype is further subdivided into intramural and endovascular trophoblasts) [30]. At a molecular level, trophoblast adhesion from the stage of implantation onwards is an integrin-dependent process [31] that takes place in a chemokine- and cytokine-rich microenvironment analogous to the blood-vascular interface. Of note, uterine expression of chemokines in humans is hormonally regulated and the blastocyst expresses chemokine receptors. In addition, oxygen tension plays an important role in guiding the differentiation process that leads to cytotrophoblast invasion of the uterus [32].

The Selectins Adhesion System

The selectins adhesion system and cadherin families are the main adhesion molecules investigated with regard to the implantation process. Selectins are a group of three carbohydrate-binding proteins that are named following the cell type expressing them (E—endothelium, P—platelets, and L—leucocytes): E-selectin is expressed on the endothelial surface; P-selectin on the surface of activated platelets; and L-selectin on lymphocytes, where it plays an essential role in the homing mechanism of these cells [27, 33, 34]. Transmigration may constitute an initial step in the implantation process. Indeed, L-selectin is strongly expressed on the blastocyst surface while, during the window of implantation, there is an upregulation in the decidual expression of the selectin oligosaccharide-based ligands, predominantly on endometrial luminal epithelium [35]. This may assist in the blastocyst decidual apposition during the implantation process. The effect of heparin on selectins during implantation is unclear. Due to its high density in negatively charged sulfates and carboxylates, heparin is able to bind the two binding sites of the natural ligand of selectin molecules (P- and L-selectins: one for the sialyl Lewis X moiety and another for the tyrosine sulfate-rich region of its native ligand P-selectin glycoprotein ligand-1 [PSGL-1]); the number of sites bonded is dependent on the length of the heparin chain. Evidence in support is presented by the study of Stevenson, Choi, and Varki [36], who investigated the effect of different unfractionated heparin and LMWH on selectin molecules in cancer cell lines [27]. Tinzaparin, with 22–36 % of its fragments greater than 8 kDa, significantly impairs L-selectin binding to its ligand; whereas enoxaparin, with 0–18 % fragments greater than 8 kDa, did not affect L-selectin expression [36]. Thus, heparins with a high proportion of fragments longer than 8 kDa may reduce inflammatory cell adhesion and homing; on the other hand, they may affect blastocyst adhesion by blocking selectin ligand binding sites. Cadherins are a group of cell adhesion proteins that mediate Ca2+-dependent cell–cell adhesion, a fundamental process required for blastocyst implantation and embryonic development [37]. E-cadherin plays an important role in maintaining cell adhesion. In cancer cells, the reduction of E-cadherin expression promotes acquisition of an invasive phenotype. Remarkably, gestational trophoblastic diseases (choriocarcinoma and complete hydatidiform mole) that are characterized by invasive trophoblast behavior have a lower E-cadherin trophoblastic expression than that of first-trimester placenta. In contrast, the trophoblast expression of E-cadherin is higher in placentas of patients with preeclampsia than in those of normal pregnant women [38]. Evidence to support the effect of heparins on trophoblast invasiveness through E-cadherin expression provides a possible mechanism by which heparin could promote trophoblast cell differentiation and motility.

Heparin-Binding EGF-Like Growth Factor

Heparin-binding epidermal growth factor (EGF)-like growth factor (HB-EGF) is a 76–86 amino acid glycosylated protein that was originally cloned from macrophage-like U937 cells. It is a member of the EGF family that stimulates growth and differentiation. HB-EGF utilizes various molecules as its "receptors." The primary receptors are in the ErbB (also named HER) system, especially ErbB1 and ErbB4 human tyrosine kinase receptors. HB-EGF is initially synthesized as a transmembrane precursor protein, similar to other members of the EGF family of growth factors. The membrane-anchored form of HB-EGF (proHB-EGF) is composed of a pro-domain followed by heparin-binding, EGF-like, juxtamembrane, transmembrane, and cytoplasmic domains. Subsequently, proHB-EGF is cleaved at the cell surface by a protease to yield the soluble form of HB-EGF (sHB-EGF) using a mechanism known as ectodomain shedding. sHB-EGF is a potent mitogen and chemoattractant for a number of different cell types. Studies of mice expressing noncleavable HB-EGF have indicated that the major functions of HB-EGF are mediated by the soluble form HB-EGF accumulates in the trophoblast [39] throughout the placenta. HB-EGF has a multiple role due to its cell-specific expression during the human endometrial cycle and early placentation, and high level expression in the first trimester [27]. The membrane active precursor functions as a juxtacrine growth factor and cell surface receptor. It has been demonstrated that HB-EGF promotes adhesion of the blastocyst to the uterine wall in a mouse in vitro system [40], suggesting a role for HB-EGF in embryo attachment to the uterine luminal epithelium. The majority of its biological functions are mediated by its mature soluble form. A major role in early stages of placentation is represented by cellular differentiation and consequent invasion of the uterine wall and vascular network. Several changes occur in the expression of adhesion molecules as cytotrophoblast differentiation proceeds, which results in pseudovasculogenesis or the adaptation by cytotrophoblasts to a molecular phenotype that mimics endothelium [41]. For example, during extravillous differentiation in vivo, integrin expression is altered from predominantly α6β4 in the villous trophoblast to α1β1 in cytotrophoblasts migrating throughout the decidual stroma [31] or engaging in endovascular invasion. Leach et al. [42] demonstrated the role of HB-EGF in regulating the conversion of human cytotrophoblasts into an invasive phenotype and the motility of these cells. This study demonstrated the ability of HB-EGF to induce "integrin switching" through intracellular signaling following ligation of HER tyrosine kinases, altering integrin gene expression to stimulate cytotrophoblast invasion at a molecular level. In addition to its effect on the invasive trophoblast phenotype, HB-EGF can affect cell motility. Indeed, cytotrophoblast motility was specifically increased by each of the EGF family members examined. The expression by cytotrophoblasts of each growth factor, as well as their receptors, suggests the possibility of an autocrine loop that advances cytotrophoblast differentiation to the extravillous phenotype. The ability of the HB-EGF molecule to prevent hypoxic-induced apoptosis plays a fundamental role in early stages of placentation.

Oxidative Stress in Early Pregnancy

During gestation, an adequate and efficient supply of nutrients and oxygen is vital for proper development of the fetus. These fetomaternal exchanges rely on adequate vascularization of both the maternal decidua and the fetus-derived placental villi [43]. In the human maternal decidua, vascular remodeling of the intramyometrial portion of the spiral arterioles occurs between the 10th and 12th week of gestation. This transformation is achieved by specialized placental cells, the cytotrophoblasts. During placentation, cytotrophoblasts that are present in anchoring villi generate multilayered columns of highly invasive extravillous trophoblasts that colonize the interstitium of the maternal decidua, the inner third of the myometrium, and the uterine blood vessels. This invasion results in the formation of the low-resistance vascular system that is essential for fetal growth [43]. This developmental period (10–12 weeks of gestation) is characterized by an important physiological switch in oxygen tension during the opening of the intervillous space. Before the ninth week of gestation, placental oxygen tension is low (20 mmHg), and after 10–12 weeks of gestation, it increases to approximately 55 mmHg [43]. At this time, the cytotrophoblast turns from a proliferative to an invasive phenotype [44]. Failure of this transition is associated with clinical complications of pregnancy, including preeclampsia, the most common cause of retarded fetal development [45]. (Fig. 2.3)

Hemochorial placentation is also dependent on the establishment and maintenance of a competent fetal placenta—a vascular network formed by branching (first and second trimesters) and nonbranching (third trimester) angiogenesis. In human placenta, branching angiogenesis is important for both the development of the villous vasculature and the formation of terminal villi. Consequently, both trophoblasts and endothelial cells are required during the early stages of placental development. Angiogenic growth factors are considered to be the main mediators of these processes. Mouse models have demonstrated the importance of two families of ligands, namely vascular endothelial growth factors (VEGFs) and angiopoietins and their tyrosine kinase receptors in fetal and placental angiogenesis [45]. Vasculogenesis starts during the third week after conception. This process is characterized by the formation of the first blood vessels from differentiation of pluripotent mesenchymal cells into hemangiogenic stem cells [45].

The subsequent step, angiogenesis, starts during the fifth week after conception and refers to the development of new vessels from preexisting vessels [45]. From day 32 to week 25 after conception, hemangioblastic cords formed by vasculogenesis develop into a richly branched villous capillary bed by two mechanisms: elongation of preexisting tubes and lateral ramification of these tubes (sprouting angiogenesis). Around week 25, this process switches from branching to nonbranching angiogenesis [45]. Nonbranching angiogenesis transpires in mid and late gestation and it is mainly characterized by endothelial cell proliferation leading to an increase in the surface of the endothelial tissue. These processes ensure the increasing supply of gas and nutrients for the growing fetus [45]. The existence of tissue-specific angiogenic factors has been postulated for many years [46], but only in the last decade has a factor, named endocrine gland-derived vascular endothelial growth factor/prokineticin 1 (EG-VEGF/PROK1), been characterized [46] as a trophoblast product.

The early placenta is poorly protected against oxidative damage. The antioxidant enzymes such as copper/zinc superoxide dismutase and mitochondrial superoxide dismutase are not expressed by the syncytiotrophoblast until approximately 8–9 weeks of gestation. The expression of the protective enzymes increases significantly after the trophoblast plugs are loosened and the placenta becomes exposed to gradually increasing levels of oxygen and consequently experiences oxidative stress [47]. At the end of the first trimester, a burst of oxidative stress is evidenced in the periphery of the early placenta. The underlying utero–placental circulation in this area is never plugged by the trophoblastic shell, allowing limited maternal blood flow to enter the placenta from 8 to 9 weeks of gestation. Focal trophoblastic

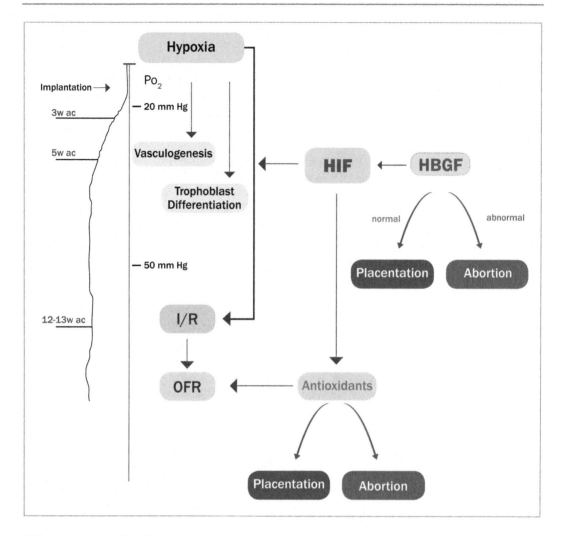

HIF - Hypoxia-Inducible Factor
I/R - Ischemia/Reperfusion
OFR - Oxygen Free Radicals

Fig. 2.3 Placental development is profoundly influenced by oxygen (O_2) tension. Human cytotrophoblasts proliferate under low O_2 conditions but differentiate at higher O_2 levels. Trophoblasts must be able to accurately sense oxygen tension hypoxia-inducible factor-1 (HIF-1). HIF-1 activates many genes involved in the cellular response to O_2 (also known as aryl hydrocarbon receptor nuclear translocator (ARNT)). HIF-1 is able to be stabilized under normoxic conditions by a variety of growth factors and cytokines including epidermal growth factor (EGF)

oxidative damage and progressive villous degeneration trigger the formation of the fetal membranes, which is an essential developmental step enabling vaginal delivery. The oxidative stress and rise in oxygenation may also stimulate the synthesis of various trophoblastic hormones, such as hCG and estrogens. The oxidizing conditions promote assembly of the hCG subunits.

Angiographic studies of the uterine vasculature have demonstrated that during normal pregnancy, flow from spiral arteries into the intervillous space is often intermittent, arising from spontaneous vasoconstriction. Placental inflow may also be compromised by external compression of the arteries during uterine contractions. Some degree of I/R (ischemia/reperfusion) stimulus may therefore be a feature of normal human pregnancy, especially toward term when the fetus and placenta are extracting large quantities of oxygen (O_2) from the intervillous space. Chronic stimulus could lead to upregulation of the anti-OFR (oxygen free radicals) defense in the placenta, reducing oxidant stress. In early pregnancy this well-controlled oxidative stress is critical in continuous placental remodeling and essential placental functions such as transport and hormonal synthesis. Miscarriages and preeclampsia could be a temporary maladaptation to a changing oxygen environment.

Independent of the cause of the miscarriage, the excessive entry of maternal blood into the intervillous space has two effects: a direct mechanical effect on the villous tissue, which becomes progressively enmeshed inside large intervillous blood thrombi, a widespread and indirect O_2-mediated trophoblastic damage; and increased apoptosis. In preeclampsia the trophoblastic invasion is sufficient to allow early pregnancy phases of placentation too shallow for complete transformation of the arterial utero–placental circulation, predisposing to a repetitive ischemia–reperfusion (I/R) phenomenon. This would impair the placentation process, leading to chronic oxidative stress in the placenta and finally to diffuse maternal endothelial cell dysfunction.

Placental development is profoundly influenced by (O_2) tension. Human cytotrophoblasts proliferate under low O_2 conditions but differentiate at higher O_2 levels. Trophoblasts must be able to accurately sense oxygen tension hypoxia-inducible factor-1. Hypoxia-inducible factor-1 (HIF-1), consisting of HIF-1 a-subunit and ARNT b-subunit (aryl hydrocarbon receptor nuclear translocator), activates many genes involved in the cellular response to O_2 deprivation. To date, three members of the HIF family of transcription factors have been identified. All the members of the HIF family consist of an inducible alpha subunit (HIF-α) and a constitutively expressed beta subunit (HIF-β, also known as aryl hydrocarbon receptor nuclear translocator (ARNT)). HIF-1 is able to be stabilized under normoxic conditions by a variety of growth factors and cytokines including epidermal growth factor (EGF), insulin, heregulin, insulin-like growth factors 1 and 2, transforming growth factor ß1, and interleukin-1ß. There is evidence that antiphospholipid syndrome associated with direct inhibition of trophoblast invasion, rather than placental thrombosis, may be the reason for pregnancy loss. Defective decidual endovascular trophoblast invasion, rather than excessive intervillous thrombosis, was the most frequent histological abnormality in antiphospholipid syndrome-associated early pregnancy loss.

Mainly performed and published in vitro studies, related to placentation and implantation, are based on a concept that these processes are similar to malignant cell invasion and expulsion into surrounding tissues and histologic structures. Migratory and invasive capacity of human endometrial stromal cells (ESCs) is now recognized as a main process in early stages of human reproduction and contributes to the intense tissue remodeling associated with embryo implantation, trophoblast invasion, and endometrial regeneration. In this part of the chapter, we concentrate on the most interesting studies and ongoing experiments that have been published in scientific journals.

A prototypical stimulus for chemokinesis is the angiogenic platelet-derived growth factor (PDGF)-BB. When applied to cells in a homogeneous solution, PDGF-BB can also act asymmetrically as a chemoattractant. The main factors in the regulation of migration are Rho family small guanosine triphosphate (GTP)-binding proteins (GTPases). They control organization of the actin cytoskeleton and the formation of cellular protrusions. More than 20 members of the Rho GTPase family have been identified, including RhoA, Rac1, and CDC42. In their active GTP-bound state, Rho GTPases perform their function through effector proteins, e.g., Rho-associated serine/threonine kinase (ROCK). Rac1 and CDC42 initiate the formation of a branched actin filament network, whereas RhoA promotes linear elongation of actin filaments [47] (Fig. 2.4). A four-step model describes two-dimensional cell migration on biological surfaces [48, 49]: (a) Protrusion of the leading edge: growing actin filaments, controlled by Rac and CDC42 activity,

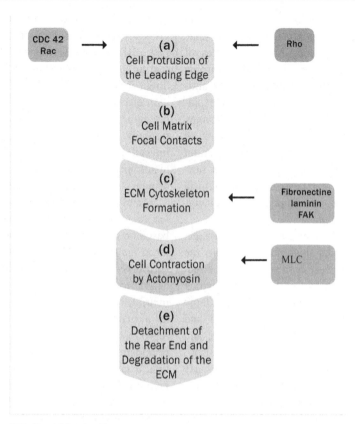

FAK - Focal Adhesion Kinase
MLC - Myosin Light Chain
ECM - Extracellular Matrix

Fig. 2.4 Protrusion of the leading edge: Growing actin filaments, controlled by Rac and CDC42 activity, push the cell membrane outward. (**b**) Cell matrix interactions and formation of focal contacts: integrins serve as receptors for ECM proteins, such as collagen, laminin, and fibronectin. Focal contacts are dynamic complexes linking ECM, integrins, and the cytoskeleton. Focal adhesion kinase (FAK) is recruited to these sites and regulates both their assembly and turnover. (**c**) Cell contraction by actomyosin: myosin light chain (MLC) is phosphorylated by MLC kinase and de-phosphorylated by MLC phosphatase. (**d**) The extent of MLC phosphorylation is regulated by RhoA through its effector ROCK, which phosphorylates and thus inhibits MLCP, resulting in actomyosin contraction. (**e**) Detachment of the rear end: focal contacts disassemble and integrins detach from the substrate. Invasion denotes cellular movement within tissues and requires degradation of (**a**)

push the cell membrane outward. (b) Cell matrix interactions and formation of focal contacts: integrins serve as receptors for ECM proteins, such as collagen, laminin, and fibronectin. Focal contacts are dynamic complexes linking ECM, integrins, and the cytoskeleton. Focal adhesion kinase (FAK) is recruited to these sites and regulates both their assembly and turnover. (c) Cell contraction by actomyosin: myosin light chain (MLC) is phosphorylated by MLC kinase and de-phosphorylated by MLC phosphatase (MLCP). The extent of MLC phosphorylation is regulated

by RhoA through its effector ROCK, which phosphorylates and thus inhibits MLCP, resulting in actomyosin contraction. (d) Detachment of the rear end: focal contacts disassemble and integrins detach from the substrate. Invasion denotes cellular movement within tissues and requires degradation of the ECM. Focalized proteolysis by surface proteases generates active soluble matrix metalloproteinases (MMPs) with selected specificities for ECM components. Invasion further involves the action of cysteine- and serine-proteases, such as kallikreins and plasminogen activators (PA), and is counteracted by tissue inhibitors of MMPs (TIMPs) and PA inhibitor secreted by cells of the invaded tissue [50].

In the pregnant uterus, the decidual compartment produces a wide array of soluble factors that can either promote or inhibit trophoblast motility [51]. Positive regulators include HB-EGF, IL-1β, and leukemia inhibitory factor (LIF). A distinct proinvasive function of IL-1β has been demonstrated in primary trophoblast cell systems. IL-1β stimulated outgrowth from villous explant cultures on collagen and migration of primary extravillous trophoblast (EVT) through fibronectin-coated inserts [52]. LIF promotes migration of the HTR-8/SVneo trophoblast cell line via induction of prostaglandin E_2 production, an effect that is enhanced by IL-1β [53]. Much evidence has been provided toward a network between HB-EGF, IL-1β, and LIF signaling pathways. Both HB-EGF and IL-1β induce LIF expression in endometrial epithelial cells [54, 55]. Migration induced by IL-1β involves cross-talk with epidermal growth factor receptor (EGFR) signaling. IL-1β stimulates MMP-9 activity and proteolytic cleavage of the transmembrane precursor of HB-EGF (tm-HB-EGF) and thus the shedding of mature HB-EGF, resulting in EGFR activation [56]. In vitro, the nontransfected or control-transfected cell EGFR levels were downregulated on treatment with HB-EGF/IL-1β/LIF, consistent with the well-characterized lysosomal degradation of EGFR induced by HB-EGF but not other EGFR ligands, such as EGF or amphiregulin [57].

Notably, HB-EGF-mediated EGFR downregulation was not seen in spheroids of si-CEACAM1 transfected AC-1 M88 cells, indicating altered EGFR trafficking, processing, and/or signaling on CEACAM1 knockdown. It was shown that overexpressed CEACAM (carcinoembryonic antigen-related cell adhesion molecules) is a direct substrate of the EGFR tyrosine kinase activity triggered by EGF binding. Phosphorylated CEACAM1 binds and sequesters the adapter protein, uncoupling EGFR from the ERK1/2 MAPK pathway, resulting in downregulation of the mitogenic activity of EGF [58]. In early pregnancy placenta, CEACAM1 is another well-known molecule expressed on activated T cells and involved in T-cell inhibition. CEACAM1 is detected in invasive extravillous trophoblast (EVT) at the implantation site but not in villous cytotrophoblasts or syncytiotrophoblasts. Cultured EVT with invasive phenotype is also positive for CEACAM1 [56]. In the AC-1M88 trophoblast cell line, CEACAM1 overexpression has been shown to enhance migration and invasiveness [59, 60]. Recently, an interactome of human implantation has been deduced from genome expression analyses of human embryos and receptive state endometrium. Among the newly identified interactors was CEACAM1, engaged in networks with annexin A2 or paxillin [61]. The function of CEACAM1 in this context is most likely based on heterotypic cell–cell interactions with endometrial cells or with the extracellular matrix (ECM) deposited by them, because no inhibitory effect of CEACAM1 silencing was seen when AC-1M88 spheroids were exposed to the factor cocktail on cell culture surface in the absence of an endometrial monolayer. The effect was apparent on laminin-1 but not on fibronectin, and was mediated by integrin-dependent signaling. Laminin expression is upregulated on in vitro decidualization of hESCs [62], and in vivo, laminins are major constituents of the decidual cell basement membrane implicated in trophoblast attachment and outgrowth [63]. Human endometrial stromal cells express very low levels of CD82 in the undifferentiated, proliferative stage. On decidualizing treatment over several days, CD82 levels increase, and this is largely due to an increase in the protein level without a corresponding induction of the encoding transcript [63]. The upregulation of CD82 is likewise seen in vivo in the secretory phase endometrium and the decidua of early pregnancy [63]. The in vitro model of decidualization properly reflects changes of the amount of CD82 within a supposedly physiological range. CD82 has been shown to directly associate with EGFR in epithelial cells, and overexpression of CD82 results in enhanced receptor endocytosis and desensitization of EGF-induced signaling [64]. On the other hand, CD82 silencing in HeLa cells promotes clathrin-dependent endocytosis of EGFR in response to EGF and diminishes EGF-mediated ERK phosphorylation within 5 min [65]. It seems that CD82 expression on decidual stromal cells (DSCs) is inhibitory to trophoblast invasion [66]. Trophoblast invasiveness was found to increase when CD82 had been silenced in the DSC monolayer. The anti-invasive function toward trophoblast cells was ascribed to decidual CD82. Based on the observation that CD82 levels were lower in endometriotic compared to normal hESCs, CD82 was assumed to be anti-invasive. Silencing of CD82 in eutopic hESCs increased their invasive potential concurrent with an upregulation of integrin β1 and a downregulation of TIMP-1 and TIMP-2 [67].

Different signaling pathways control directed migration in a gradient (chemotaxis) versus random motility in a uniform (chemokinesis) signal. Involvement of ERK1/2, p38, and phosphoinositide 3-kinase (PI3K)/AKT signaling in chemotaxis, whereas chemokinesis depended primarily on PI3K/AKT activation were described [68]. The latter signaling pathway thus does not appear to be perturbed by CD82 silencing, or other, as-yet-unidentified, compensatory pathways are activated by the factor cocktail. Implantation of a blastocyst or expansion of trophoblast spheroid on endometrial stromal cells depends on motility of the stromal cells that align around the implanting entity. This is facilitated by inhibition of ROCK signaling, which promotes chemokinesis [69–71].

By proteome profiling for cytokines and angiogenesis two factors were identified as trophoblast products: PlGF and PDGF-AA. PlGF is a member of the VEGF family and binds to the VEGFR1 receptor [72]. Although it has been characterized as a chemoattractant for various cell types [73, 74], it did not exhibit such activity on T-HESC in our study. On the other hand, PDGF-AA elicited a chemotactic response in T-HESC, and by the use of a neutralizing antibody, we could demonstrate that PDGF-AA is a chemoattractive constituent of trophoblast-conditioned medium. This observation may have implications in the earliest stages of blastocyst implantation because PDGF-AA expression has been identified in the trophectoderm of Day 5 implantation competent blastocysts, while the corresponding receptor PDGFRα is expressed by the receptive endometrium [75]. The impact of primary trophoblast supernatant on endometrial

stromal cell gene expression has been assessed by gene expression profiling [76]. Among the most highly upregulated endometrial genes in response to trophoblast supernatant were IL6 and CXCL1. It was detected that IL-6 and CXCL1 as proteins were highly induced on decidualization in T-HESC. The trophoblast signals are likely to enhance the decidualizing reaction of the stromal compartment and support a feed-forward loop to promote the dynamic interactions at the invasion front. Conversely, effects of decidualized endometrial stromal cell-derived factors on trophoblast invasiveness and on the profile of invasive trophoblast membrane and secreted proteins have been described, implying a role for decidual cells in the regulation of implantation and placentation [77, 78]. Decidualizing hESCs have been shown to respond to cultured developmentally impaired human blastocysts by reduced secretion of HB-EGF and IL-1β. This does not occur in the presence of normal blastocysts and underscores the concept of decidualized stromal cells serving as biosensors for embryo quality.

The quality control mechanism might be based partly on motile processes, as migration of hESCs from fertile control women toward low-quality embryos was reportedly inhibited compared to migration in the presence of high-quality embryos [79]. Moreover, the hESCs isolated from women with recurrent pregnancy loss failed to discriminate between high- and low-quality embryos in their migratory response [79]. It has been shown that recurrent pregnancy loss coincides with impaired decidualization of hESCs in these subjects, perturbing embryo-maternal interactions [8]. It was hypothesized that stimulation of motility between decidualizing endometrial stromal and trophoblast cells reduces not only invasiveness of trophoblasts but also motility of decidualizing endometrial stromal cells and contributes to tissue remodeling on blastocyst implantation and formation of the placenta. PDGF-AA was identified as a novel trophoblast-derived chemoattractant for endometrial stromal cells. CD82 and CEACAM1 are cell surface molecules that participate in promoting migration in response to soluble and matrix-dependent triggers in endometrial stromal and trophoblast cells, respectively.

Summary

In early placental development, there are at least two possible fates for the interstitial extravillous trophoblast cells migrating into the endometrium: apoptosis and giant cell transformation. Both processes may serve to limit trophoblast invasion of the increasing fetal demands for nutrient and gas exchange leading to the main disorders of pregnancy—miscarriage, preeclampsia, growth restriction RPL, and IUFD—rooted in defective placentation caused, at least in part, by maternal factors.

The two compartments of placenta—the trophoblast and uterine endometrium—are equally involved and responsible regarding the fate of the specific pregnancy. The trophoblast has an intrinsic and carefully timed differentiation program designed to enable placentation to meet the requirements of the developing fetus. The maternal decidual is specialized to allow not only meeting but also accepting the fetal allograft trophoblast-derived biological molecules in biochemical contact and signaling systems controlled by the maternal compartment to allow a normal pregnancy to end with a normal and healthy newborn child.

References

1. Practice Committee of American Society for Reproductive Medicine. Definitions of infertility and recurrent pregnancy loss: a committee opinion. Fertil Steril. 2013;99(1):63.
2. Lessey BA. Endometrial receptivity and the window of implantation. Baillieres Best Pract Res Clin Obstet Gynaecol. 2000;14(5):775–88. Review.
3. Macklon NS, Geraedts JP, Fauser BC. Conception to ongoing pregnancy: the 'black box' of early pregnancy loss. Hum Reprod Update. 2002;8(4):333–43. Review.
4. Gargett CE, Nguyen HP, Ye L. Endometrial regeneration and endometrial stem/progenitor cells. Rev Endocr Metab Disord. 2012;13(4):235–51. doi:10.1007/s11154-012-9221-9. Review.
5. Teklenburg G, Salker M, Molokhia M, Lavery S, Trew G, Aojanepong T, et al. Natural selection of human embryos: decidualizing endometrial stromal cells serve as sensors of embryo quality upon implantation. PLoS One. 2010;5, e10258.
6. Aplin JD, Hey NA, Li TC. MUC1 as a cell surface and secretory component of endometrial epithelium: reduced levels in recurrent miscarriage. Am J Reprod Immunol. 1996;35:261–6.
7. Quenby S, Vince G, Farquharson R, Aplin J. Recurrent miscarriage: a defect in nature's quality control? Hum Reprod. 2002;17:1959–63.
8. Salker M, Teklenburg G, Molokhia M, Lavery S, Trew G, Aojanepong T, et al. Natural selection of human embryos: impaired decidualization of endometrium disables embryo-maternal interactions and causes recurrent pregnancy loss. PLoS One. 2010;5, e10287.
9. Teklenburg G, Salker M, Heijnen C, Macklon NS, Brosens JJ. The molecular basis of recurrent pregnancy loss: impaired natural embryo selection. Mol Hum Reprod. 2010;16:886–95.
10. Wilcox AJ, Baird DD, Weinberg CR. Time of implantation of the conceptus and loss of pregnancy. N Engl J Med. 1999;340:1796–9.
11. Achache H, Revel A. Endometrial receptivity markers, the journey to successful embryo implantation. Hum Reprod Update. 2006;12(6):731–46. Epub 2006 Sep 18.
12. Gellersen B, Brosens IA, Brosens JJ. Decidualization of the human endometrium: mechanisms, functions, and clinical perspectives. Semin Reprod Med. 2007; 25(6):445–53. Review.
13. Leitao R, Rodriguez A. Inhibition of Plasmodium sporozoites infection by targeting the host cell. Exp Parasitol. 2010;126(2):273–7. doi:10.1016/j.exppara.2010.05.012. Epub 2010 May 21.
14. Verma S, Hiby SE, Loke YW, King A. Human decidual natural killer cells express the receptor for and respond to the cytokine interleukin 15. Biol Reprod. 2000;62(4):959–68.
15. Dimitriadis E, White CA, Jones RL, Salamonsen LA. Cytokines, chemokines and growth factors in endometrium related to implantation. Hum Reprod Update. 2005;11(6):613–30. Epub 2005 Jul 8. Review.
16. Hanna N, Bonifacio L, Weinberger B, Reddy P, Murphy S, Romero R, Sharma S. Evidence for interleukin-10-mediated inhibition of cyclo-oxygenase-2 expression and prostaglandin production in preterm human placenta. Am J Reprod Immunol. 2006;55(1):19–27.
17. Gellersen B, Brosens J. Cyclic AMP and progesterone receptor cross-talk in human endometrium: a decidualizing affair. J Endocrinol. 2003;178(3):357–72.
18. Salker MS, Nautiyal J, Steel JH, Webster Z, Sućurović S, Nicou M, et al. Disordered IL-33/ST2 activation in decidualizing stromal cells prolongs uterine receptivity in women with recurrent pregnancy loss. PLoS One. 2012;7(12), e52252. doi:10.1371/journal.pone.0052252. Epub 2012 Dec 27.
19. Lockwood GM, Ledger WL, Barlow DH, Groome NP, Muttukrishna S. Measurement of inhibin and activin in early human pregnancy: demonstration of fetoplacental origin and role in prediction of early-pregnancy outcome. Biol Reprod. 1997;57(6):1490–4.

20. Brosens JJ, Hodgetts A, Feroze-Zaidi F, Sherwin JR, Fusi L, Salker MS, et al. Proteomic analysis of endometrium from fertile and infertile patients suggests a role for apolipoprotein A-I in embryo implantation failure and endometriosis. Mol Hum Reprod. 2010;16(4):273–85. doi:10.1093/molehr/gap108. Epub 2009 Dec 14.

21. Nancy P, Tagliani E, Tay CS, Asp P, Levy DE, Erlebacher A. Chemokine gene silencing in decidual stromal cells limits T cell access to the maternal-fetal interface. Science. 2012;336(6086):1317–21. doi:10.1126/science.1220030.

22. Burney RO, Giudice LC. Pathogenesis and pathophysiology of endometriosis. Fertil Steril. 2012; 98(3):511–9. doi:10.1016/j.fertnstert.2012.06.029. Epub 2012 Jul 20. Review.

23. Maheshwari A, Pandey S, Shetty A, Hamilton M, Bhattacharya S. Obstetric and perinatal outcomes in singleton pregnancies resulting from the transfer of frozen thawed versus fresh embryos generated through in vitro fertilization treatment: a systematic review and meta-analysis. Fertil Steril. 2012;98(2): 368–77, e1–9. doi:10.1016/j.fertnstert.2012.05.019. Epub 2012 Jun 13. Review.

24. Petrie RJ, Doyle AD, Yamada KM. Random versus directionally persistent cell migration. Nat Rev Mol Cell Biol. 2009;10(8):538–49. doi:10.1038/nrm2729. Epub 2009 Jul 15. Review.

25. Dey SK, Lim H, Das SK, Reese J, Paria BC, Daikoku T, Wang H. Molecular cues to implantation. Endocr Rev. 2004;25(3):341–73. Review.

26. Lopata A, Bentin-Ley U, Enders A. "Pinopodes" and implantation. Rev Endocr Metab Disord. 2002;3(2): 77–86. Review. No abstract available.

27. Quaranta M, Erez O, Mastrolia SA, Koifman A, Leron E, Eshkoli T, et al. The physiologic and therapeutic role of heparin in implantation and placentation. Peer J. 2015;3, e691. doi:10.7717/peerj.691. eCollection2015. Review.

28. Hoozemans DA, Schats R, Lambalk CB, Homburg R, Hompes PG. Human embryo implantation: current knowledge and clinical implications in assisted reproductive technology. Reprod Biomed Online. 2004; 9(6):692–715. Review.

29. Jauniaux E. Design, beauty and differentiation: the human fetus during the first trimester of gestation. Reprod Biomed Online. 2000;1(3):107–8.

30. Hertig AT, Rock J, Adams EC. A description of 34 human ova within the first 17 days of development. Am J Anat. 1956;98(3):435–93.

31. Damsky CH, Fitzgerald ML, Fisher SJ. Distribution patterns of extracellular matrix components and adhesion receptors are intricately modulated during first trimester cytotrophoblast differentiation along the invasive pathway, in vivo. J Clin Invest. 1992;89(1): 210–22.

32. Lash GE, Hornbuckle J, Brunt A, Kirkley M, Searle RF, Robson SC, et al. Effect of low oxygen concentrations on trophoblast-like cell line invasion. Placenta. 2007;28(5-6):390–8. Epub 2006 Aug 14.

33. Rosen SD. Ligands for L-selectin: homing, inflammation, and beyond. Annu Rev Immunol. 2004;22:129–56. Review.

34. Rosen SD. Homing in on L-selectin. J Immunol. 2006;177(1):3–4.

35. Genbacev OD, Prakobphol A, Foulk RA, Krtolica AR, Ilic D, Singer MS, et al. Trophoblast L-selectin-mediated adhesion at the maternal-fetal interface. Science. 2003;299(5605):405–8.

36. Stevenson JL, Choi SH, Varki A. Differential metastasis inhibition by clinically relevant levels of heparins--correlation with selectin inhibition, not antithrombotic activity. Clin Cancer Res. 2005;11(19 Pt 1):7003–11.

37. Frenette PS, Wagner DD. Adhesion molecules—Part II: Blood vessels and blood cells. N Engl J Med. 1996;335(1):43–5.

38. Li R, Hao G. Local injury to the endometrium: its effect on implantation. Curr Opin Obstet Gynecol. 2009; 21(3):236–9. doi:10.1097/GCO.0b013e32832a0654. Review.

39. Cha J, Sun X, Dey SK. Mechanisms of implantation: strategies for successful pregnancy. Nat Med. 2012; 18(12):1754–67. doi:10.1038/nm.3012.

40. Raab G, Klagsbrun M. Heparin-binding EGF-like growth factor. Biochim Biophys Acta. 1997;1333(3): F179–99. Review.

41. Zhou Y, Damsky CH, Fisher SJ. Preeclampsia is associated with failure of human cytotrophoblasts to mimic a vascular adhesion phenotype. One cause of defective endovascular invasion in this syndrome? J Clin Invest. 1997;99(9):2152–64.

42. Leach RE, Kilburn B, Wang J, Liu Z, Romero R, Armant DR. Heparin-binding EGF-like growth factor regulates human extravillous cytotrophoblast development during conversion to the invasive phenotype. Dev Biol. 2004;266(2):223–37.

43. Hoffmann P, Feige J-J, Alfaidy N. Expression and oxygen regulation of endocrine gland-derived vascular endothelial growth factor/prokineticin-1 and its receptors in human placenta during early pregnancy. Endocrinology. 2006;147(4):1675–84. doi:10.1210/en.2005-0912.

44. Caniggia I, Mostachfi H, Winter J, Gassmann M, Lye SJ, Kuliszewski M, et al. Hypoxia-inducible factor-1 mediates the biological effects of oxygen on human trophoblast differentiation through TGFβ3. J Clin Invest. 2000;105(5):577–87.

45. Shibuya M. Vascular endothelial growth factor (VEGF) and its receptor (VEGFR) signaling in angiogenesis. A crucial target for anti- and Pro-angiogenic therapies. Genes Cancer. 2011;2(12):1097–105.

46. Brouillet S, Hoffmann P, Benharouga M, Salomon A, Schaal JP, Feige J-J, et al. Molecular characterization of EG-VEGF-mediated angiogenesis: differential effects on microvascular and macrovascular endothelial cells. Mol Biol Cell. 2010;21(16):2832–43.

47. Jaffe AB, Hall A. Rho GTPases: biochemistry and biology. Annu Rev Cell Dev Biol. 2005;21:247–69. Review.

48. Lauffenburger DA, Horwitz AF. Cell migration: a physically integrated molecular process. Cell. 1996; 84(3):359–69. Review.
49. Mitra AK, Del Core MG, Agrawal DK. Cells, cytokines and cellular immunity in the pathogenesis of fibroproliferative vasculopathies. Can J Physiol Pharmacol. 2005;83(8-9):701–15. Review.
50. Salamonsen LA. Role of proteases in implantation. Rev Reprod. 1999;4(1):11–22. Review.
51. Knöfler M, Pollheimer J. IFPA award in placentology lecture: molecular regulation of human trophoblast invasion. Placenta. 2011;33(Suppl):S55–62.
52. Prutsch N, Fock V, Haslinger P, Haider S, Fiala C, Pollheimer J, et al. The role of interleukin-1β in human trophoblast motility. Placenta. 2012;33: 696–703.
53. Horita H, Kuroda E, Hachisuga T, Kashimura M, Yamashita U. Induction of prostaglandin E2 production by leukemia inhibitory factor promotes migration of first trimester extravillous trophoblast cell line, HTR-8/SVneo. Hum Reprod. 2007;22:1801–9.
54. Lessey BA, Gui Y, Apparao KB, Young SL, Mulholland J. Regulated expression of heparin-binding EGF-like growth factor (HB-EGF) in the human endometrium: a potential paracrine role during implantation. Mol Reprod Dev. 2002;62:446–55.
55. Perrier d'Hauterive S, Charlet-Renard C, Berndt S, Dubois M, Munaut C, Goffin F, et al. Human chorionic gonadotropin and growth factors at the embryonic-endometrial interface control leukemia inhibitory factor (LIF) and interleukin 6 (IL-6) secretion by human endometrial epithelium. Hum Reprod. 2004;19:2633–43.
56. Gellersen B, Wolf A, Kruse M, Schwenke M, Bamberger A-M. Human endometrial stromal cell-trophoblast interactions: mutual stimulation of chemotactic migration and promigratory roles of cell surface molecules CD82 and CEACAM1. Biol Reprod. 2013;88(3):80.
57. Roepstorff K, Grandal MV, Henriksen L, Knudsen SL, Lerdrup M, Grovdal L, et al. Differential effects of EGFR ligands on endocytic sorting of the receptor. Traffic. 2009;10:1115–27.
58. Abou-Rjaily GA, Lee SJ, May D, Al-Share QY, Deangelis AM, Ruch RJ, et al. CEACAM1 modulates epidermal growth factor receptor--mediated cell proliferation. J Clin Invest. 2004;114:944–52.
59. Ebrahimnejad A, Streichert T, Nollau P, Horst AK, Wagener C, Bamberger AM, et al. CEACAM1 enhances invasion and migration of melanocytic and melanoma cells. Am J Pathol. 2004;165:1781–7.
60. Briese J, Oberndörfer M, Pätschenik C, Schulte HM, Makrigiannakis A, Löning T, et al. Osteopontin (OPN) is colocalized with the adhesion molecule CEACAM1 in the extravillous trophoblast of the human placenta and enhances invasion of CEACAM1-expressing placental cells. J Clin Endocrinol Metab. 2005;90:5407–13.
61. Altmäe S, Reimand J, Hovatta O, Zhang P, Kere J, Laisk T, et al. Research resource: interactome of human embryo implantation: identification of gene expression pathways, regulation, and integrated regulatory networks. Mol Endocrinol. 2012;26:203–17.
62. Irwin JC, de las Fuentes L, Giudice LC. Growth factors and decidualization in vitro. Ann N Y Acad Sci 1994; 734: 7-18. 65 Aplin JD. Adhesion molecules in implantation. Rev Reprod. 1997;2:84–93.
63. Kimber SJ. Blastocyst implantation: the adhesion cascade. In: Aplin JD, Fazelabas AT, Glasser SR, Giudice LC, editors. The endometrium: molecular, cellular & clinical perspectives. 2nd ed. London: Informa Healthcare; 2008. p. 331–51.
64. Gellersen B, Briese J, Oberndörfer M, Redlin K, Samalecos A, Richter D-U, et al. Expression of the metastasis suppressor KAI-1 in decidual cells at the human maternal fetal interface: Regulation and functional implications. Am J Pathol. 2007;170:126–39.
65. Odintsova E, Sugiura T, Berditchevski F. Attenuation of EGF receptor signaling by a metastasis suppressor, the tetraspanin CD82/KAI-1. Curr Biol. 2000;10: 1009–12.
66. Danglot L, Chaineau M, Dahan M, Gendron MC, Boggetto N, Perez F, et al. Role of TI-VAMP and CD82 in EGFR cell-surface dynamics and signaling. J Cell Sci. 2010;123:723–35.
67. Li MQ, Hou XF, Shao J, Tang CL, Li DJ. The DSCs-expressed CD82 controls the invasiveness of trophoblast cells via integrinβ1/MAPK/MAPK3/1 signaling pathway in human first-trimester pregnancy. Biol Reprod. 2010;82:968–79.
68. Li MQ, Hou XF, Lv SJ, Meng YH, Wang XQ, Tang CL, et al. CD82 gene suppression in endometrial stromal cells leads to increase of the cell invasiveness in the endometriotic milieu. J Mol Endocrinol. 2011; 47:195–208.
69. Schwenke M, Knöfler M, Velicky P, Weimar CHE, Kruse M, Samalecos A, et al. Control of human endometrial stromal cell motility by PDGF-BB, HBEGF and trophoblast-secreted factors. PLoS One. 2013;8(1), e54336.
70. Grewal S, Carver JG, Ridley AJ, Mardon HJ. Implantation of the human embryo requires Rac1-dependent endometrial stromal cell migration. Proc Natl Acad Sci U S A. 2008;105:16189–94.
71. Grewal S, Carver J, Ridley AJ, Mardon HJ. Human endometrial stromal cell Rho GTPases have opposing roles in regulating focal adhesion turnover and embryo invasion in vitro. Biol Reprod. 2010;83: 75–82.
72. Yamazaki Y, Morita T. Molecular and functional diversity of vascular endothelial growth factors. Mol Divers. 2006;10:515–27.
73. Fiedler J, Leucht F, Waltenberger J, Dehio C, Brenner RE. VEGF-A and PlGF-1 stimulate chemotactic migration of human mesenchymal progenitor cells. Biochem Biophys Res Commun. 2005;334:561–8.

74. Fischer C, Mazzone M, Jonckx B, Carmeliet P. FLT1 and its ligands VEGFB and PlGF: drug targets for anti-angiogenic therapy? Nat Rev Cancer. 2008;8: 942–56.

75. Haouzi D, Dechaud H, Assou S, Monzo C, de Vos J, Hamamah S. Transcriptome analysis reveals dialogues between human trophectoderm and endometrial cells during the implantation period. Hum Reprod. 2011;26:1440–9.

76. Hess AP, Hamilton AE, Talbi S, Dosiou C, Nyegaard M, Nayak N, et al. Decidual stromal cell response to paracrine signals from the trophoblast: amplification of immune and angiogenic modulators. Biol Reprod. 2007;76:102–17.

77. Godbole G, Suman P, Gupta SK, Modi D. Decidualized endometrial stromal cell derived factors promote trophoblast invasion. Fertil Steril. 2011;95:1278–83.

78. Menkhorst EM, Lane N, Winship AL, Li P, Yap J, Meehan K, et al. Decidual-secreted factors alter invasive trophoblast membrane and secreted proteins implying a role for decidual cell regulation of placentation. PLoS One. 2012;7, e31418.

79. Weimar CHE, Kavelaars A, Brosens JJ, Gellersen B, de Vreeden-Elbertse JMT, Heijnen CJ, et al. Endometrial stromal cells of women with recurrent miscarriage fail to discriminate between high and low-quality human embryos. PLoS One. 2012;7, e41424.

Part II

Causes of Recurrent Pregnancy Loss

Neta Benshalom-Tirosh, Dan Tirosh, Naama Steiner, and Asher Bashiri

Progesterone, Luteal Phase Deficiency, and Recurrent Pregnancy Loss

Progestins and Progesterone Receptors

In addition to progesterone, the natural progestin, there are several different classes of progestins, such as retro-progesterone (dydrogesterone), and several progesterone derivatives. Several synthetic supplements act as prodrugs and need to be metabolized in order to become biologically active. The progestogenic effect, inducing characteristic changes in the estrogen-primed endometrium, is common for all progestins, but there is a wide range of additional biologic effects, which vary between different progestins [1]. Dydrogesterone is a retro-progesterone, a stereoisomer of progesterone with additional carbon.

It is highly selective as a progestin and due to its structure, it binds almost exclusively to the progesterone receptor, with a lower affinity than that of progesterone, but perhaps a better bioavailability [1].

The biological effect of progesterone is mediated by two types of human progesterone receptor (hPR-A and hPR-B). In most cell contexts, hPR-B functions as a transcriptional activator of progesterone-responsive genes, whereas hPR-A functions as a transcriptional inhibitor. It has been demonstrated that alteration in expression of progesterone receptor subtypes may alter progesterone's biologic effect in different target tissues [2]. Other factors affecting the activity of progesterone may be the result of polymorphism in progesterone receptors [3]; however, further research is required concerning this issue.

Progesterone-Induced Blocking Factor

The trophoblast tissue has special characteristics, inducing an immunomodulation process, actively protecting itself from the maternal immune system. Maternal progesterone and its interaction with progesterone receptors at the level of the decidua seem to have a major role in this defense mechanism [4]. Progesterone-induced blocking factor (PIBF), a protein that can block natural killer (NK) cell-mediated lysis

N. Benshalom-Tirosh, M.D. • D. Tirosh, M.D.
A. Bashiri, M.D. (✉)
Department of Obstetrics and Gynecology, Faculty of Health Sciences, Soroka University Medical Center, Ben-Gurion University of the Negev,
Be'er Sheva, Israel
e-mail: abashiri@bgu.ac.il

N. Steiner, M.D.
Recurrent Pregnancy Loss Clinic, Department of Obstetrics and Gynecology, Soroka Medical Center, Be'er Sheva, Israel

© Springer International Publishing Switzerland 2016
A. Bashiri et al. (eds.), *Recurrent Pregnancy Loss*, DOI 10.1007/978-3-319-27452-2_3

of certain tumor cells, has been identified in pregnant women [5]. PIBF is thought to have an anti-abortive effect that may be related to a shift from Th1 to Th2 cytokines. Studies have shown that there is a Th1 tendency in RPL [4]. In a study by Raghuphaty et al. [6] studying 24 women with a history of successful pregnancies and 23 women with a history of unexplained RPL, the Th1/Th2 cytokines ratio was higher in the RPL group whereas there was a clear Th2 bias during the first trimester in the successful pregnancy group. Another suggested role for PIBF in protecting the trophoblast is through changes in NK cells activity [4]. Even though the role of these cells in normal pregnancy is still controversial, there have been reports of alteration of the subtypes of noncytotoxic NK cells in the decidua of a first trimester pregnancy [7, 8]. The relative proportion of these cells is increased in normal pregnancy compared with that of a nonpregnant uterus. However their activity is lower in the normal pregnancy compared to a nonpregnant uterus or to women with RPL [9].

In a study by Kalinka et al. [10], 27 women with threatened miscarriage were treated for 10 days with dydrogesterone (30–40 mg/day). Serum progesterone and estradiol concentrations, along with urine PIBF concentrations, were measured by ELISA. The results were compared to those of 16 healthy pregnant controls who received no treatment. There were no statistical differences between pregnancy outcomes in dydrogesterone-treated women with threatened miscarriage and healthy controls. Serum progesterone concentrations in the control patients increased as the pregnancy progressed, but not in the threatened miscarriage group. However, following dydrogesterone treatment, a statistically significant rise in the initially low PIBF levels was observed in the miscarriage group, reaching a comparable PIBF level to the healthy control group. This suggests that dydrogesterone might improve pregnancy success rates in threatened miscarriage by inducing PIBF production.

Luteal Phase Deficiency

The luteal phase is the later phase of the menstrual cycle, beginning with ovulation and the formation of the corpus luteum and ending in either pregnancy or lysis of the corpus luteum. The main hormone associated with this phase is progesterone, produced in large amounts by the corpus luteum and playing a critical role in increasing endometrium receptiveness for implantation of the blastocyst. The corpus luteum receives a signal to continue producing progesterone through the secretion of human chorionic gonadotropin (hCG) by the trophoblast, which also secretes estradiol, estrone, and relaxin. Removal of the corpus luteum prior to the completion of 8 weeks gestation results in miscarriage [11]. Luteal phase deficiency (LPD) is affected by several factors, including stress, exercise, weight loss, hyperprolactinemia, and menstrual cycles at the onset of puberty or perimenopause [12]; however, the exact mechanism for this disorder is unclear. Several hypotheses have been proposed to establish this mechanism. It could be associated with decreased levels of follicle stimulating hormone (FSH) and luteinizing hormone (LH) that may cause the corpus luteum to undergo atrophy. Other suggested mechanisms for LPD include decreased response to progesterone by the endometrium or failure of progesterone production secondary to abnormal follicle formation, along with a poor quality of the oocyte [12].

Even though the exact mechanism of LPD is unclear, there is no debate regarding the crucial role progesterone has in maintaining the early pregnancy. One possible mechanism is through the inhibition of oxytocin-induced myometrial activity around the time of ovulation [13]. Another suggested pathway is through inhibition of prostaglandin excitation, and diversity in prostaglandin E_2 (PGE2)-induced changes in glycosaminoglycan (GAG) synthesis by human fibroblasts of the cervix during pregnancy [14]. Other than its role in the luteal phase, progesterone also has an immunosuppressive effect, which helps maintain the pregnancy, and it also helps relax the uterine muscles, possibly by inhibiting prostaglandins and thus preventing uterine contractions [15, 16].

LPD can be diagnosed by measuring serum progesterone or by performing an endometrial biopsy. Although histologic dating of the endometrium after timed biopsy has been the historical gold standard for the diagnosis of LPD, the value and reproducibility of this modality is currently under debate. In a study of timed endometrial biopsies examining 130 fertile women, Murray and colleagues [17] found that histologic endometrial dating had neither the accuracy nor the precision to diagnose LPD and did not influence the clinical management of these patients. Luteal phase serum progesterone levels between 2 and 10 ng/ml and serum progesterone levels below 15 ng/ml in the first 10 weeks of gestation are considered diagnostic of corpus luteum dysfunction [6]. However, one should keep in mind that serum progesterone levels are not predictive of pregnancy outcome [4].

Recommendations for Progesterone Treatment in Women with Recurrent Pregnancy Loss

There are several studies supporting the administration of progesterone supplements to women with unexplained RPL. In a study by Zibdeh et al. [18], 180 women with unexplained RPL were randomized to receiving oral dydrogesterone, intramuscular hCG, or no treatment (controls). Treatment was started as soon as possible after confirmation of pregnancy and continued until the 12th gestational week. Pregnancy loss was significantly less common in the dydrogesterone group (13.4 %) than in the control group (29 %). There were no differences between the groups with respect to pregnancy complications or congenital abnormalities. This study demonstrated that hormonal support with dydrogesterone can increase the chances of a successful pregnancy in women with a history of RPL. In a systematic review conducted by Carp et al. [19] assessing whether dydrogesterone lowers the incidence of subsequent miscarriage in women with RPL, 509 women who fulfilled the criteria for meta-analysis

were included. The number of subsequent miscarriages or continuing pregnancies per woman was compared between women receiving dydrogesterone and women managed by standard bed rest or placebo intervention. There was a 10.5 % miscarriage rate after dydrogesterone administration compared to 23.5 % in control women (OR for miscarriage 0.29 [CI 0.13–0.65]) and a 13 % absolute reduction in the miscarriage rate. The results of this study show a significant reduction of 29 % in the odds for miscarriage when dydrogesterone is compared to standard care, indicating an actual treatment effect.

In a Cochrane database review published in 2013 [20], a subgroup analysis of women with RPL (defined as 3 or more consecutive miscarriages) treated with progesterone demonstrated a statistically significant decrease in miscarriage rate compared to placebo or no treatment (OR 0.39; 95 % CI 0.21–0.72); no statistically significant differences were found between the routes of administration of progesterone—oral, vaginal, or intramuscular (see Fig. 3.1).

Even though the studies regarding progesterone supplementation in RPL are scarce and not always statistically significant, the majority of them promote the use of progesterone in women with unexplained RPL. Further research in this area is recommended and is currently being conducted.

Recommendations based on current evidence state that progesterone supplementation may be of benefit in cases of RPL, especially when the etiology is unexplained [21, 22]. In our experience the use of progesterone up until 12 weeks of gestation should be considered for women with RPL, and that is the common practice in our clinic.

Prolactin and Recurrent Pregnancy Loss

Measurement of prolactin levels is part of the endocrinologic evaluation of RPL.

Hyperprolactinemia affects the hypothalamic-pituitary-ovarian axis and may cause insufficient folliculogenesis and oocyte maturation and/or

Study or subgroup	Progestogen n/N	Placebo n/N	Peto Odds Ratio Peto,Fixed,95% CI	Weight	Peto Odds Ratio Peto,Fixed,95% CI
I Women with a history of 3 or more prior miscarriages					
El-Zibdeh 2005	11/82	14/48		7.4 %	0.37 [0.15, 0.90]
Goldzieher 1964	2/8	4/10		1.6 %	0.53 [0.08, 3.59]
Le Vine 1964	4/15	8/15		2.9 %	0.34 [0.08, 1.44]
Swyer 1953	7/27	9/20		4.1 %	0.44 [0.13, 1.46]
Subtotal (95% CI)	**132**	**93**		**16.1 %**	**0.39 [0.21, 0.72]**

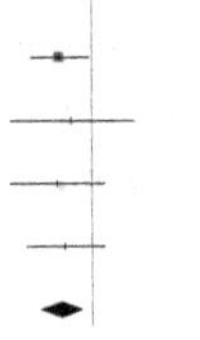

Fig. 3.1 Progestogen versus placebo/no treatment. Outcome 3 miscarriages (women with previous recurrent miscarriage only). [Adapted from Haas DM, Ramsey PS. Progestogen for preventing miscarriage. Cochrane Database Syst Rev. Has 2008;10:CD003511. With permission from John Wiley & Sons, Inc]

a short luteal phase. Increased circulating prolactin levels stimulate a generalized increase in hypothalamic dopaminergic neural activity, intended to suppress prolactin secretion but also inhibiting GnRH neurons. The end result is anovulation or an even more profound hypogonadotropic hypogonadism, depending on the extent to which gonadotropin secretion is suppressed. Mild hyperprolactinemia (20–50 ng/mL) may cause only a short luteal phase, resulting from poor preovulatory follicular development. Moderate hyperprolactinemia (50–100 ng/mL) frequently causes oligomenorrhea or amenorrhea, and higher prolactin levels (>100 ng/mL) typically result in frank hypogonadism with low estrogen levels and their clinical consequences [23].

Nevertheless, the association between hyperprolactinemia and RPL is debatable. In a case–control study, Bussen et al. evaluated the frequency of endocrine abnormalities during the follicular phase in women with a history of RPL. The concentration of prolactin in the study group of 42 women with RPL (three or more consecutive miscarriages) was significantly higher compared to the control group (42 nulligravid females with tubal or male factor infertility without miscarriage) ($p = 0.015$). They concluded that RPL is associated with abnormalities in prolactin secretion during the follicular phase [24].

Hirahara et al. found that treating with bromocriptine to achieve appropriate circulating levels of prolactin in women with RPL and prolactin disorder may improve subsequent pregnancy outcomes. The percentage of successful pregnancies was higher in the bromocriptine-treated group

than in the group that was not treated with bromocriptine (85.7 % vs. 52.4 %, $p < 0.05$), and the serum prolactin levels during early pregnancy were significantly higher in patients who miscarried (31.8–55.3 ng/mL) than in patients whose pregnancies were successful [25]. On the other hand, Li et al. measured some endocrine function in the early follicular phase (days 3–5) in 144 women with unexplained recurrent (≥ 3) miscarriages. No association was found between recurrent miscarriage and hyperprolactinemia [26].

Although the association between hyperprolactinemia and RPL is somewhat controversial, we recommend, as do others [21], to screen for prolactin levels as part of RPL evaluation.

Polycystic Ovary Syndrome and Recurrent Pregnancy Loss

Definition and Diagnosis

Polycystic ovary syndrome (PCOS) is a complex and multifactorial disorder, first described in 1935 by Stein and Leventhal [27]. The syndrome is a combination of hyperandrogenism, ovulatory dysfunction, and polycystic ovaries. The prevalence of PCOS is 4–7 % of women of reproductive age [28–30].

In recent years several expert groups addressed the issue of defining uniform diagnostic criteria for PCOS [31], i.e., the National Institutes of Health (NIH) criteria [32], the Rotterdam criteria [33], and the Androgen Excess Society [34]. These different criteria stressed the fact that the definition for PCOS is controversial and it has a wide spectrum of clinical presentation. The most widespread diagnostic criteria are the Rotterdam criteria, which require the presence of 2 out of 3 criteria for establishing a diagnosis: (1) Oligo- or anovulation, (2) Clinical and/or biochemical signs of hyperandrogenism, (3) Polycystic ovaries (presence of 12 or more follicles in each ovary measuring 2–9 mm in diameter, and/or increased ovarian volume >10 mL) [33].

All of these diagnostic criteria require the exclusion of other etiologies (e.g., congenital adrenal hyperplasia, androgen secreting tumors, Cushing's syndrome).

A large proportion of women with PCOS have some degree of ovulatory dysfunction, which results in oligomenorrhea or amenorrhea, and subsequent decreased infertility [35]. Hyperinsulinemia and insulin resistance are also common features among women with PCOS and are thought to have an important role in the pathophysiology of the syndrome [36]; however, it is not included in the diagnostic criteria. Moreover, in several studies that evaluated the prevalence of impaired glucose metabolism, it was found that 30–35 % of women with PCOS had impaired glucose tolerance and 7–10 % had type 2 diabetes mellitus [35, 37, 38].

Association with RPL

The prevalence of PCO morphology among women with RPL is thought to be as high as 40 % [39], although there are reports about higher prevalence [40]. Using a combination of clinical findings and ultrasound (US) or biochemical features, Yang et al. found that the prevalence of PCOS among women with RPL was even as high as 56 % [41]. On the other hand, Li et al. found that the prevalence of hyperandrogenemia in RPL was 14.6 % while ultrasound features of PCO existed in only 7.8 % [26]. This wide range is probably the result of the use of nonuniform definitions for PCOS. Cocksedge et al. examined PCOS prevalence among women with RPL, using the current recommended Rotterdam crite-

ria for diagnosis. The study investigated a total of 300 women with RPL and found that about 10 % of women had PCOS [42].

The Mechanism for Recurrent Pregnancy Loss Among Women with Polycystic Ovary Syndrome

The exact mechanisms that may cause RPL in PCOS patients are obscure. Several etiologies have been proposed, related to the pathophysiology, endocrinology, and metabolic disturbances in PCOS. Among these are obesity, insulin resistance or hyperinsulinemia, thrombophilia-associated disorders, elevated LH, and hyperandrogenism [39, 43, 44].

Elevated BMI

Many women with PCOS suffer from obesity and various comorbidities related to it (diabetes, HTN, coronary heart disease) [35]. A body mass index greater than 30 kg/m^2 increases the risk for RPL (OR: 3.5) [44, 45]. It has also been demonstrated that there is some correlation between PCOS, BMI, and RPL [46]. Weight loss among women with elevated BMI is associated with decreased pregnancy loss rates [47]. However, to date, no study has evaluated the association between weight loss and reduction in the risk for additional miscarriage in RPL patients [44].

Insulin Resistance and Hyperinsulinemia

In recent years there has been increasing interest in the role of insulin resistance and hyperinsulinemia linked to PCOS and RPL. Several studies have evaluated insulin resistance and RPL [48, 49]. In a population of women with RPL, there was found to be a higher prevalence of insulin resistance when compared with matched controls (OR: 3.55; 95 % CI 1.4–9.0) [48].

These findings were supported by studies showing that treatment with an insulin-sensitizing agent (metformin) reduced subsequent risk for miscarriage in women with RPL. Metformin lowers hepatic glucose production and increases insulin sensitivity and thereby lowers insulin blood levels. A retrospective cohort study has shown that the use of metformin during pregnancy is associated with a reduction in the miscarriage rate in women with RPL and PCOS [50]. Thereafter, a small prospective case–control clinical trial showed benefit of metformin treatment among PCOS women with RPL and abnormal glucose tolerance test [51]. Nawaz and Rizvi demonstrated, in a case–control study, that among infertile women treated with metformin there was significant decrease in the rate of pregnancy loss among women with RPL (12 % vs. 49 %; $p < 0.001$) [52]. However, to date, there are no randomized controlled trials assessing the role of metformin in women with RPL.

The only systematic review of randomized controlled trials concerning metformin and pregnancy loss among women with PCOS found that there was no improvement in pregnancy loss risk with metformin treatment [53].

Currently, routine metformin treatment during pregnancy is not recommended for women with PCOS [21, 31, 54].

Thrombophilic-Associated Disorders

Hyperinsulinemia and elevated activity of plasminogen activator inhibitor-1 (PAI-1) have been linked to increased incidence of miscarriage observed among women with PCOS [48, 55–57]. PAI-1 inhibits plasmin formation during plasminogen activation and subsequent fibrinolysis and has been reported to be elevated in women with PCOS. Elevated levels of PAI have been reported to be an independent risk factor for early spontaneous pregnancy loss [56]. In addition to its effects on insulin resistance, metformin lowers circulating levels of plasminogen activator inhibitor (PAI) [58].

Hyperhomocysteinemia is a common finding in women with PCOS [59] and was found to be associated with both RPL and PCOS [60]. It was shown that combined treatment with aspirin and low molecular weight heparin (LMWH) in women with hyperhomocysteinemia improved successful pregnancy rates [61]. In a small (~20 women) nonrandomized controlled study investigating women with PCOS with a history of one or more previous spontaneous miscarriages, who also had thrombophilia and/or hypofibrinolysis, it was found that the use of low molecular weight heparin along with metformin reduced pregnancy loss by 4.4-fold compared to previous gestations without treatment [62, 63].

Elevated LH and Hyperandrogenism

Hyperandrogenism and elevated LH are considered a part of the biochemical features of PCOS and have classically served a significant role in diagnosis of women with PCOS [35, 64]. In recent years, their significance in the diagnosis of PCOS has decreased, and since LH is released in pulses, abnormal levels are generally not used in order to diagnose PCOS [35].

Although elevated follicular phase LH and hyperandrogenism have been linked to RPL [39, 43], routine testing for LH and free-T in order to diagnose PCOS in patients with RPL is not recommended, since it did not predict subsequent miscarriage [65]. There was no difference in subsequent pregnancy outcome in women with prior RPL with high LH and elevated testosterone, compared to those with normal values [39, 66]. Suppressing LH secretion did not improve the outcome of pregnancy [67, 68].

PCOS is a complex entity, which encompasses a spectrum of endocrinologic and metabolic phenomena. When reviewing the literature dealing with RPL and its relation to PCOS, we may conclude that the relation of PCOS and RPL is weak; the different mechanisms suggested are just other supporting evidence for that. We can single out insulin resistance as one of the leading possible connections between PCOS and RPL, which may lead us to the notion that glucose metabolism, rather than PCOS per se, is more strongly related to the etiology of RPL.

When searching for an etiology for RPL in an index case, we should not try to reach the diagnosis of PCOS unless specific clinical features strongly suggest this entity, and aim at testing this woman's glucose tolerance.

Treatment Options

In the committee opinion of the American Society for Reproductive Medicine (ASRM) dealing with the recommended evaluation and treatment of RPL, PCOS is mentioned to have controversial scientific evidence for its association with pregnancy loss [21].

The recommendations for PCOS women with RPL should include weight reduction when BMI is elevated, and consider metformin in a specific population of women with elevated levels of both insulin and androgen.

Weight Loss

Life style modification, specifically weight loss, has a beneficial effect on several medical conditions related to obesity and PCOS. An additional benefit of the medical recommendation for BMI reduction for obese PCOS patients might be in lowering the incidence of RPL (see Chap. 9).

Metformin Supplementation

Metformin use during pregnancy does not appear to be linked to teratogenicity or developmental disorders among exposed children studied during their first 18 months of life [62]. There is insufficient evidence to evaluate the effect of metformin in pregnancy to prevent early pregnancy loss in women with RPL. Empirical treatment may be offered only in the context of clinical trial [43].

The use of LMWH may reduce the incidence of RPL in a selected group of women with PCOS and thrombophilia [62, 63] and needs additional research before we can recommend its use as part of treatment guidelines in those patients.

Thyroid Disorders and Recurrent Pregnancy Loss

Thyroid disorders are among the most common endocrine disorders in women of childbearing age. Thyroid disorders are divided into (1) Hyperthyroidism—excess activity resulting in increased level of thyroid hormones (T3 triiodothyronine and T4 thyroxine) and decreased levels of TSH (thyroid-stimulating hormone), and (2) Hypothyroidism—decrease in the level of thyroid hormones with elevated TSH.

Thyroid disorders have been associated with several early pregnancy and obstetric adverse outcomes such as infertility (or subfertility), early pregnancy loss, preeclampsia, stillbirth, and preterm labor and delivery [69–71]. A certain degree of impairment in neurocognitive development has also been described in relation to overt hypothyroidism [72].

There is evidence that pregnant women express different levels of TSH and free T4, and therefore measurements of thyroid functions may require gestation-specific reference ranges, according to the pregnancy trimester [73]. This is also reinforced by the observation that in women requiring thyroid replacement therapy during pregnancy, there is an increase in levothyroxine requirement starting as early as the first trimester, and a need for close monitoring of thyroid functions throughout pregnancy [74, 75].

Hypothyroidism and Pregnancy Loss

Hypothyroidism is the second most common endocrinopathy during pregnancy, and its incidence ranges from 2 to 5 %. Autoimmune thyroiditis (also known as Hashimoto's thyroiditis) and iatrogenic thyroid gland destruction as a therapeutic measure for hyperthyroidism are the most common etiologies for this endocrinopathy in pregnant women [74, 76, 77]. Disorders of hypothyroidism can be divided into overt and subclinical hypothyroidism, the latter usually presenting with elevated TSH and normal levels of thyroid hormones.

Observational studies have described an increased rate of first trimester pregnancy loss in women with overt and subclinical hypothyroidism. It has been shown that the risk of child loss (composite outcome for miscarriage and fetal and neonatal death) was significantly increased with the increase in TSH levels during early pregnancy, even within normal range. There was no such association between FT4 levels and the risk of child loss in the same population [78]. It has also been shown that women with subclinical hypothyroidism have a lower gestational age at miscarriage [79].

In euthyroid women, negative to thyroid autoantibodies, the rate of pregnancy loss was found to be significantly higher in women with TSH between 2.5 and 5.0 mIU/L compared to women with TSH level below 2.5 mIU/L [80]. This finding raises questions about redefining the normal range of TSH during pregnancy, especially in the first trimester, influencing risk for miscarriage.

Treatment with thyroid replacement therapy (levothyroxine), when adequate, results in a lower miscarriage rate. In a population of women diagnosed with hypothyroidism, when levothyroxine treatment was inadequate, the outcome of pregnancy was miscarriage in 60 % of overtly hypothyroid women and in 71.4 % of subclinically hypothyroid women ($p < 0.006$). When treatment was adequate, term pregnancy was achieved in 100 % of overtly hypothyroid women and 90.5 % of subclinically hypothyroid women ($p < 0.006$) [69].

Hypothyroidism and Recurrent Pregnancy Loss

Several studies have described the relationship between hypothyroidism and RPL. The prevalence of hypothyroidism among women with a history of RPL ranges from 4 to 10 % [79, 81, 82]. The rate of subclinical hypothyroidism in the RPL population has a wider range between 7 and 29 % [82–85]. This rate is also influenced by the TSH threshold for defining subclinical hypothyroidism [80, 85].

In one observational cohort study examining over 200 women with a history of RPL, no statistically significant difference was shown with regard to the subsequent live birth rate between the subclinical hypothyroidism and euthyroid groups, nor in the treated and untreated subclinical hypothyroidism subgroups [82].

Hyperthyroidism

The prevalence of hyperthyroidism during pregnancy ranges from 0.1 to 1 %, with Graves' disease accounting for most of the cases [74, 86]. The prevalence of hyperthyroidism among women with a history of RPL in one study was shown to be 3 % [82].

The relationship between pregnancy loss and hyperthyroidism was described mainly in reports of small numbers of subjects, and hyperthyroidism is generally not considered a major risk factor for miscarriage. Maternal hyperthyroidism before and during pregnancy was associated with a higher prevalence of spontaneous miscarriages, even when these women were treated [87]. One report of a specific familial disorder showed a higher rate of miscarriage in women affected by familial resistance to thyroid hormones (high serum concentration of free thyroxine and triiodothyronine without suppressed thyrotropin) compared to unaffected relatives [88]. Currently, there is no recommendation to routinely evaluate hyperthyroidism in women with RPL [21, 68].

Positive Anti-thyroid Peroxidase and Anti-thyroid Thyroglobulin in Women with Pregnancy Loss

In recent years, there has been a rise in interest in the effect of thyroid autoantibodies on first trimester pregnancy loss, and more specifically recurrent pregnancy loss. It is thought that anti-thyroid antibodies exert their effect in both a TSH-dependent and a TSH-independent manner [85–89].

The prevalence of anti-thyroid antibodies in females of childbearing age is 10–18 % [83, 84, 90, 91]. In one study less than 20 % of the women with anti-thyroid antibodies were clinically hypothyroid [83]. The prevalence of anti-thyroid antibodies in women with RPL is significantly higher, between 19 and 30 % [83, 84, 91, 92].

Although in some studies the presence of thyroid autoantibodies did not affect the future risk of pregnancy loss in the population of women with RPL [92], a meta-analysis of 22 studies showed a clear association between thyroid autoimmunity and miscarriage with a pooled odds ratio of 2.5 in eight case–control studies and a pooled relative risk of 2.3 in 14 cohort studies [93]. A second meta-analysis of 31 studies published around the same time evaluated linkage between anti-thyroid antibodies and miscarriage, with 28 studies showing a positive association. When dividing the meta-analysis to cohort and case–control studies, the data in the cohort showed an odds ratio of 3.9 for miscarriage with the presence of thyroid autoantibodies. The odds ratio of miscarriage for women with RPL with positive thyroid autoantibodies was 4.22. For case–control studies the odds ratio for miscarriage was 1.8, and slightly higher in women with RPL (OR 1.86, $p = 0.008$) [94].

The antibodies most frequently associated with pregnancy loss and RPL are anti-thyroid-peroxidase (anti-TPO) and anti-thyroglobulin (anti-TG) [84, 91, 95]. Several studies have demonstrated that women with RPL positive for anti-thyroid antibodies also have a higher rate of other autoimmune antibodies (up to 90 %), suggesting a more general maternal immune system abnormality leading to RPL (see Fig. 3.2) [89, 91, 95].

Treatment with thyroid replacement therapy in early pregnancy has been suggested in women with positive antibodies regardless of thyroid functions. In one study, in women positive for anti-TPO antibodies there was no difference in the prevalence of miscarriage between hypothyroid and euthyroid groups after treatment with L-thyroxine [84].

Screening Recommendation for Women with Recurrent Pregnancy Loss

TSH measurement, with or without thyroid hormone levels, is an inexpensive and sensitive tool for evaluation of thyroid function abnormalities. As such, it has been recommended by several clinical societies as a part of the preliminary evaluation for women with RPL [21, 22]. However, some authors recommend considering TSH measurement for the evaluation of RPL only for women with clinical signs or symptoms of thyroid abnormalities [96]. Notably, recent studies have advocated a change in the threshold for subclinical hypothyroidism, suggesting that TSH values above 2.5 mIU/L might be considered outside the normal range [21, 80].

Universal screening of thyroid functions for pregnant women is currently not recommended, since it did not result in a decrease in adverse outcomes when compared with case findings according to risk factors [97].

Recommendations for screening for thyroid autoantibodies are still inconclusive. Currently, societies dealing with reproductive medicine conclude that there is insufficient data to recommend routine screening of antibodies, especially when TSH is measured in the normal range [21, 68]. Recent clinical practice guidelines cosponsored by the American Association of Clinical Endocrinologists and the American Thyroid Association state that anti-TPO measurement should be considered when evaluating patients with RPL, regardless of infertility [98].

Several studies have shown some advantage in a measurement of TSH values after a short TRH stimulation test, where abnormal response or the expression of higher TSH values are thought to be related to early pregnancy loss and RPL [99, 100]. However, this test is not commonly accepted as part of RPL evaluation.

In view of the recent literature, our recommendation is that baseline TSH levels (with or without thyroxine levels) should be measured in all patients presenting with RPL, and that measurement of anti-TPO and anti-TG should be considered in patients in whom thyroid dysfunction is suspected in view of clinical signs and symptoms or abnormal TSH/thyroxine levels. Establishing the presence of thyroid autoantibodies in this population may also contribute to further research in search of a better understanding of the association between thyroid autoimmunity and RPL.

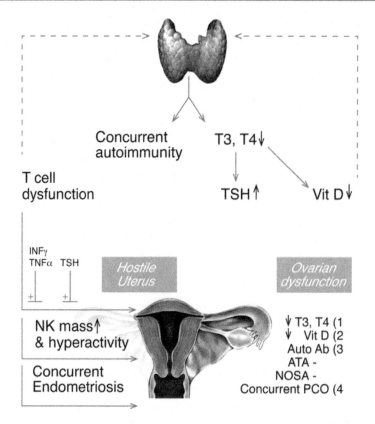

Fig. 3.2 Schematic illustration of the pathophysiological mechanisms that underlie infertility and pregnancy loss in women with hypothyroid autoimmunity. *Dashed lines* denote factors that potentially contribute to thyroid auto-immunity in addition to their effect on infertility (vitamin D and T cell dysfunction). For clarity, mechanisms are grouped into those that are primarily associated with hostile uterine environment and ovarian dysfunction. Concurrent autoimmunity is frequently seen in women with thyroid hypothyroidism and is associated with non-organ–specific antibodies (NOSA) in addition to autoim-mune thyroid antibodies (ATA; other indirect effects are not indicated). Concurrent endometriosis and polycystic ovary are indicated due to their increased association with thyroid autoimmunity. Thyroxine, T4; Triiodothyronine, T3; Vit D, Vitamin D; TSH, Thyroid-stimulating hormone; Interferon-g, INFg; Tumor necrosis factor-a, TNF-a; Natural killer cells, NK; PCO, polycystic ovaries. [Reprinted from Twig G, Shina A, Amital H, Shoenfeld Y. Pathogenesis of infertility and recurrent pregnancy loss in thyroid autoimmunity. J Autoimmun. 2012;38(2-3):J275-81. With permission from Elsevier]

Treatment Recommendation for Women with Recurrent Pregnancy Loss

Currently the standard of care for pregnant women or women trying to conceive is treatment with thyroid replacement therapy in order to achieve a euthyroid state [75]. It has been shown that adequate treatment of hypothyroid state during gestation minimizes the risks of many possible adverse outcomes, including the risk for pregnancy loss [22, 68, 69].

In regard to patients with positive autoantibodies who are euthyroid, there is insufficient evidence as to the need for thyroid replacement therapy [84]. The clinical practice guidelines cosponsored by the American Association of Clinical Endocrinologists and the American Thyroid Association state that treatment with L-thyroxine should be considered in women of childbearing age with normal serum TSH levels when they are pregnant or planning a pregnancy if they have or have had positive levels of serum anti-TPO, particularly when there is a history of miscarriage or past history of hypothyroidism [98].

Due to the relationship between thyroid autoimmunity and the presence of other autoantibodies in women with RPL, several studies have evaluated the use of intravenous immunoglobulin (IVIG) in thyroid autoantibodies positive patients. This treatment is not common, especially since thyroid replacement therapy appears to be more effective than IVIG in preventing a new miscarriage in a population with RPL [101].

In conclusion, thyroid replacement therapy should be initiated for every woman with RPL and abnormal thyroid function tests. As for euthyroid women with positive autoantibodies, the initiation of treatment is not well established and should be tailored according to individual patient characteristics pending further research in this area.

Uncontrolled Diabetes and Recurrent Pregnancy Loss

Women with poorly controlled pregestational diabetes, reflected by hemoglobin A1c (HbA1c) levels higher than 8 %, seem to have higher rates of spontaneous abortion in early pregnancy compared to women without diabetes. Diabetic women with good metabolic control are no more likely to experience pregnancy loss compared with nondiabetic women [102]. A direct correlation exists between HbA1c levels, the incidence of pregnancy loss, and congenital malformations, even in nondiabetic patients [103]. Therefore it is recommended in ASRM guidelines to assess HbA1c for women with RPL [21].

One of the possible mechanisms for the increased rate of pregnancy loss in women with elevated HbA1c is an increase in congenital malformations. A meta-analysis conducted by Ray et al. [104] compared levels of HbA1c of diabetic pregnant women with preconception care to those without any care. In 14 cohort studies reviewed, the pooled rate of major anomalies was lower among preconception care recipients (2.1 %) than in nonrecipients (6.5 %) (RR 0.36, 95 % CI 0.22–0.59), and this finding was linked by the authors to a significantly lower first tri-

mester HbA1c in women who received preconception care.

The level of HbA1c related to an increase in first trimester pregnancy loss is also an important study issue. Greene et al. conducted a study of 303 pregnant type 1 DM patients; the risk of spontaneous abortion was found to be 12.4 % with first trimester HbA1c ≤ 9.3 %, and 37.5 % with HbA1c > 14.4 % (risk ratio (RR) 3.0, 95 % CI 1.3–7.0) [105]. In an observational study conducted by Temple et al. [106], women were divided into two groups according to their HbA1c concentration upon their first visit. Women with values <7.5 % (mean of normal range plus 5 standard deviations) were defined as having fair-control and those with values ≥ 7.5 % were defined as having poor control. There were 242 pregnancies in 158 women; 32 pregnancies had an adverse outcome, with 18 (7 %) spontaneous miscarriages. Adverse outcome was significantly higher in the poor-control group than the fair-control group (RR 4.3, 95 % CI 1.8–10). Also, when comparing the spontaneous miscarriage rate, the poor-control group had a fourfold increase in the spontaneous miscarriage rate compared with the fair-control group (RR 4.0, 95 % CI 1.2–13.1). Therefore, it can be concluded that to prevent most pregnancy losses in diabetic women, the recommended level of HbA1c should be ≤ 7.5.

Finally, screening for diabetes mellitus should be done to patients with RPL at least by fasting glucose. However, as was mention before, it is recommended in the ASRM guidelines to assess HbA1c for women with RPL [21].

References

1. Schindler AE, Campagnoli C, Druckmann R, Huber J, Pasqualini JR, Schweppe KW, et al. Classification and pharmacology of progestins. Maturitas. 2003;46 Suppl 1:S7–16.
2. Wen DX, Xu YF, Mais DE, Goldman ME, McDonnell DP. The A and B isoforms of the human progesterone receptor operate through distinct signaling pathways within target cells. Mol Cell Biol. 1994;14(12):8356–64.
3. Su MT, Lee IW, Chen YC, Kuo PL. Association of progesterone receptor polymorphism with idiopathic

recurrent pregnancy loss in Taiwanese Han population. J Assist Reprod Genet. 2011;28(3):239–43.

4. Druckmann R, Druckmann MA. Progesterone and the immunology of pregnancy. J Steroid Biochem Mol Biol. 2005;97:389–96.

5. Faust Z, Laskarin G, Rukavina D, Szekeres-Bartho J. Progesterone-induced blocking factor inhibits degranulation of natural killer cells. Am J Reprod Immunol. 1999;42(2):71–5.

6. Raghupathy R, Makhseed M, Azizieh F, Omu A, Gupta M, Farhat R. Cytokine production by maternal lymphocytes during normal human pregnancy and in unexplained recurrent spontaneous abortion. Hum Reprod. 2000;15(3):713–8.

7. Shemesh A, Tirosh D, Sheiner E, Tirosh NB, Brusilovsky M, Segev R, et al. First trimester pregnancy loss and the expression of alternatively spliced NKp30 isoforms in maternal blood and placental tissue. Front Immunol. 2015;6:189.

8. Lachapelle MH, Miron P, Hemmings R, Roy DC. Endometrial T, B, and NK cells in patients with recurrent spontaneous abortion. Altered profile and pregnancy outcome. J Immunol. 1996;156(10): 4027–34.

9. Chao KH, Yang YS, Ho HN, Chen SU, Chen HF, Dai HJ, et al. Decidual natural killer cytotoxicity decreased in normal pregnancy but not in anembryonic pregnancy and recurrent spontaneous abortion. Am J Reprod Immunol. 1995;34(5):274–80.

10. Kalinka J, Szekeres-Bartho J. The impact of dydrogesterone supplementation on hormonal profile and progesterone-induced blocking factor concentrations in women with threatened abortion. Am J Reprod Immunol. 2005;53(4):166–71.

11. Csapo AI, Pulkkinen M. Indispensability of the human corpus luteum in the maintenance of early pregnancy. Luteectomy evidence. Obstet Gynecol Surv. 1978;33(2):69–81.

12. Luisi SLL, Genazzani AR. Endocrinology of pregnancy loss. In: Carp HJA, editor. Recurrent pregnancy loss, causes, controversies and treatment. Boca Raton: Taylor and Francis Group; 2008. p. 79–87.

13. Csapo AI, Pinto-Dantas CA. The effect of progesterone on the human uterus. Proc Natl Acad Sci U S A. 1965;54(4):1069–76.

14. Carbonne B, Dallot E, Haddad B, Ferre F, Cabrol D. Effects of progesterone on prostaglandin E(2)-induced changes in glycosaminoglycan synthesis by human cervical fibroblasts in culture. Mol Hum Reprod. 2000;6(7):661–4.

15. Tan H, Yi L, Rote NS, Hurd WW, Mesiano S. Progesterone receptor-A and -B have opposite effects on proinflammatory gene expression in human myometrial cells: implications for progesterone actions in human pregnancy and parturition. J Clin Endocrinol Metab. 2012;97(5):E719–30.

16. Szekeres-Bartho J, Halasz M, Palkovics T. Progesterone in pregnancy; receptor-ligand inter-

action and signaling pathways. J Reprod Immunol. 2009;83(1-2):60–4.

17. Murray MJ, Meyer WR, Zaino RJ, Lessey BA, Novotny DB, Ireland K, et al. A critical analysis of the accuracy, reproducibility, and clinical utility of histologic endometrial dating in fertile women. Fertil Steril. 2004;81(5):1333–43.

18. El-Zibdeh MY. Dydrogesterone in the reduction of recurrent spontaneous abortion. J Steroid Biochem Mol Biol. 2005;97(5):431–4.

19. Carp H. A systematic review of dydrogesterone for the treatment of recurrent miscarriage. Gynecol Endocrinol. 2015;1–9.

20. Haas DM, Ramsey PS. Progestogen for preventing miscarriage. Cochrane Database Syst Rev. 2013;10, CD003511.

21. Medicine PCotASfR. Evaluation and treatment of recurrent pregnancy loss: a committee opinion. Fertil Steril. 2012;98(5):1103–11.

22. Jauniaux E, Farquharson RG, Christiansen OB, Exalto N. Evidence-based guidelines for the investigation and medical treatment of recurrent miscarriage. Hum Reprod. 2006;21(9):2216–22.

23. Speroff L, Fritz MA. Clinical gynecologic endocrinology and infertility. 8th ed. Philadelphia: Lippincott Williams & Wilkins; 2011.

24. Bussen S, Sütterlin M, Steck T. Endocrine abnormalities during the follicular phase in women with recurrent spontaneous abortion. Hum Reprod. 1999;14(1):18–20.

25. Hirahara F, Andoh N, Sawai K, Hirabuki T, Uemura T, Minaguchi H. Hyperprolactinemic recurrent miscarriage and results of randomized bromocriptine treatment trials. Fertil Steril. 1998;70(2):246–52.

26. Li TC, Spuijbroek MD, Tuckerman E, Anstie B, Loxley M, Laird S. Endocrinological and endometrial factors in recurrent miscarriage. BJOG. 2000;107(12):1471–9.

27. Stein IFLM. Amenorrhea associated with bilateral polycystic ovaries. Am J Obstet Gynecol. 1935;29:181.

28. Knochenhauer ES, Key TJ, Kahsar-Miller M, Waggoner W, Boots LR, Azziz R. Prevalence of the polycystic ovary syndrome in unselected black and white women of the southeastern United States: a prospective study. J Clin Endocrinol Metab. 1998;83(9):3078–82.

29. Asunción M, Calvo RM, San Millán JL, Sancho J, Avila S, Escobar-Morreale HF. A prospective study of the prevalence of the polycystic ovary syndrome in unselected Caucasian women from Spain. J Clin Endocrinol Metab. 2000;85(7):2434–8.

30. Azziz R, Woods KS, Reyna R, Key TJ, Knochenhauer ES, Yildiz BO. The prevalence and features of the polycystic ovary syndrome in an unselected population. J Clin Endocrinol Metab. 2004;89(6):2745–9.

31. Bulletins--Gynecology ACoP. ACOG Practice Bulletin No. 108: Polycystic ovary syndrome. Obstet Gynecol. 2009;114(4):936–49.

32. Dunaif AGJ, Haseltine FP, Merriam GR. Polycystic ovary syndrome. Boston: Blackwell Scientific Publications; 1992.

33. Group REA-SPCW. Revised 2003 consensus on diagnostic criteria and long-term health risks related to polycystic ovary syndrome. Fertil Steril. 2004;81(1):19–25.

34. Azziz R, Carmina E, Dewailly D, Diamanti-Kandarakis E, Escobar-Morreale HF, Futterweit W, et al. Positions statement: criteria for defining polycystic ovary syndrome as a predominantly hyperandrogenic syndrome: an Androgen Excess Society guideline. J Clin Endocrinol Metab. 2006;91(11): 4237–45.

35. Ehrmann DA. Polycystic ovary syndrome. N Engl J Med. 2005;352(12):1223–36.

36. Dunaif A. Insulin resistance and the polycystic ovary syndrome: mechanism and implications for pathogenesis. Endocr Rev. 1997;18(6):774–800.

37. Ehrmann DA, Barnes RB, Rosenfield RL, Cavaghan MK, Imperial J. Prevalence of impaired glucose tolerance and diabetes in women with polycystic ovary syndrome. Diabetes Care. 1999;22(1):141–6.

38. Legro RS, Kunselman AR, Dodson WC, Dunaif A. Prevalence and predictors of risk for type 2 diabetes mellitus and impaired glucose tolerance in polycystic ovary syndrome: a prospective, controlled study in 254 affected women. J Clin Endocrinol Metab. 1999;84(1):165–9.

39. Rai R, Backos M, Rushworth F, Regan L. Polycystic ovaries and recurrent miscarriage--a reappraisal. Hum Reprod. 2000;15(3):612–5.

40. Watson H, Kiddy DS, Hamilton-Fairley D, Scanlon MJ, Barnard C, Collins WP, et al. Hypersecretion of luteinizing hormone and ovarian steroids in women with recurrent early miscarriage. Hum Reprod. 1993;8(6):829–33.

41. Yang CJ, Stone P, Stewart AW. The epidemiology of recurrent miscarriage: a descriptive study of 1214 prepregnant women with recurrent miscarriage. Aust N Z J Obstet Gynaecol. 2006;46(4):316–22.

42. Cocksedge KA, Saravelos SH, Metwally M, Li TC. How common is polycystic ovary syndrome in recurrent miscarriage? Reprod Biomed Online. 2009;19(4):572–6.

43. Cocksedge KA, Li TC, Saravelos SH, Metwally M. A reappraisal of the role of polycystic ovary syndrome in recurrent miscarriage. Reprod Biomed Online. 2008;17(1):151–60.

44. Sugiura-Ogasawara M. Recurrent pregnancy loss and obesity. Best Pract Res Clin Obstet Gynaecol. 2015;29(4):489–97.

45. Lashen H, Fear K, Sturdee DW. Obesity is associated with increased risk of first trimester and recurrent miscarriage: matched case-control study. Hum Reprod. 2004;19(7):1644–6.

46. Al-Azemi M, Omu FE, Omu AE. The effect of obesity on the outcome of infertility management in women with polycystic ovary syndrome. Arch Gynecol Obstet. 2004;270(4):205–10.

47. Clark AM, Ledger W, Galletly C, Tomlinson L, Blaney F, Wang X, et al. Weight loss results in significant improvement in pregnancy and ovulation rates in anovulatory obese women. Hum Reprod. 1995;10(10):2705–12.

48. Craig LB, Ke RW, Kutteh WH. Increased prevalence of insulin resistance in women with a history of recurrent pregnancy loss. Fertil Steril. 2002;78(3): 487–90.

49. Chakraborty P, Goswami SK, Rajani S, Sharma S, Kabir SN, Chakravarty B, et al. Recurrent pregnancy loss in polycystic ovary syndrome: role of hyperhomocysteinemia and insulin resistance. PLoS One. 2013;8(5), e64446.

50. Jakubowicz DJ, Iuorno MJ, Jakubowicz S, Roberts KA, Nestler JE. Effects of metformin on early pregnancy loss in the polycystic ovary syndrome. J Clin Endocrinol Metab. 2002;87(2):524–9.

51. Zolghadri J, Tavana Z, Kazerooni T, Soveid M, Taghieh M. Relationship between abnormal glucose tolerance test and history of previous recurrent miscarriages, and beneficial effect of metformin in these patients: a prospective clinical study. Fertil Steril. 2008;90(3):727–30.

52. Nawaz FH, Rizvi J. Continuation of metformin reduces early pregnancy loss in obese Pakistani women with polycystic ovarian syndrome. Gynecol Obstet Invest. 2010;69(3):184–9.

53. Palomba S, Falbo A, Orio F, Zullo F. Effect of preconceptional metformin on abortion risk in polycystic ovary syndrome: a systematic review and meta-analysis of randomized controlled trials. Fertil Steril. 2009;92(5):1646–58.

54. Mathur R, Alexander CJ, Yano J, Trivax B, Azziz R. Use of metformin in polycystic ovary syndrome. Am J Obstet Gynecol. 2008;199(6):596–609.

55. Atiomo WU, Bates SA, Condon JE, Shaw S, West JH, Prentice AG. The plasminogen activator system in women with polycystic ovary syndrome. Fertil Steril. 1998;69(2):236–41.

56. Glueck CJ, Wang P, Fontaine RN, Sieve-Smith L, Tracy T, Moore SK. Plasminogen activator inhibitor activity: an independent risk factor for the high miscarriage rate during pregnancy in women with polycystic ovary syndrome. Metabolism. 1999;48(12):1589–95.

57. Glueck CJ, Wang P, Bornovali S, Goldenberg N, Sieve L. Polycystic ovary syndrome, the G1691A factor V Leiden mutation, and plasminogen activator inhibitor activity: associations with recurrent pregnancy loss. Metabolism. 2003;52(12):1627–32.

58. Palomba S, Orio F, Falbo A, Russo T, Tolino A, Zullo F. Plasminogen activator inhibitor 1 and miscarriage after metformin treatment and laparoscopic ovarian drilling in patients with polycystic ovary syndrome. Fertil Steril. 2005;84(3):761–5.

59. Wijeyaratne CN, Nirantharakumar K, Balen AH, Barth JH, Sheriff R, Belchetz PE. Plasma homocysteine in polycystic ovary syndrome: does it correlate with insulin resistance and ethnicity? Clin Endocrinol (Oxf). 2004;60(5):560–7.

60. Kazerooni T, Ghaffarpasand F, Asadi N, Dehkhoda Z, Dehghankhalili M, Kazerooni Y. Correlation between thrombophilia and recurrent pregnancy loss in patients with polycystic ovary syndrome: a comparative study. J Chin Med Assoc. 2013;76(5): 282–8.

61. Chakraborty P, Banerjee S, Saha P, Nandi SS, Sharma S, Goswami SK, et al. Aspirin and low-molecular weight heparin combination therapy effectively prevents recurrent miscarriage in hyperhomocysteinemic women. PLoS One. 2013;8(9), e74155.

62. Glueck CJ, Goldenberg N, Pranikoff J, Loftspring M, Sieve L, Wang P. Height, weight, and motor-social development during the first 18 months of life in 126 infants born to 109 mothers with polycystic ovary syndrome who conceived on and continued metformin through pregnancy. Hum Reprod. 2004;19(6):1323–30.

63. Ramidi G, Khan N, Glueck CJ, Wang P, Goldenberg N. Enoxaparin-metformin and enoxaparin alone may safely reduce pregnancy loss. Transl Res. 2009;153(1):33–43.

64. Kumar A, Woods KS, Bartolucci AA, Azziz R. Prevalence of adrenal androgen excess in patients with the polycystic ovary syndrome (PCOS). Clin Endocrinol (Oxf). 2005;62(6):644–9.

65. Sugiura-Ogasawara M, Sato T, Suzumori N, Kitaori T, Kumagai K, Ozaki Y. The polycystic ovary syndrome does not predict further miscarriage in Japanese couples experiencing recurrent miscarriages. Am J Reprod Immunol. 2009;61(1):62–7.

66. Nardo LG, Rai R, Backos M, El-Gaddal S, Regan L. High serum luteinizing hormone and testosterone concentrations do not predict pregnancy outcome in women with recurrent miscarriage. Fertil Steril. 2002;77(2):348–52.

67. Clifford K, Rai R, Watson H, Franks S, Regan L. Does suppressing luteinising hormone secretion reduce the miscarriage rate? Results of a randomised controlled trial. BMJ. 1996;312(7045):1508–11.

68. 17 RCoOaGRG-TGN. The investigation and treatment of couples with recurrent first-trimester and second-trimester miscarriage. April 2011.

69. Abalovich M, Gutierrez S, Alcaraz G, Maccallini G, Garcia A, Levalle O. Overt and subclinical hypothyroidism complicating pregnancy. Thyroid. 2002; 12(1):63–8.

70. Poppe K, Glinoer D. Thyroid autoimmunity and hypothyroidism before and during pregnancy. Hum Reprod Update. 2003;9(2):149–61.

71. van den Boogaard E, Vissenberg R, Land JA, van Wely M, van der Post JA, Goddijn M, et al. Significance of (sub)clinical thyroid dysfunction and thyroid autoimmunity before conception and in early pregnancy: a systematic review. Hum Reprod Update. 2011;17(5):605–19.

72. Haddow JE, Palomaki GE, Allan WC, Williams JR, Knight GJ, Gagnon J, et al. Maternal thyroid deficiency during pregnancy and subsequent neuropsychological development of the child. N Engl J Med. 1999;341(8):549–55.

73. Lambert-Messerlian G, McClain M, Haddow JE, Palomaki GE, Canick JA, Cleary-Goldman J, et al. First- and second-trimester thyroid hormone reference data in pregnant women: a FaSTER (First- and Second-Trimester Evaluation of Risk for aneuploidy) Research Consortium study. Am J Obstet Gynecol. 2008;199(1):62.e1–6.

74. LeBeau SO, Mandel SJ. Thyroid disorders during pregnancy. Endocrinol Metab Clin North Am. 2006;35(1):117–36. vii.

75. Alexander EK, Marqusee E, Lawrence J, Jarolim P, Fischer GA, Larsen PR. Timing and magnitude of increases in levothyroxine requirements during pregnancy in women with hypothyroidism. N Engl J Med. 2004;351(3):241–9.

76. Nambiar V, Jagtap VS, Sarathi V, Lila AR, Kamalanathan S, Bandgar TR, et al. Prevalence and impact of thyroid disorders on maternal outcome in asian-Indian pregnant women. J Thyroid Res. 2011; 2011:429097.

77. Casey BM, Dashe JS, Spong CY, McIntire DD, Leveno KJ, Cunningham GF. Perinatal significance of isolated maternal hypothyroxinemia identified in the first half of pregnancy. Obstet Gynecol. 2007;109(5):1129–35.

78. Benhadi N, Wiersinga WM, Reitsma JB, Vrijkotte TG, Bonsel GJ. Higher maternal TSH levels in pregnancy are associated with increased risk for miscarriage, fetal or neonatal death. Eur J Endocrinol. 2009;160(6):985–91.

79. De Vivo A, Mancuso A, Giacobbe A, Moleti M, Maggio Savasta L, De Dominici R, et al. Thyroid function in women found to have early pregnancy loss. Thyroid. 2010;20(6):633–7.

80. Negro R, Schwartz A, Gismondi R, Tinelli A, Mangieri T, Stagnaro-Green A. Increased pregnancy loss rate in thyroid antibody negative women with TSH levels between 2.5 and 5.0 in the first trimester of pregnancy. J Clin Endocrinol Metab. 2010;95(9):E44–8.

81. Rao VR, Lakshmi A, Sadhnani MD. Prevalence of hypothyroidism in recurrent pregnancy loss in first trimester. Indian J Med Sci. 2008;62(9):357–61.

82. Bernardi LA, Cohen RN, Stephenson MD. Impact of subclinical hypothyroidism in women with recurrent early pregnancy loss. Fertil Steril. 2013;100(5): 1326–31.

83. Kutteh WH, Yetman DL, Carr AC, Beck LA, Scott RT. Increased prevalence of antithyroid antibodies identified in women with recurrent pregnancy loss but not in women undergoing assisted reproduction. Fertil Steril. 1999;71(5):843–8.

84. Lata K, Dutta P, Sridhar S, Rohilla M, Srinivasan A, Prashad GR, et al. Thyroid autoimmunity and obstetric outcomes in women with recurrent miscarriage: a case-control study. Endocr Connect. 2013;2(2): 118–24.

85. Liu H, Shan Z, Li C, Mao J, Xie X, Wang W, et al. Maternal subclinical hypothyroidism, thyroid autoimmunity, and the risk of miscarriage: a prospective cohort study. Thyroid. 2014;24(11):1642–9.

86. Carlé A, Pedersen IB, Knudsen N, Perrild H, Ovesen L, Rasmussen LB, et al. Epidemiology of subtypes of hyperthyroidism in Denmark: a population-based study. Eur J Endocrinol. 2011;164(5):801–9.

87. Andersen SL, Olsen J, Wu CS, Laurberg P. Spontaneous abortion, stillbirth and hyperthyroidism: a danish population-based study. Eur Thyroid J. 2014;3(3):164–72.

88. Anselmo J, Cao D, Karrison T, Weiss RE, Refetoff S. Fetal loss associated with excess thyroid hormone exposure. JAMA. 2004;292(6):691–5.

89. Twig G, Shina A, Amital H, Shoenfeld Y. Pathogenesis of infertility and recurrent pregnancy loss in thyroid autoimmunity. J Autoimmun. 2012;38(2-3):J275–81.

90. Bagis T, Gokcel A, Saygili ES. Autoimmune thyroid disease in pregnancy and the postpartum period: relationship to spontaneous abortion. Thyroid. 2001;11(11):1049–53.

91. Ticconi C, Giuliani E, Veglia M, Pietropolli A, Piccione E, Di Simone N. Thyroid autoimmunity and recurrent miscarriage. Am J Reprod Immunol. 2011;66(6):452–9.

92. Rushworth FH, Backos M, Rai R, Chilcott IT, Baxter N, Regan L. Prospective pregnancy outcome in untreated recurrent miscarriers with thyroid autoantibodies. Hum Reprod. 2000;15(7):1637–9.

93. Chen L, Hu R. Thyroid autoimmunity and miscarriage: a meta-analysis. Clin Endocrinol (Oxf). 2011;74(4):513–9.

94. Thangaratinam S, Tan A, Knox E, Kilby MD, Franklyn J, Coomarasamy A. Association between thyroid autoantibodies and miscarriage and preterm birth: meta-analysis of evidence. BMJ. 2011;342: d2616.

95. Marai I, Carp H, Shai S, Shabo R, Fishman G, Shoenfeld Y. Autoantibody panel screening in recurrent miscarriages. Am J Reprod Immunol. 2004; 51(3):235–40.

96. Christiansen OB, Nybo Andersen AM, Bosch E, Daya S, Delves PJ, Hviid TV, et al. Evidence-based investigations and treatments of recurrent pregnancy loss. Fertil Steril. 2005;83(4):821–39.

97. Negro R, Schwartz A, Gismondi R, Tinelli A, Mangieri T, Stagnaro-Green A. Universal screening versus case finding for detection and treatment of thyroid hormonal dysfunction during pregnancy. J Clin Endocrinol Metab. 2010;95(4): 1699–707.

98. Garber JR, Cobin RH, Gharib H, Hennessey JV, Klein I, Mechanick JI, et al. Clinical practice guidelines for hypothyroidism in adults: cosponsored by the American Association of Clinical Endocrinologists and the American Thyroid Association. Thyroid. 2012;22(12):1200–35.

99. Lazzarin N, Moretti C, De Felice G, Vaquero E, Manfellotto D. Further evidence on the role of thyroid autoimmunity in women with recurrent miscarriage. Int J Endocrinol. 2012;2012:717185.

100. Dal Lago A, Vaquero E, Pasqualetti P, Lazzarin N, De Carolis C, Perricone R, et al. Prediction of early pregnancy maternal thyroid impairment in women affected with unexplained recurrent miscarriage. Hum Reprod. 2011;26(6):1324–30.

101. Vaquero E, Lazzarin N, De Carolis C, Valensise H, Moretti C, Ramanini C. Mild thyroid abnormalities and recurrent spontaneous abortion: diagnostic and therapeutical approach. Am J Reprod Immunol. 2000;43(4):204–8.

102. Mills JL, Simpson JL, Driscoll SG, Jovanovic-Peterson L, Van Allen M, Aarons JH, et al. Incidence of spontaneous abortion among normal women and insulin-dependent diabetic women whose pregnancies were identified within 21 days of conception. N Engl J Med. 1988;319(25):1617–23.

103. Jovanovic L, Knopp RH, Kim H, Cefalu WT, Zhu XD, Lee YJ, et al. Elevated pregnancy losses at high and low extremes of maternal glucose in early normal and diabetic pregnancy: evidence for a protective adaptation in diabetes. Diabetes Care. 2005;28(5):1113–7.

104. Ray JG, O'Brien TE, Chan WS. Preconception care and the risk of congenital anomalies in the offspring of women with diabetes mellitus: a meta-analysis. QJM. 2001;94(8):435–44.

105. Greene MF, Hare JW, Cloherty JP, Benacerraf BR, Soeldner JS. First-trimester hemoglobin A1 and risk for major malformation and spontaneous abortion in diabetic pregnancy. Teratology. 1989;39(3):225–31.

106. Temple R, Aldridge V, Greenwood R, Heyburn P, Sampson M, Stanley K. Association between outcome of pregnancy and glycaemic control in early pregnancy in type 1 diabetes: population based study. BMJ. 2002;325(7375):1275–6.

Genetics of Recurrent Pregnancy Loss

4

Arie Koifman, David Chitayat, and Asher Bashiri

Introduction

The Genetic Proportion of RPL

Clinically recognized pregnancy loss is common, occurring in approximately 15–25 % of documented pregnancies [1, 2]. While the majority of sporadic losses before 10 weeks' gestation result from random aneuploidy [3], recurrent pregnancy loss (RPL) is a distinct disorder defined by two or more miscarriages under 20 weeks of gestation in clinical pregnancies. RPL is a relatively rare event with estimated prevalence of 5 % in women experiencing two consecutive miscarriages, and 1 % in women with three or more miscarriages.

A. Koifman, MD (✉)
Institute of Human Genetics, Department of Obstetrics and Gynecology, Soroka University Medical Center, Faculty of Health Sciences, Ben-Gurion University of the Negev, Be'er-Sheva, Israel
e-mail: ariek@bgu.ac.il

D. Chitayat, MD, FABMG, FACMG, FCCMG, FRCPC
Department of Obstetrics and Gynecology, The Prenatal Diagnosis and Medical Genetics Program, Mount Sinai Hospital, Toronto, ON, Canada

A. Bashiri, MD
Director Maternity C and Recurrent Pregnancy Loss Clinic, Department of Obstetrics and Gynecology, Soroka University Medical Center, Faculty of Health Sciences, Ben-Gurion University of the Negev, Be'er Sheva, Israel

In this review we discuss the genetic factors involved in RPL, the recommended work-up and management, and future directions in clinical practice and research.

The Modern Era of Genetics

The involvement of medical genetics in all medical specialties has changed dramatically the approach to clinical practice. Rapid advances in genetics technology allowed clinicians to use, understand, and research more disorders within a short time and with a smaller expense.

The Importance of Genetics Work-Up in RPL Assessment

At least 50 % of the RPL cases are considered idiopathic. However, a genetic role in RPL has been established by several studies. Christiansen et al. [4] noticed two- to sevenfold increased prevalence of recurrent miscarriages (RM) among first-degree relatives compared to the background population, and further studies showed that overall frequency of miscarriage among the siblings of patients with idiopathic RPL is approximately doubled compared to that in the general population [5, 6].

Unexplained RM is a stressful condition for a couple and supportive care is currently the only assistance that can be offered. However, early

© Springer International Publishing Switzerland 2016
A. Bashiri et al. (eds.), *Recurrent Pregnancy Loss*, DOI 10.1007/978-3-319-27452-2_4

recognition of an increased risk for miscarriages and systematic monitoring has a beneficial effect for those couples and studies even reported increasing live births [7–9]. Genetic and genomic studies of RPL potentially have the benefit of understanding the mechanism underlying the cause of RPL, producing a risk estimation for the couple in the future and may suggest a treatment.

A Brief Introduction to Genetics

In order to understand our current knowledge in genetics it is important to clarify some basic terms and nomenclature that we will be using in this review.

It was Gregor Johann Mendel, an Austrian botanist monk (1822–1884), who defined the single-gene inheritance (thus, "Mendelian"). Traditionally genetics was studied through relatively rare, single-gene, diseases. However, a steadily growing body of evidence suggests that genetics has an impact on the vast majority of medical conditions. In fact, if neoplastic diseases are included, up to 91 % of the general population will be affected by a condition with a genetic component.

Current clinical concepts with some technological advances are used to understand the etiology and pathogenesis of diseases with the future aim to use this knowledge to diagnose, treat, or prevent diseases.

Chromosomes, Karyotype, Chromosome Rearrangements

Historically, identification of numerical and structural chromosomal abnormalities were the main aim in prenatal diagnosis. However, currently cells may also be cultured and used for biochemical studies and molecular analyses. Understanding genetic principles and applying accurate patient counseling is an essential tool in contemporary practice.

Basic chromosome structure consists of a short arm (p), a long arm (q), and a centromere in between.

Each chromosome arm is divided into one to four major regions, depending on chromosomal length; each band, positively or negatively stained, is given a number, which rises as the distance from the centromere increases. For example, 1q23 designates the chromosome number (1), the long arm (q), the second region distal to the centromere (2), and the third band (3) in that region.

Karyotyping

Cells are cultured in the laboratory to stimulate cell division. Colchicine is then added to arrest mitosis during metaphase, when each chromosome has replicated to two chromatids attached at the centromere. The cells, which are spread onto microscope slides, and stained with giemsa (G) or fluorescent (Q) dye and computer imaging, are being used to produce a visual display of the chromosomes.

Additional staining procedures and techniques for extending chromosome length have greatly increased the precision of cytogenetic analysis and diagnosis.

Structural Abnormalities
Translocations

Reciprocal Translocations. A reciprocal or double-segment translocation is a rearrangement of chromosomal material in which breaks occur in two different chromosomes, and the fragments are exchanged. The rearranged chromosomes are called *derivative (der) chromosomes* [10]. If no chromosomal material is gained or lost in this process, it is called apparently *balanced translocation. Which means that under the microscope we do not see a gain or loss of a genetic material.* However, a submicroscopic deletion or duplication can happen and can be detected using other molecular methods. Thus, only if the person carrying the translocation has no obvious abnormality, the translocation can be called. Offspring who inherit either the two normal chromosomes or the two translocated chromosomes also usually have a normal phenotype. Carriers of a balanced translocation can produce unbalanced gametes that result in abnormal offspring (Fig. 4.1a).

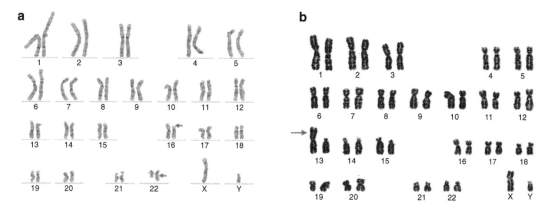

Fig. 4.1 (a) An example of a reciprocal translocation involving chromosomes 16 and 22. The carrier parent can transmit an unbalanced translocation to the fetus. (b) An example of a Robertsonian translocation involving chromosome 13

Robertsonian translocation (ROB) is a form of chromosomal rearrangement that involves one of the short-arm five acrocentric chromosome pairs, namely 13, 14, 15, 21, and 22 [11, 12]. They are named after the American biologist William Rees Brebner Robertson (1881–1941), who first described a Robertsonian translocation in grasshoppers in 1916 [13] (Fig. 4.1b).

Robertsonian translocations result in a loss of part or all of the short arms and fusion of the long arms of the chromosome involved keeping one or two centromeres in between. The short arms of these chromosomes (also called satellites) are lost but since they contain redundant DNA their loss does not cause harm. A Robertsonian translocation in balanced form causes no health issues. In unbalanced forms, Robertsonian translocations can result in trisomies or monosomies. While some trisomies may survive (21, 18, or 13), at least through pregnancy all autosomal monosomies are lethal and will usually result in a first-trimester miscarriage.

Inversions

Inversion is caused by two breaks occurring in the same chromosome with the intervening genetic material inverted before the breaks are repaired. Although, in a balanced situation, no genetic material is lost or duplicated, the rearrangement may alter gene function, if the break is in a gene or its promoter. The inversion can be paracentric, when the two breaks are in one of the arms with a 180° rotation of the segment involved or pericentric if the breaks are in each of the chromosome arms with a 180° rotation around the centromere [14, 15].

Carriers of a paracentric inversion make either balanced gametes or gametes with acentric and dicentric gametes, the products of which are usually lethal. Thus the risk of abnormal offspring is extremely low. Carriers of a *pericentric* inversions can form unbalanced gametes with duplication and deletion of the segment involved and is thus at high risk to produce abnormal gametes and thus abnormal offspring.

Techniques and Methods

FISH Analysis

This technique provides a rapid method for identifying a microscopic or submicroscopic deletion and/or duplication of a segment of a chromosome or a whole chromosome. In this technique a segment of a chromosome called a probe is being stained with a fluorescent dye and is being allowed to hybridize to the karyotype. The probe will hybridize to its corresponding segment on the karyotype which is being tested. The karyotype in an interphase or a metaphase state is being checked with a fluorescent microscope to see if the segment is deleted or duplicated [16, 17].

Chromosomal Micro Array Analysis

Chromosomal micro array (CMA) is designed and utilized to detect copy number variants (CNVs), i.e., deletions or duplications (and in some platforms, loss of heterozygosity (LOH) and thus uniparental disomy (UPD)).

CNVs consist of up to 12 % of the human genome. Many of the CNVs are considered polymorphic and/or familial and these are usually nonpathogenic. However, many are pathogenic and thus associated with abnormalities/mental retardation (MR) or predisposition to abnormalities/MR. CMA has a substantially higher resolution than microscopic chromosome abnormality and can thus identify submicroscopic deletion/duplication which cannot be identified by the traditional chromosome analysis.

The evolution of CMAs was rapid and directed toward new clinical targets and fields. Genomic PCR products, bacterial artificial chromosomes (BACs), and oligonucleotides all were used in comparative genomic hybridization CGH analysis (a type of CMA) [18–20]. While the validity and use of CMA were emerging, array designs were addressing the question of coverage and resolution. Probe coverage on chromosomal backbone is variable and needed for method validation and accuracy. Disease-targeted probes were located according to known loci and interpretable regions. The use of such a high-resolution/high-coverage arrays contributed significantly to the detection discovery of new copy variants related to clinical conditions and to the delineation of many others.

Single-nucleotide polymorphism (SNP) array is a type of CMA which uses polymorphisms within a population. There are around 50 million SNPs that have been identified in the human genome [21]. An SNP array is a useful tool for studying variations between whole genomes. SNP arrays can be used for determining disease susceptibility, measuring the efficacy of drug therapies, etc. An SNP array is also being used to determine CNVs (submicroscopic deletions and duplications). A significant advantage of SNP array over CGH array is the ability to report on regions of LOH and thus identify cases with UPD, consanguinity, and products of incest relationship. A significant drawback of all CMAs is the inability to detect balanced changes such as balanced translocation (reciprocal or Robertsonian).

Next-Generation Sequencing and WES/WGS

The *polymerase chain reaction* (*PCR*) is a technology used to amplify a single copy or a few copies of a piece of DNA across several orders of magnitude, generating thousands to millions of copies of a particular DNA sequence [22].

DNA sequencing is the process of determining the precise order of nucleotides within a DNA molecule. The first DNA sequences were obtained in the early 1970s. While at first the task was extremely time consuming and laborious, development of fluorescence-based sequencing methods with automated analysis has made DNA sequencing [23] easier and substantially faster [24].

Several new methods for DNA sequencing were developed in the mid to late 1990s and were implemented in commercial DNA sequencers almost a decade later.

Basically, all the methods use a random surface-PCR arraying method coupled to "base-by-base" sequencing method. Later, several commercial companies begun to market "massively parallel signature sequencing," or MPSS. This method incorporated a parallelized, adapter/ligation-mediated, bead-based sequencing technology and served as the first commercially available "next-generation" sequencing (NGS) method [25]. Sharply reduced costs and increased availability began a new era for massive sequencing, and genome-wide association studies (GWAS) emerged. Dealing with common diseases, GWAS' approach was to seek genomic variants "that will be able to assist in to mapping risk groups." In the investigation of single-gene disorders "whole-genome or whole-exome sequencing" facilitated the detection of new genes and expanded the spectrum of many known genetic customized NGS panels were developed, by which a parallel sequencing of several genes that may be involved in a common phenotype is being carried out. This approach is accurate and a relatively inexpensive option for identifying a causative gene in diseases with known genetic etiology.

MicroRNA Analysis

MicroRNAs constitute a recently discovered class of noncoding RNAs that play key roles in the regulation of gene expression [26–29]. Acting at the posttranscriptional level, these small molecules fine-tune the expression of up to 30 % of all mammalian protein-encoding genes. Mature microRNAs are short, single-stranded RNA molecules approximately 22 nucleotides in length. MicroRNAs are encoded by multiple loci, some of which are organized in tandemly co-transcribed clusters. MicroRNA genes are transcribed by RNA polymerase II as large primary transcripts (pri-microRNA) that are processed by a protein complex containing the RNase III enzyme Drosha, to form an approximately 70-nucleotide precursor microRNA (pre-microRNA). This precursor is subsequently transported to the cytoplasm where it is processed by a second RNase III enzyme, Dicer, to form a mature microRNA of approximately 22 nucleotides. The mature microRNA is then incorporated into a ribonuclear particle to form the RNA-induced silencing complex, RISC, which mediates gene silencing. MicroRNAs usually induce gene silencing by binding to target sites found within the 3′UTR of the targeted mRNA. This interaction prevents protein production by suppressing protein synthesis and/or by initiating mRNA degradation. Since most target sites on the mRNA have only partial base complementarity with their corresponding microRNA, individual microRNAs may target as many as 100 different mRNAs. Moreover, individual mRNAs may contain multiple binding sites for different microRNAs, resulting in a complex regulatory network. MicroRNAs have been shown to be involved in a wide range of biological processes such as cell cycle control, apoptosis, and several developmental and physiological processes including stem cell differentiation, hematopoiesis, hypoxia, cardiac and skeletal muscle development,

neurogenesis, insulin secretion, cholesterol metabolism, aging, immune responses, and viral replication. In addition, highly tissue-specific expression and distinct temporal expression patterns during embryogenesis suggest that microRNAs play a key role in the differentiation and maintenance of tissue identity. In addition to their important roles in healthy individuals, microRNAs have also been implicated in a number of diseases including a broad range of cancers, heart disease, and neurological disorders. Consequently, microRNAs are intensely studied as candidates for diagnostic and prognostic biomarkers and predictors of drug response.

Genetic Basis of Miscarriage

Prospective cohort studies demonstrated that only around one-third of conceptions progress to a live birth [30, 31]. The incidence of early clinical pregnancy loss is estimated to be 15 %, and is (mainly maternal) age dependent; late losses between 12 and 22 weeks occur less frequently and constitute around 4 % [5].

The prevalence of RPL is much lower and the reported prevalence varies by inclusion criteria. If only clinical pregnancies are included, the prevalence is 0.8–1.4 %, while if preclinical pregnancies are included as well the prevalence can be high as 3 % [32]. As defined by The Practice Committee of the American Society for Reproductive Medicine, RPL is etiologically a heterogeneous condition. In the literature, a multifactorial background of RPL is accepted at the population level, but at the individual level of a specific couple, RPL is considered to be monofactorial. However, none of the reported causes exhibit high sensitivity or specificity regarding RPL, meaning etiologic causes of RPL may occur in couples with RPL as well as in couples with normal fecundity [33].

In about 50 % of the cases, miscarriage is the result of chromosome abnormalities. About 50 % of these are the result of trisomies and 50 % are non-trisomies, mainly monosomy X and triploidy. Thus, most cases are not inherited and caused by de novo numerical chromosome aberrations (monosomies, polyploidies, and trisomies) originating in the gametes prior to fertilization or occurring after fertilization. Usually those tend to be nonrecurring abnormalities with some associated with maternal age. Less frequently the miscarriage is a result of a gamete with an unbalanced chromosomal translocation inherited from a parent carrying a balanced chromosome rearrangement.

Recessive genes or interactions of several genes may also cause lethal malformations in the fetus/embryo; however the incidence of miscarriages caused by genes with an autosomal recessive mode of inheritance is uncertain and probably low.

Fetal Aneuploidy

In the general population, the risk of miscarriage due to fetal aneuploidy increases with maternal age. The risk of trisomy is known to increase with maternal age, but translocations do not seem to be age-related.

This age-related risk of miscarriage also applies to RPL [34]. Most miscarriages with aneuploidies are de novo, with a recurrence risk being low, and the risk is being determined by the mother's age-related risk. In fact, several reports demonstrated that the recurrence risk of a miscarriage seems to be higher following a miscarriage of a chromosomally normal conceptus than after a chromosomally abnormal miscarriage [32, 35].

In a series of 167 cases Carp et al. [32] described the chromosomal abnormalities in 36 cases of RPL and showed that the most common chromosomal abnormality was trisomy, found in 24 of the 36 chromosomally abnormal embryos. Trisomy 21 was the most common aberration, appearing in 5 of the 24 trisomies followed by trisomies 16 and 18, triploidy, monosomy X, and unbalanced translocations. The authors concluded that karyotyping the abortuses allows the patient to be given a more accurate diagnosis and more useful prognostic information regarding subsequent pregnancy outcomes. A patient who

miscarried an aneuploid embryo had a better chance for a subsequent live birth than the patient with a euploid miscarriage (OR = 3.11). This finding was also found by Ogasawara et al. [36] and was statistically significant. Warburton et al. [37] reported on 273 women who had two abortuses karyotyped. They concluded that there is no increased risk of trisomy after a previous trisomic miscarriage, and that the prognosis is favorable for these patients. This may not be the case in euploid miscarriages. Carp et al. [32] reported that all 11 patients with a euploid miscarriage who had a repeat karyotypically normal loss had a higher recurrence with another euploid fetus, suggesting an alternative cause of miscarriage. Philipp et al. [38] explored in several studies the correlation between embryonic disorganization detected by embryoscopy and chromosome abnormalities. In their report from 2003, fetal malformations were observed in 85 % of cases presenting with early clinical miscarriage. The same study also demonstrated that 75 % of the fetuses had an abnormal karyotype. Only a small proportion of fetuses with chromosomal aberration can survive to term. Even trisomy 21, the most common trisomy observed in neonates at term, has demise in 80 % in utero or in the neonatal period [35, 39]. Ven der Berg [40] summarized six studies [34, 36, 38, 41–45] describing cytogenetic abnormalities in RPL. Of the 1359 successfully karyotyped miscarriage samples, 39 % had an abnormal karyotype. The spectrum of chromosome abnormalities included 90 % numerical abnormalities, 3 % structural abnormalities, and 13 % other chromosome abnormalities (mosaicism, double, triple, and quadruple trisomies, and autosomal monosomy; some samples had more than one abnormality). Most cases of chromosomal abnormalities are due to maternal non-disjunction of Meiosis I.

Balanced parental rearrangements are found in 3–6 % of RPL cases [8] and the most commonly encountered parental chromosome rearrangements include balanced translocations and inversions. This risk of miscarriage in these cases is influenced by the size and the genetic content of the rearranged chromosomal segments.

Cryptic CNVs

Some of the miscarriages may be due to submicroscopic chromosomal changes [38]. The introduction of CMA enabled a search for CNVs associated with RPL.

Since CMA does not require cell culture, it provides us with more accurate information regarding the incidence and type of chromosome abnormalities associated with miscarriages. Rosenfeld et al. [46] showed that using CMA and excluding cases referred with known microscopic abnormal karyotypes, clinically significant abnormalities were identified in 12.8 % (64/499) of the miscarriages/stillborn. Detection rates were significantly higher with earlier gestational age and clinically significant abnormalities were identified in 6.9 % (20/288) of cases with normal karyotypes. This detection rate did not significantly vary with gestational age, suggesting that, unlike aneuploidy, the contribution of submicroscopic chromosome abnormalities to fetal demise does not vary with gestational age. SNP analysis detected abnormalities of potential clinical significance, including female triploidy, in an additional 6.5 % (7/107).

Different reports affirmed the value of CMA in cases where obtaining tissue for karyotype was difficult or unavailable (e.g., culture failure) [47–49].

As published by Reddy (as a part of the Stillbirth Collaborative Research Network), of the 51 samples with pathologic CNVs, only 43.1 % (n 22) were detected by karyotype [50]. Only a few reports regarding the use of CMA in recurrent pregnancy loss could be identified. Although the detection rates using CMA are higher than in karyotype the interpretation of the findings is more complex especially when inherited [51].

The literature regarding CNVs in sporadic miscarriage as well as RPL is sparse. van der Berg [40] summarized data from seven studies reporting findings of CMA for detecting submicroscopic genetic abnormalities in sporadic miscarriage samples; those studies refer to 362 miscarriages in total. These combined studies suggest that in 5 % of all sporadic miscarriages CNVs are found that cannot be detected by conventional cytogenetic analysis. In their report, Warren et al. reported CMA results in one-third (8/25) of their cohort presenting with RPL. Four de novo submicroscopic chromosome abnormalities were found by two different arrays (Xp22.31, 12q33.3, 5p15.33, and Xp22.31); three were duplications and one deletion. None of the CNVs seem to have gene content reported that correlates to pregnancy loss [49].

The clinical relevance of these CNVs is still being learned and no conclusive findings are yet available. Issues like inherited versus de novo, size and location, variable expressivity and penetrance, and parental origin are all important aspects of CNV interpretation. A small number of cases are reported with parental testing, allowing only limited conclusions to be drawn [51, 52]. Further studies are needed to determine the size and distribution of the de novo CNVs in this group and whether these CNVs have an etiologic role in the miscarriages.

Role of MiRNAs in Miscarriage

MicroRNA (miRNA) has a function in post-transcriptional regulation of gene expression by targeting mRNAs for degradation and/or translational repression [53], and thus has a role in the repression of protein expression. Thus there might be a role for miRNA in RPL.

In patients with recurrent implantation failure some miRNAs were differently expressed. The affected pathways are of Wnt signaling and cell cycle and formation of adhesion molecules [54]. Hu et al. [55] reported two single-nucleotide polymorphisms (SNPs) within the pri-miR-125a in 217 Han Chinese patients with RPL compared with 431 controls. This SNP is downregulated in pre- and mature-miR-125a, leading to reduction in miR-125a and to less efficient inhibition of target genes, LIFR and ERBB2, which play important roles in the embryo implantation and decidualization. Other miRNAs associated with RPL were reported by Jeon et al. [56] in their study; miR-196a2CC, miR-499AG+GG, and the miR-196a2CC/miR-499AG+GG combination was associated with increased risk of idiopathic

RPL, indicating that the functions of those miR-NAs and their target genes may be important in the etiology of RPL.

The assumption that the miRNA can profile to explain or predict RPL (or an ongoing pregnancy) is appealing, but more studies are required to consolidate the data.

The Genetic Work-Up of RPL

Parental

Traditionally, chromosome analysis has been recommended for couples with RPL although some controversy is still surrounding this recommendation. Those in favor of routine chromosome analysis suggest that it should be included in the counseling provided to couples with RPL regarding the recurrence risk and the chance of having a fetus/newborn with unbalanced chromosomal rearrangement. Those who oppose offering routine karyotyping for couples with RPL refer to a study pointing out that carrier couples with at least two previous miscarriages had the same chance of having a healthy child as non-carrier couples with at least two miscarriages (83 % and 84 %, respectively), and more importantly a low risk (0.8 %) of pregnancies with an unbalanced karyotype surviving into the second trimester [57].

However current clinical guidelines do recommend parental karyotyping as part of the evaluation of couples with RPL, especially if the maternal age is low at the second miscarriage, or if there is a history of two or more miscarriages in first-degree relatives.

De Jong et al. [58] stated that knowing the result of the fetal karyotype does not predict anything for the next pregnancy, since usually the value of this knowledge is in explaining to the parents the reason for the specific miscarriage in case of an abnormal fetal karyotype. There may be another advantage of such knowledge. In their original paper, Mevorach-Zussman et al. [59] stated that anxiety is a major component in RPL couples. In their cohort supportive care was not sufficient, so may be solid medical knowledge

can actually contribute to relieving the anxiety of RPL couples.

Routine chromosomal microarray for couples with RPL is controversial and should be based on the results of CMA done on the product of conception. Couples with RPL due to inherited chromosome abnormality will most probably have balanced chromosome rearrangement which cannot be detected by CMA.

miRNA analysis has not been recommended in the routine investigation recommended to couples with RPL. As in many other medical fields, miRNA seems to be a promising direction for the developing medications targeting the regulation of gene expression.

Aiming to improve pregnancy outcomes, and achieving a healthy newborn, assisted reproductive technologies (ARTs) have been used for couples with RPL. Preimplantation genetic diagnosis (PGD) can be used to target on known chromosomal aberrations or preimplantation genetic screening used to screen for chromosomal aberrations (PGS) [60]. Both methods select the best suitable (without chromosomal abnormality) fertilized egg to be transferred to the uterus.

The second possibility is assuming that the etiology lies within the embryonic environment, aka the uterus, and thus placing the embryo in a surrogate uterus.

PGS is CMA done on a cell obtained from the blastocyst. PGS can only be performed in conjunction with an in vitro fertilization (IVF). In contrast, PGD is done to evaluate the embryos for a single-gene disorder carried by the couple, such as sickle cell disease or cystic fibrosis, where carrier status has been documented in each of the parents [61].

In high-risk patients for an aneuploid embryo, such as advanced maternal age, recurrent miscarriage, repeated implantation failure, and severe male factor patients [62–64], PGS was suggested as a method to improve pregnancy success rate. Because the majority of data was collected by karyotyping of products of conception, many PGS cycles were focused on common aneuploidies, mainly utilizing fluorescence in situ hybridization (FISH) approaches. Unfortunately, results from this approach were disappointing.

Mastenbroek et al. [65] concluded that PGS significantly reduced the rates of pregnancies and live births following IVF in women with advanced maternal age. A renewed interest in PGS was noted with the introduction of microarray technologies. To date the data from studies is limited by the methodology limitations and the small number of patients included in these studies and only a few randomized controlled trials addressing the question of whether or not PGS should be used in RPL patients [64] are available.

Several studies have shown that PGD for familial translocations reduced miscarriage rates from >90 to <15 % [66–69]. The same reduction rates were noted in RPL patients [70].

Christiansen [71] referred to available studies regarding PGS in PRL cases. Comparing four observational studies on RPL to seven studies on natural conception, live birth rates were 35 % and 41 %, respectively; miscarriage rate for the PGS group was 9 %, and 28 % in the natural conception group. It was suggested that since conception after PGS is expected to take longer than natural conception, the most appropriate way to compare pregnancy outcome after PGS versus natural conception is to register the live birth rate per time unit.

Surrogacy remains an option for couples with RPL of an unknown etiology although the data is sparse and inconsistent. It is important to emphasize the caution one must take while solid data is still missing.

Cost-Effectiveness

Foyouzi et al. [72] reported a cost analysis comparing cytogenetic analysis of POC following two miscarriages with a standard RPL work-up. The authors showed a substantial economic advantage relative to the common approach to RPL with an increased advantage.

As discussed, different guidelines for the management of RM recommend parental chromosome analysis in couples with RM to identify if one of the parents is a carrier of a balanced structural chromosome rearrangement [7, 57]. Once a chromosome rearrangement has been detected in a member of a couple, invasive prenatal diagnosis can be offered in subsequent pregnancies to diagnose unbalanced chromosomal abnormalities in the fetus. Van Leeuwen et al. [73] looked at the economic aspect in the genetic work-up of couples with RPL. In this study, by using a theoretical economic analysis, the authors showed that, in the vast majority of couples with RM, amniocentesis in all ongoing pregnancies without knowing the carrier status is less expensive than parental chromosome analysis followed by amniocentesis in case of carrier status in one of the parents.

Bernardi et al. suggested that a selective karyotyping of the miscarriage is cost effective, as opposed to a nonselective approach [74].

In order to assess the cost-effectiveness of PGS to achieve a live born, in comparison to expectant management in RPL couples [75], a decision analytical model comparing costs and clinical outcomes study was undertaken. In this study, the authors found that PGS was not a cost-effective strategy for increasing live birth, and the PGS live birth rate needs to be 91 % to be cost effective compared with expectant management.

Concluding Remarks

In summary approximately 2–4 % of RPL is associated with a parental balanced structural chromosome rearrangement, most commonly balanced reciprocal or Robertsonian translocations as well as chromosomal inversions, insertions, and mosaicism. Single-gene defects are seldom associated with RPL.

CMA done on the POC as well as parental karyotyping should be included in the investigation of RPL and genetic counseling should be offered in all cases of RPL associated with parental chromosomal abnormalities. Therapy may include in vitro fertilization with preimplantation genetic screening or diagnosis. The use of donor gametes may be suggested in cases involving parental chromosome rearrangement and surrogate mother may be discussed when the etiology cannot be delineated.

Data available to date is summarized in Fig. 4.2.

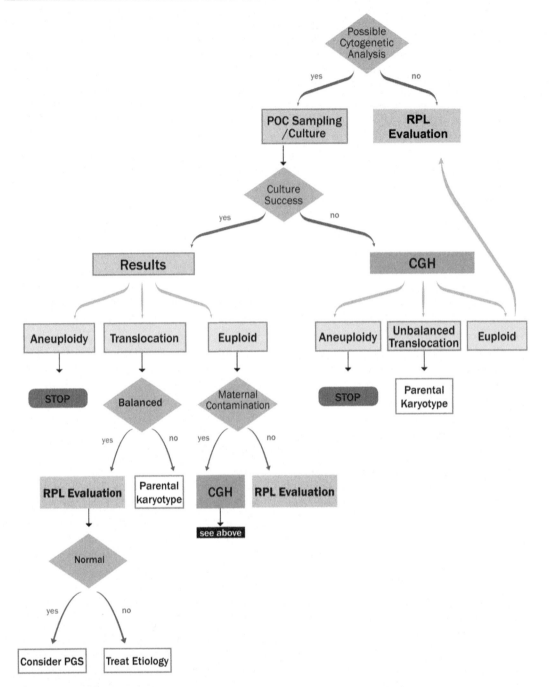

RPL - Recurrent Pregnancy Loss
CGH - Chromosomal Micro Array
POC - Product of Conception
PGS - Preimplantation Genetic Screening

Fig. 4.2 Flowchart showing recent data regarding RPL work-up

References

1. Stephenson M, Kutteh W. Evaluation and management of recurrent early pregnancy loss. Clin Obstet Gynecol. 2007;50(1):132–45. doi:10.1097/GRF.0b013e31802f1c28.
2. Practice Committee of the American Society for Reproductive Medicine. Evaluation and treatment of recurrent pregnancy loss: a committee opinion. Fertil Steril. 2012;98(5):1103–11. doi:10.1016/j.fertnstert.2012.06.048.
3. Stirrat GM. Recurrent miscarriage. II: clinical associations, causes, and management. Lancet. 1990;336(8717):728–33.
4. Christiansen OB. A fresh look at the causes and treatments of recurrent miscarriage, especially its immunological aspects. Hum Reprod Update. 1996;2(4):271–93.
5. Andersen A, Wohlfahrt J, Christens P, Olsen J. Maternal age and fetal loss: population based register linkage study. BMJ. 2000;320(7251):1708–12.
6. Kolte AM, Nielsen HS, Moltke I, et al. A genome-wide scan in affected sibling pairs with idiopathic recurrent miscarriage suggests genetic linkage. Mol Hum Reprod. 2011;17(6):379–85. doi:10.1093/molehr/gar003.
7. Jauniaux E, Farquharson RG, Christiansen OB, Exalto N. Evidence-based guidelines for the investigation and medical treatment of recurrent miscarriage. Hum Reprod. 2006;21(9):2216–22. doi:10.1093/humrep/del150.
8. Branch DW, Gibson M, Silver RM. Recurrent miscarriage. N Engl J Med. 2010;363(18):1740–7. doi:10.1056/NEJMcp1005330.
9. Musters AM, Taminiau-Bloem EF, van den Boogaard E, van der Veen F, Goddijn M. Supportive care for women with unexplained recurrent miscarriage: patients' perspectives. Hum Reprod. 2011;26(4):873–7. doi:10.1093/humrep/der021.
10. Zackai EH, Emanuel BS, Optiz JM. Site-specific reciprocal translocation, t(11;22) (q23;q11), in several unrelated families with 3:1 meiotic disjunction. Am J Med Genet. 1980;7(4):507–21. doi:10.1002/ajmg.1320070412.
11. Martin RH. Cytogenetic analysis of sperm from a male heterozygous for a 13;14 Robertsonian translocation. Hum Genet. 1988;80(4):357–61. doi:10.1007/BF00273651.
12. Ogur G, Van Assche E, Vegetti W, et al. Chromosomal segregation in spermatozoa of 14 Robertsonian translocation carriers. Mol Hum Reprod. 2006;12(3):209–15. doi:10.1093/molehr/gah253.
13. Vikraman SK, et al. A rare balanced parental t (21q;21q) Robertsonian translocation that results in Down syndrome in all viable pregnancies. Int J Reprod Contracept Obstet Gynecol. 2015;4(2):514–7.
14. Sankoff D. Short inversions and conserved gene clusters. New York, NY: ACM; 2002. p. 164–7. doi:10.1145/508791.508825.
15. Schreurs A, Legius E, Meuleman C, Fryns J-P, D'Hooghe TM. Increased frequency of chromosomal abnormalities in female partners of couples undergoing in vitro fertilization or intracytoplasmic sperm injection. Fertil Steril. 2000;74(1):94–6. doi:10.1016/S0015-0282(00)00558-6.
16. Wilkinson DG. In situ hybridization: a practical approach. Oxford: Oxford University Press; 1998.
17. Levsky JM, Singer RH. Fluorescence in situ hybridization: past, present and future. J Cell Sci. 2003;116(Pt 14):2833–8. doi:10.1242/jcs.00633.
18. Lucito R, Healy J, Alexander J, Reiner A. Representational oligonucleotide microarray analysis: a high-resolution method to detect genome copy number variation. Genome Res. 2003;13(10):2291–3053.
19. Peiffer DA, Le JM, Steemers FJ, Chang W. High-resolution genomic profiling of chromosomal aberrations using Infinium whole-genome genotyping. Genome Res. 2006;16(9):1136–48.
20. Bejjani BA, Saleki R, Ballif BC, et al. Use of targeted array-based CGH for the clinical diagnosis of chromosomal imbalance: is less more? Am J Med Genet A. 2005;134(3):259–67. doi:10.1002/ajmg.a.30621.
21. Sachidanandam R, Weissman D, Schmidt SC, et al. A map of human genome sequence variation containing 1.42 million single nucleotide polymorphisms. Nature. 2001;409(6822):928–33. doi:10.1038/35057149.
22. Wagener C, Epplen JT, Erlich H, Peretz H, Vihko P. Molecular biology techniques in the diagnosis of monogenic diseases. Clin Chim Acta. 1994;225(1):S35–50. doi:10.1016/0009-8981(94)90035-3.
23. Olsvik O, Wahlberg J, Petterson B, et al. Use of automated sequencing of polymerase chain reaction-generated amplicons to identify three types of cholera toxin subunit B in Vibrio cholerae O1 strains. J Clin Microbiol. 1993;31(1):22–5.
24. Pettersson E, Lundeberg J, Ahmadian A. Generations of sequencing technologies. Genomics. 2009;93(2):105–11. doi:10.1016/j.ygeno.2008.10.003.
25. Brenner S, Johnson M, Bridgham J, Golda G. Gene expression analysis by massively parallel signature sequencing (MPSS) on microbead arrays. Nature. 2000;18(6):630–4.
26. Winter J, Jung S, Keller S, Gregory RI, Diederichs S. Many roads to maturity: microRNA biogenesis pathways and their regulation. Nat Cell Biol. 2009;11(3):228–34. doi:10.1038/ncb0309-228.
27. Bushati N, Cohen SM. microRNA Functions. http://dxdoiorg/101146/annurevcellbio23090506123406. 2007;23(1):175–205. doi:10.1146/annurev.cellbio.23.090506.123406.
28. Zeng Y. Principles of micro-RNA production and maturation. Oncogene. 2006;25(46):6156–62. doi:10.1038/sj.onc.1209908.
29. McManus MT, Petersen CP, Haines BB, Chen J, Sharp PA. Gene silencing using micro-RNA designed hairpins. RNA. 2002;8(6):842–50.
30. Wilcox AJ, Weinberg CR, O'Connor JF, et al. Incidence of early loss of pregnancy. N Engl J Med. 1988;319(4):189–94. doi:10.1056/NEJM198807283190401.

31. Wang X, Chen C, Wang L, Chen D, Guang W, French J. Conception, early pregnancy loss, and time to clinical pregnancy: a population-based prospective study. Fertil Steril. 2003;79(3):577–84.

32. Carp H. Karyotype of the abortus in recurrent miscarriage. Fertil Steril. 2001;75(4):678–82. doi:10.1016/S0015-0282(00)01801-X.

33. Nielsen HS, Christiansen OB. Prognostic impact of anticardiolipin antibodies in women with recurrent miscarriage negative for the lupus anticoagulant. Hum Reprod. 2005;20(6):1720–8. doi:10.1093/humrep/deh790.

34. Stephenson MD, Awartani KA, Robinson WP. Cytogenetic analysis of miscarriages from couples with recurrent miscarriage: a case-control study. Hum Reprod. 2002;17(2):446–51.

35. Jacobs PA. Retrospective and prospective epidemiological studies of 1,500 karyotyped spontaneous human abortions. Birth Defects Res A Clin Mol Teratol. 2013;97(7):487–8. doi:10.1002/bdra.23145.

36. Ogasawara M, Aoki K, Okada S, Suzumori K. Embryonic karyotype of abortuses in relation to the number of previous miscarriages. Fertil Steril. 2000;73(2):300–4.

37. Warburton D, Kline J, Stein Z, Hutzler M, Chin A, Hassold T. Does the karyotype of a spontaneous abortion predict the karyotype of a subsequent abortion? Evidence from 273 women with two karyotyped spontaneous abortions. Am J Hum Genet. 1987;41(3):465–83.

38. Philipp T, Philipp K, Reiner A, Beer F, Kalousek DK. Embryoscopic and cytogenetic analysis of 233 missed abortions: factors involved in the pathogenesis of developmental defects of early failed pregnancies. Hum Reprod. 2003;18(8):1724–32. doi:10.1093/humrep/deg309.

39. Morris JK, Wald NJ, Watt HC. Fetal loss in down syndrome pregnancies. Prenat Diagn. 1999;19(2):142–5. doi:10.1002/(SICI)1097-0223(199902)19:2<142::AID-PD486>3.0.CO;2-7.

40. van den Berg MMJ, van Maarle MC, van Wely M, Goddijn M. Genetics of early miscarriage. Biochimica et Biophysica Acta (BBA). 2012;1822(12):1951–9. doi:10.1016/j.bbadis.2012.07.001.

41. Stern JJ, Dorfmann AD, Gutierrez-Najar AJ, Cerrillo M, Coulam CB. Frequency of abnormal karyotypes among abortuses from women with and without a history of recurrent spontaneous abortion. Fertil Steril. 1996;65(2):250–3.

42. Sullivan AE, Silver RM, LaCoursiere DY, Porter TF, Branch DW. Recurrent fetal aneuploidy and recurrent miscarriage. Obstet Gynecol. 2004;104(4):784–8. doi:10.1097/01.AOG.0000137832.86727.e2.

43. Carp HJA. Recurrent miscarriage: genetic factors and assessment of the embryo. Isr Med Assoc J. 2008;10(3):229–31.

44. Lomax B, Tang S, Separovic E, et al. Comparative genomic hybridization in combination with flow cytometry improves results of cytogenetic analysis of spontaneous abortions. Am J Hum Genet. 2000;66(5):1516–21. doi:10.1086/302878.

45. Halder A, Fauzdar A. Skewed sex ratio & low aneuploidy in recurrent early missed abortion. Indian J Med Res. 2006;124(1):41–50.

46. Rosenfeld JA, Tucker ME, Escobar LF, et al. Diagnostic utility of microarray testing of pregnancy losses. Ultrasound Obstet Gynecol. 2015. doi:10.1002/uog.14866.

47. Benkhalifa M, Kasakyan S, Clement P, et al. Array comparative genomic hybridization profiling of first-trimester spontaneous abortions that fail to grow in vitro. Prenat Diagn. 2005;25(10):894–900. doi:10.1002/pd.1230.

48. Schaeffer AJ, Chung J, Heretis K, Wong A, Ledbetter DH, Lese MC. Comparative genomic hybridization-array analysis enhances the detection of aneuploidies and submicroscopic imbalances in spontaneous miscarriages. Am J Hum Genet. 2004;74(6):1168–74. doi:10.1086/421250.

49. Warren JE, Turok DK, Maxwell TM, Brothman AR, Silver RM. Array comparative genomic hybridization for genetic evaluation of fetal loss between 10 and 20 weeks of gestation. Obstet Gynecol. 2009;114(5):1093–102. doi:10.1097/AOG.0b013e3181bc6ab0.

50. Reddy U. Stillbirth collaborative research network: genetic changes identified in stillbirths using molecular cytogenetic technology. Am J Obstet Gynecol. 2011. doi:10.1111/j.1538-7836.2005.01581.x/full.

51. Rajcan-Separovic E, Qiao Y, Tyson C, et al. Genomic changes detected by array CGH in human embryos with developmental defects. Mol Hum Reprod. 2010;16(2):125–34. doi:10.1093/molehr/gap083.

52. Rajcan-Separovic E, Diego-Alvarez D, Robinson WP, et al. Identification of copy number variants in miscarriages from couples with idiopathic recurrent pregnancy loss. Hum Reprod. 2010;25(11):2913–22. doi:10.1093/humrep/deq202.

53. Bartel DP, Chen C-Z. Micromanagers of gene expression: the potentially widespread influence of metazoan microRNAs. Nat Rev Genet. 2004;5(5):396–400. doi:10.1038/nrg1328.

54. Revel A, Achache H, Stevens J, Smith Y, Reich R. MicroRNAs are associated with human embryo implantation defects. Hum Reprod. 2011;26(10):2830–40. doi:10.1093/humrep/der255.

55. Hu Y, Liu C-M, Qi L, et al. Two common SNPs in pri-miR-125a alter the mature miRNA expression and associate with recurrent pregnancy loss in a Han-Chinese population. RNA Biol. 2011;8(5):861–72. doi:10.4161/rna.8.5.16034.

56. Jeon YJ, Choi YS, Rah H, et al. Association study of microRNA polymorphisms with risk of idiopathic recurrent spontaneous abortion in Korean women. Gene. 2012;494(2):168–73. doi:10.1016/j.gene.2011.12.026.

57. Franssen MTM, Korevaar JC, van der Veen F, Leschot NJ, Bossuyt PMM, Goddijn M. Reproductive outcome after chromosome analysis in couples with two

or more miscarriages: index [corrected]-control study. BMJ. 2006;332(7544):759–63. doi:10.1136/bmj.38735.459144.2F.

58. de Jong PG, Goddijn M. Testing for inherited thrombophilia in recurrent miscarriage. Semin Reprod Med. 2011;29(6):540–7.

59. Mevorach-Zussman N, Bolotin A, Shalev H, Bilenko N, Mazor M, Bashiri A. Anxiety and deterioration of quality of life factors associated with recurrent miscarriage in an observational study. J Perinat Med. 2012;40(5):495–501.

60. Rubio C, Simón C, Vidal F, et al. Chromosomal abnormalities and embryo development in recurrent miscarriage couples. Hum Reprod. 2003;18(1): 182–8.

61. Brezina PR, Brezina DS, Kearns WG. Preimplantation genetic testing. BMJ. 2012;345, e5908.

62. Vialard F, Boitrelle F, Molina-Gomes D, Selva J. Predisposition to aneuploidy in the oocyte. Cytogenet Genome Res. 2011;133(2-4):127–35. doi:10.1159/000324231.

63. Fragouli E, Wells D, Whalley KM, Mills JA, Faed MJW, Delhanty JDA. Increased susceptibility to maternal aneuploidy demonstrated by comparative genomic hybridization analysis of human MII oocytes and first polar bodies. Cytogenet Genome Res. 2006;114(1):30–8. doi:10.1159/000091925.

64. Brezina PR, Ke RW, Kutteh WH. Preimplantation genetic screening: a practical guide. Clin Med Insights Reprod Health. 2013;7(7):37–42. doi:10.4137/CMRH.S10852.

65. Mastenbroek S, Twisk M, van Echten-Arends J, et al. In vitro fertilization with preimplantation genetic screening. N Engl J Med. 2007;357(1):9–17. doi:10.1056/NEJMoa067744.

66. Munné S, Sandalinas M, Escudero T, Fung J, Gianaroli L, Cohen J. Outcome of preimplantation genetic diagnosis of translocations. Fertil Steril. 2000;73(6):1209–18.

67. Verlinsky Y, Tur-Kaspa I, Cieslak J, et al. Preimplantation testing for chromosomal disorders improves reproductive outcome of poor-prognosis patients. Reprod Biomed Online. 2005;11(2):219–25.

68. Kyu Lim C, Hyun Jun J, Mi Min D, et al. Efficacy and clinical outcome of preimplantation genetic diagnosis using FISH for couples of reciprocal and Robertsonian translocations: the Korean experience. Prenat Diagn. 2004;24(7):556–61. doi:10.1002/pd.923.

69. Otani T, Roche M, Mizuike M, Colls P. Preimplantation genetic diagnosis significantly improves the pregnancy outcome of translocation carriers with a history of recurrent miscarriage and unsuccessful pregnancies. Reprod Biomed Online. 2006;13(6): 869–74.

70. Garrisi JG, Colls P, Ferry KM, Zheng X, Garrisi MG. Effect of infertility, maternal age, and number of previous miscarriages on the outcome of preimplantation genetic diagnosis for idiopathic recurrent pregnancy loss. Fertil Steril. 2009;92(1):288–95.

71. Christiansen OB, Steffensen R, Nielsen HS, Varming K. Multifactorial etiology of recurrent miscarriage and its scientific and clinical implications. Gynecol Obstet Invest. 2008;66(4):257–67. doi:10.1159/000149575.

72. Foyouzi N, Cedars MI, Huddleston HG. Cost-effectiveness of cytogenetic evaluation of products of conception in the patient with a second pregnancy loss. Fertil Steril. 2012;98(1):151–155.e153. doi:10.1016/j.fertnstert.2012.04.007.

73. van Leeuwen M, Vansenne F, Korevaar JC, van der Veen F, Goddijn M, Mol BWJ. Economic analysis of chromosome testing in couples with recurrent miscarriage to prevent handicapped offspring. Hum Reprod. 2013;28(7):1737–42. doi:10.1093/humrep/det067.

74. Bernardi LA, Plunkett BA, Stephenson MD. Is chromosome testing of the second miscarriage cost saving? A decision analysis of selective versus universal recurrent pregnancy loss evaluation. Fertil Steril. 2012;98(1): 156–61. doi:10.1016/j.fertnstert.2012.03.038.

75. Murugappan G, Ohno MS, Lathi RB. Cost-effectiveness analysis of preimplantation genetic screening and in vitro fertilization versus expectant management in patients with unexplained recurrent pregnancy loss. Fertil Steril. 2015;103(5): 1215–20.

Inherited and Acquired Thrombophilias and Adverse Pregnancy Outcomes

William H. Kutteh

Introduction

Three decades ago antiphospholipid antibodies (aPL) were proposed to have a causal association with recurrent pregnancy loss (RPL), suspected due to placental clots that were observed after pregnancy loss with subsequent positive serum aPLs. Following the hypothesis-inducing investigations, an association was found between aPL and RPL. However, it was not until 1996 that Kutteh et al. found that treatment of pregnant women who have aPL syndrome with heparin and aspirin increased live birth rate to 80 % [1].

With a causal role of aPL established [2], research was driven by further hypotheses that inherited thrombophilias may cause pregnancy losses via their resulting hypercoagulability, and expanded to also include other adverse pregnancy outcomes, including effects on preeclampsia, intrauterine growth restriction (IUGR), placental abruption, and stillbirth. The various case control trials that resulted have yielded conflicting conclusions regarding inherited thrombophilias and adverse pregnancy outcomes, and randomized controlled trials are lacking. No causal role has been established to date [3]. Our group performed a survey of the screening and treatment patterns for thrombophilia in pregnancy among obstetricians (OBs) and reproductive endocrinologists (REIs) regarding thrombophilias in pregnancy [4]. We found that many physicians may still screen and treat for inherited thrombophilias beyond the recommendations. This chapter provides an overview of the pathophysiology of the most common inherited thrombophilias, and historical findings of their relationships to adverse pregnancy outcomes. It also summarizes the current recommendations for screening and treatment of inherited thrombophilias [5].

Overview

Inherited thrombophilia is defined as a genetic predisposition to venous thromboembolism (VTE), usually a genetic deletion or alteration of a functional protein in the coagulation cascade.

The most common inherited thrombophilias include factor V Leiden (FVL G1691A) mutation, prothrombin gene mutation (prothrombin G20210A), protein C deficiency (PCD), protein S deficiency (PSD), methyltetrahydrofolate reductase (MTHFR) mutation, and antithrombin III (AT) deficiency. Each of these has a common role in inducing a hypercoagulable state via direct or indirect augmentation of prothrombin to thrombin, its active clot-inducing form (Fig. 5.1). Since hypercoagulability with inherited thrombophilias has been well established, screening of

W.H. Kutteh, MD, PhD, HCLD (✉)
Department of Obstetrics and Gynecology, Vanderbilt University, 80 Humphreys Center, Memphis, TN 38120, USA
e-mail: wkutteh@fertilitymemphis.com

© Springer International Publishing Switzerland 2016
A. Bashiri et al. (eds.), *Recurrent Pregnancy Loss*, DOI 10.1007/978-3-319-27452-2_5

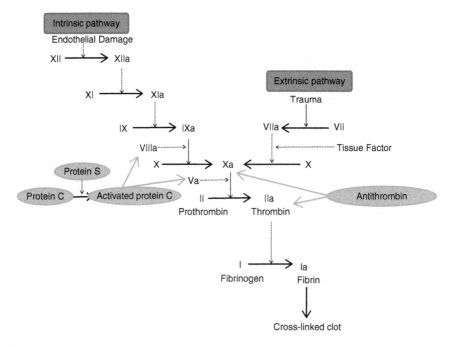

Fig. 5.1 Cascade of thrombus formation. Intrinsic pathway (*left side*) starts with endothelial damage. Extrinsic pathway (*right side*) starts with trauma

pregnant women with a personal history of VTE has been generally well accepted in practice, with the purpose of providing thromboembolic prophylaxis if needed. This practice is supported by the most recent guidelines, and its acceptance confirmed in our survey findings of physicians' practices [4]. Screening in the presence of a family history of VTE has also historically been accepted, but has recently been challenged as not being founded on evidence [6–9]. Subsequently, the practice is being reassessed currently, with some evidence against screening in women with a positive family history of VTE [9].

A larger controversy has existed in the recent past around the utility of screening for inherited thrombophilias in women with a history of adverse pregnancy outcome or loss. Several strong arguments exist against screening in this population. Perhaps most importantly, only weak associations have been found between hypercoagulability and pregnancy outcomes, and no causative relationship has been established [3]. Even more, many inherited thrombophilias are common in the general population, and most of these women have normal pregnancy outcomes

[10]. From the standpoint of thromboembolism prevention, some argue that inherited genetic aberrations in clotting proteins are less likely to be significant in the absence of a thromboembolic event history, and that screening this population is akin to screening the general population, which has shown to be cost ineffective [11]. Due to these positions, recommendations are against screening women in this group.

Despite the above arguments and published recommendations regarding the utility of screening in pregnant women with a history of loss or adverse outcome, our findings have suggested that many physicians continue to screen this population. These convictions are not unfounded, and several historical studies support this stance. Most studies in support of this practice hypothesize microthrombi, thrombosis, and infarction of the placenta as a contributing etiology of pregnancy complications or loss [1, 11, 12]. In addition, an argument exists that women with any type of thromboembolic defect have a higher prevalence of pregnancy complications [13]. Following is a summary of the available evidence regarding each inherited thrombophilia in relation to adverse pregnancy outcomes and risk of VTE. All data reported here is assuming an absence of personal or family history of VTE.

Factor V Leiden

Activated factor V is a clotting protein that works in conjunction with activated factor X to directly convert prothrombin to thrombin. A specific mutant form of this protein, factor V Leiden (F5 c.1691G>A; and p.Arg506Gln), is resistant to inactivation, leading to higher amounts of activated factor V, more thrombin formation, and thus a hypercoagulable state (Fig. 5.1). Although its heterozygous form is the most common inherited thrombophilia, its prevalence is still low in the general population [4]. Less than 0.3 % of these heterozygotes will have a VTE in pregnancy [5].

Concerning adverse fetal outcomes, two recent comprehensive reviews of the literature have determined that carriers of FVL G1691A have an increased relative risk for RPL (OR 1.52, 95 % CI: 1.06–2.19; and OR 2.02, 95 % CI: 1.60–2.55) [14, 15]. However, the maternal-fetal medicine (MFM) network also emphasized a low absolute risk (4.2 %) of pregnancy loss in women with FVL G1691A [15]. No significant association exists between FVL G1691A and preeclampsia or small gestational age [15, 16]. Associations between placental abruption and FVL G1691A are also lacking [17–19]. However, a more recent MFM network case–control study, while confirming a lack of association with placental abruption, did find an increase in fetal hypoxia-inducing factors in the placentas of mothers with FVL G1691A compared with age-matched controls [20]. Current guidelines agree that evidence is inadequate to recommend screening for factor V Leiden in women with adverse pregnancy outcomes of any kind [5, 9, 11, 14].

Prothrombin

Prothrombin G20210A substitution mutation (F2 c.20210G>A) is the second most common inherited thrombophilia, second only to heterozygous factor V Leiden. A mutated form causes a deficiency in thrombin, with a resulting increase in concentration of prothrombin in the plasma (Fig. 5.1). VTE incidence with prothrombin G20210A is low, with one early study suggesting prothrombin G20210A heterozygotes to have an absolute risk of <0.5 %, and homozygotes to only reach 2–3 %. Concerning RPL, Bradley's comprehensive literature review suggested that women with this mutation were overall twice as likely to have RPL as those without the prothrombin G20210A mutation (OR 2.07, 95 % CI, 1.59–2.7), but the MFM network determined no association in their case–control study and meta-analysis [14, 15, 21]. Both literature reviews stated that no definitive conclusion could be made about RPL and prothrombin G20210A due to a paucity of studies. There is consensus among all published reviews of literature that no association exists between prothrombin G20210A and preeclampsia or IUGR [15, 16, 22]. One study has suggested a correlation with placental abruption, but most have found no correlation between prothrombin G20210A and placental abruption [16, 21, 23]. Accordingly, the American Congress of Obstetricians and Gynecologists (ACOG) recommends against screening for prothrombin G20210A in women with any history of adverse pregnancy outcomes [5].

Protein C and Protein S Deficiencies

Protein S and activated protein C, in combination, are necessary for the activation of factors V and VIII, as summarized in Fig. 5.1. Therefore, a deficiency in either of these proteins can result in a hypercoagulable state. Whereas the risk of VTE during pregnancy with either protein deficiency is up to 7 % in the presence of a personal or family history of VTE, the absolute risk of VTE in the absence of such history is 0.1 % and 0.1–0.8 %, respectively [4]. Further, the prevalence of the disorders is only 0.2–0.3 % in the general population. No studies have found an association between either PCD or PSD and early pregnancy loss, IUGR, or placental abruption. A review of literature from 2002 that included only 3–5 pertinent studies found an increased risk of preeclampsia with PCD (OR 21.5, CI 4.4–414.4) and PSD (OR 12.7, CI 4–39.7), with an absolute risk of 1.4 % and 12.3 %, respectively. The same study suggested an increase in stillbirth among those with PSD (OR 16.2, CI 5–52.3), with an absolute risk of 6 % [23]. However, due to the small number of studies with relatively few participants, ACOG currently does not recommend screening for protein S or protein C deficiency in women with any history of adverse pregnancy outcomes [5].

Antithrombin Deficiency

Antithrombin is a small protein that inactivates both factor Xa and thrombin, and serves as a regulator of clot formation (Fig. 5.1). A rare deficiency in this protein results in severe coagulopathy, increasing the risk up to 25 times those with normal antithrombin levels. Women with antithrombin III deficiency do indeed have an increased risk of embryonic demise and fetal death compared with the general population [24–27]. However, due to the low prevalence (1/2500), screening is not recommended in those with a prior pregnancy loss. Studies observing its effects on other adverse pregnancy outcomes are lacking, also due to low prevalence.

MTHFR

MTHFR is one of the three enzymes that is essential for the metabolism of folic acid, and is responsible for directly converting homocysteine to methionine. A mutation in this enzyme can cause increased levels of substrate homocysteine. Hyperhomocysteinemia debatably can result in a hypercoagulable state at the endothelium, and has historically been associated with RPL [28]; but its relationship to thrombosis is only theoretical [29]. Two predominant mutations exist, MTHFR C677T and A1298C. Most recently, however, evidence has suggested that homocysteine is only a marker for thrombosis rather than a cause, and that it must be combined with other thrombophilias to present any significant risk of VTE [29–33]. Existing data suggests an absence of any correlation with preeclampsia, IUGR, or placental abrup-

tion. However, ACOG and the MFM network has determined that data is insufficient to determine the correlation [20, 22, 34]. Accordingly, ACOG does not recommend screening women for MTHFR with any history of adverse fetal outcomes or with a history of VTE [5].

MTHFR polymorphisms are also associated with an increased risk of neural tube defects (NTDs) due to low-serum folic acid [35]. Women delivering a baby with an NTD have more than twice the incidence of having an MTHFR C677T polymorphism [36]. In addition, the combination of MTHFR C677T polymorphism with MTHFR A1298C polymorphism may further increase the risk of NTD [37]. Therefore, we think it is prudent to treat these patients with amounts of folic acid similar to those used to treat patients who had a prior infant with an NTD [36–38].

Combined Defects

Most studies have only observed VTE risks on pregnancy outcomes with individual thrombophilias. However, a few have assessed combinations of these disorders, such as FVL G1691A/prothrombin G20210A double heterozygosity, and FVL G1691A in the presence of an MTHFR mutation, concluding that an additive or a synergistic effect is present [26, 39–44]. This distinction should be made, although further exploration of this topic is beyond the scope of our review.

Acquired Thrombophilias

Due to their non-genetic preponderance, acquired thrombophilias are classified separately from inherited thrombophilias, and will be summarized only briefly for the purpose of contrast since these disorders are also beyond the scope of this review. The most common acquired thrombophilia involves the presence of aPL. The presence of these antibodies has been associated with second-trimester as well as first-trimester pregnancy loss [45, 46]. As such, it is recommended to screen for the most common of these antibodies (lupus anticoagulant, anticardiolipin, and anti-beta2 glycoprotein) in women with a history of more than two or three first-trimester losses, and in women with one or more loss after 20 weeks with no alternative explanation [5, 11]. It is also well established that treating these thrombophilias with heparin and aspirin improves pregnancy outcomes [1, 2].

Treatment of Inherited Thrombophilias

Given the current lack of evidence to support an association between adverse pregnancy outcomes and inherited thrombophilias, it is currently not recommended to treat inherited thrombophilias with adverse pregnancy outcomes alone in mind [4]. However, treatment is justifiable in some patients with known thrombophilias who are at increased risk of VTE during pregnancy [47]. The ACOG

treatment recommendations have been abbreviated and summarized in Table 5.1. They specifically address thresholds at which to begin anticoagulants, which can be used to treat all known inherited thrombophilias except MTHFR mutations. Guidelines do not address the treatment of known MTHFR mutations for VTE prevention, but the traditional treatment has been vitamin B and folate. However, evidence now suggests that vitamin B supplementation does not reduce VTE incidence [32, 48]. Therefore, if one decides to test for and treat these mutations, folate alone may be the best choice.

Discussion

The most recent ACOG recommendations indicate that evidence is insufficient to screen for thrombophilias based on previous adverse preg-

Table 5.1 Recommended thromboprophylaxis for pregnancies complicated by inherited thrombophilias

Clinical scenario	Antepartum management	Postpartum management
Low-risk thrombophilia[a] without previous VTE	Surveillance only or prophylactic heparin	Surveillance only if no risk factors; postpartum anticoagulation if risk factors[b]
Low-risk thrombophilia[a] with a single previous episode of VTE—not receiving long-term anticoagulation therapy	Surveillance only or prophylactic heparin	Postpartum anticoagulation therapeutic or intermediate-dose heparin
High-risk thrombophilia[c] without previous VTE	Prophylactic heparin	Postpartum anticoagulation therapy
High-risk thrombophilia[c] with a single previous episode of VTE—not receiving long-term anticoagulation therapy	Prophylactic, intermediate-dose, or adjusted-dose heparin	Postpartum anticoagulation therapy or intermediate or adjusted-dose heparin
Thrombophilia or no thrombophilia with two or more episodes of VTE—not receiving long-term anticoagulation therapy	Prophylactic or therapeutic-dose heparin	Postpartum anticoagulation therapy or Therapeutic-dose heparin for 6 weeks
Thrombophilia or no thrombophilia with two or more episodes of VTE—receiving long-term anticoagulation therapy	Therapeutic-dose heparin	Resumption of long-term anticoagulation therapy

Based on data from Ref. [47]
[a]Low-risk thrombophilia: factor V Leiden heterozygous; prothrombin G20210A heterozygous; protein C or protein S deficiency
[b]First-degree relative with a history of a thrombotic episode before age 50 years, or other major thrombotic risk factors (e.g., obesity, prolonged immobility)
[c]High-risk thrombophilia: antithrombin deficiency; double heterozygous for prothrombin G20210A mutation and factor V Leiden; factor V Leiden homozygous or prothrombin G20210A mutation homozygous

nancy outcomes (intrauterine growth restriction, stillbirth, abruption, or pregnancy loss) alone in the absence of additional risk factors for thrombosis [5]. However, around 40 % of physicians treated these women, suggesting that many are still following older literature, which suggests that inherited thrombophilias are associated with adverse pregnancy outcomes [4]. Nevertheless, the authors agree that evidence is not adequate to make a definitive association between these pregnancy outcomes and inherited thrombophilias.

For those who meet appropriate criteria for inherited thrombophilia screening, ACOG recommends that the following tests be ordered: factor V Leiden, prothrombin G20210A, protein C and S, and antithrombin III [5]. Most physicians currently order all of the above, but greater than 40 % of physicians reported also ordering MTHFR and homocysteine levels in their thrombophilia screen, both of which are not considered part of the recommended thrombophilia evaluation according to ACOG. However, some of these decisions may have been based on the well-supported association of MTHFR polymorphisms with neural tube defects [36–38].

Concerning treatment, ACOG recommends that only acquired thrombophilias (antiphospholipid antibody syndrome) be treated for RPL, and then with heparin and aspirin [5, 49]. While over half of physicians appropriately treat these antibodies, a large percentage still only use heparin or aspirin, which has been shown to be inferior to combination therapy [1, 2]. The majority of physicians who treat inherited thrombophilias appropriately use heparin with or without aspirin [4].

Summary of Current State of Research and Future Direction

Overall, discrepancies in the literature do still exist concerning appropriate screening and management of those with prior adverse pregnancy outcomes. Large prospective, multicentered trials and evaluation of national databases, which are currently being conducted, will be required to clearly determine the risks associated with inherited thrombophilias in this regard. Until these

data are available, physicians should compare their current practice patterns for thrombophilia screening to the guidelines in the ACOG Practice Bulletin, with an emphasis on individualizing their management where data is not sufficient.

References

1. Kutteh WH. Antiphospholipid antibody-associated recurrent pregnancy loss: treatment with heparin and low-dose aspirin is superior to low-dose aspirin alone. Am J Obstet Gynecol. 1996;174(5):1584–9.
2. Rai R et al. Randomised controlled trial of aspirin and aspirin plus heparin in pregnant women with recurrent miscarriage associated with phospholipid antibodies (or antiphospholipid antibodies). BMJ. 1997; 314(7076):253–7.
3. Rodger MA et al. Inherited thrombophilia and pregnancy complications revisited. Obstet Gynecol. 2008;112(2 Pt 1):320–4.
4. Davenport WB, Kutteh WH. Inherited thrombophilias and adverse pregnancy outcomes: a review of screening patterns and recommendations. Obstet Gynecol Clin N Am. 2014;41:133–44.
5. Lockwood C, Wendel G. Practice bulletin no. 124: inherited thrombophilias in pregnancy. Obstet Gynecol. 2011;118(3):730–40.
6. Wichers IM et al. Assessment of coagulation and fibrinolysis in families with unexplained thrombophilia. Thromb Haemost. 2009;101(3):465–70.
7. Villani M et al. Risk of obstetric and thromboembolic complications in family members of women with previous adverse obstetric outcomes carrying common inherited thombophilias. J Thromb Haemost. 2012;10(2):223–8.
8. Lussana F et al. Pregnancy-related venous thromboembolism: risk and the effect of thromboprophylaxis. Thromb Res. 2012;129(6):673–80.
9. Horton AL et al. Family history of venous thromboembolism and identifying factor V Leiden carriers during pregnancy. Obstet Gynecol. 2010;115(3):521–5.
10. Branch DW. The truth about inherited thrombophilias and pregnancy. Obstet Gynecol. 2010;115(1):2–4.
11. Bates SM et al. Venous thromboembolism, thrombophilia, antithrombotic therapy, and pregnancy: American College of Chest Physicians evidence-based clinical practice guidelines (8th edn). Chest. 2008;133(6 Suppl):844S–86.
12. Dizon-Townson DS et al. Fetal carriers of the factor V Leiden mutation are prone to miscarriage and placental infarction. Am J Obstet Gynecol. 1997;177(2):402–5.
13. Rey E et al. Thrombophilic disorders and fetal loss: a meta-analysis. Lancet. 2003;361(9361):901–8.
14. Bradley LA et al. Can factor V Leiden and prothrombin G20210A testing in women with recurrent pregnancy loss result in improved pregnancy outcomes?

Results from a targeted evidence-based review. Genet Med. 2012;14(1):39–50.

15. Rodger MA et al. The association of factor V leiden and prothrombin gene mutation and placenta-mediated pregnancy complications: a systematic review and meta-analysis of prospective cohort studies. PLoS Med. 2010;7(6), e1000292.

16. Howley HE, Walker M, Rodger MA. A systematic review of the association between factor V Leiden or prothrombin gene variant and intrauterine growth restriction. Am J Obstet Gynecol. 2005;192(3):694–708.

17. Dizon-Townson D et al. The relationship of the factor V Leiden mutation and pregnancy outcomes for mother and fetus. Obstet Gynecol. 2005;106(3):517–24.

18. Jaaskelainen E et al. M385T polymorphism in the factor V gene, but not Leiden mutation, is associated with placental abruption in Finnish women. Placenta. 2004;25(8-9):730–4.

19. Prochazka M et al. Factor V Leiden in pregnancies complicated by placental abruption. BJOG. 2003;110(5):462–6.

20. Rogers BB et al. Avascular villi, increased syncytial knots, and hypervascular villi are associated with pregnancies complicated by factor V Leiden mutation. Pediatr Dev Pathol. 2010;13(5):341–7.

21. Silver RM et al. Prothrombin gene G20210A mutation and obstetric complications. Obstet Gynecol. 2010;115(1):14–20.

22. Infante-Rivard C et al. Absence of association of thrombophilia polymorphisms with intrauterine growth restriction. N Engl J Med. 2002;347(1):19–25.

23. Alfirevic Z, Roberts D, Martlew V. How strong is the association between maternal thrombophilia and adverse pregnancy outcome? A systematic review. Eur J Obstet Gynecol Reprod Biol. 2002;101(1):6–14.

24. Di Nisio M, Middeldorp S, Buller HR. Direct thrombin inhibitors. N Engl J Med. 2005;353(10): 1028–40.

25. Blumenfeld Z, Brenner B. Thrombophilia-associated pregnancy wastage. Fertil Steril. 1999;72(5):765–74.

26. Preston FE et al. Increased fetal loss in women with heritable thrombophilia. Lancet. 1996;348(9032):913–6.

27. Sanson BJ et al. The risk of abortion and stillbirth in antithrombin-, protein C-, and protein S-deficient women. Thromb Haemost. 1996;75(3):387–8.

28. Peng F et al. Single nucleotide polymorphisms in the methylenetetrahydrofolate reductase gene are common in US Caucasian and Hispanic American populations. Int J Mol Med. 2001;8(5):509–11.

29. Krabbendam I, Dekker GA. Pregnancy outcome in patients with a history of recurrent spontaneous miscarriages and documented thrombophilias. Gynecol Obstet Invest. 2004;57(3):127–31.

30. den Heijer M et al. Hyperhomocysteinemia and venous thrombosis: a meta-analysis. Thromb Haemost. 1998;80(6):874–7.

31. Eichinger S. Homocysteine, vitamin B6 and the risk of recurrent venous thromboembolism. Pathophysiol Haemost Thromb. 2003;33(5-6):342–4.

32. den Heijer M et al. Homocysteine lowering by B vitamins and the secondary prevention of deep vein thrombosis and pulmonary embolism: a randomized, placebo-controlled, double-blind trial. Blood. 2007;109(1):139–44.

33. Bezemer ID et al. No association between the common MTHFR 677C → T polymorphism and venous thrombosis: results from the MEGA study. Arch Intern Med. 2007;167(5):497–501.

34. Nurk E et al. Associations between maternal methylenetetrahydrofolate reductase polymorphisms and adverse outcomes of pregnancy: the Hordaland Homocysteine Study. Am J Med. 2004;117(1):26–31.

35. Molloy AM et al. Folate status and neural tube defects. Biofactors. 1999;10(2-3):291–4.

36. Ceyhan ST et al. Thrombophilia-associated gene mutations in women with pregnancies complicated by fetal neural tube defects. Int J Gynaecol Obstet. 2008;101(2):188–9.

37. Akar N et al. Spina bifida and common mutations at the homocysteine metabolism pathway. Clin Genet. 2000;57(3):230–1.

38. Molloy AM, Weir DG, Scott JM. Homocysteine, folate enzymes and neural tube defects. Haematologica. 1999;84(Suppl EHA-4):53–6.

39. Coulam CB et al. Multiple thrombophilic gene mutations rather than specific gene mutations are risk factors for recurrent miscarriage. Am J Reprod Immunol. 2006;55(5):360–8.

40. Kutteh WH, Triplett DA. Thrombophilias and recurrent pregnancy loss. Semin Reprod Med. 2006;24(1):54–66.

41. Brenner B et al. Thrombophilic polymorphisms are common in women with fetal loss without apparent cause. Thromb Haemost. 1999;82(1):6–9.

42. Sarig G et al. Thrombophilia is common in women with idiopathic pregnancy loss and is associated with late pregnancy wastage. Fertil Steril. 2002;77(2):342–7.

43. Kupferminc MJ et al. Increased frequency of genetic thrombophilia in women with complications of pregnancy. N Engl J Med. 1999;340(1):9–13.

44. Castoldi E et al. Combinations of 4 mutations (FV R506Q, FV H1299R, FV Y1702C, PT 20210G/A) affecting the prothrombinase complex in a thrombophilic family. Blood. 2000;96(4):1443–8.

45. Infante-Rivard C et al. Lupus anticoagulants, anticardiolipin antibodies, and fetal loss. A case-control study. N Engl J Med. 1991;325(15):1063–6.

46. Lockshin MD. Pregnancy loss in the antiphospholipid syndrome. Thromb Haemost. 1999;82(2):641–8.

47. Lockwood C, Wendel G, Silverman N. ACOG Practice Bulletin no. 138. Thromboembolism in Pregnancy. Obstet Gynecol 2013;122(3);706–16.

48. Lonn E et al. Homocysteine lowering with folic acid and B vitamins in vascular disease. N Engl J Med. 2006;354(15):1567–77.

49. Kutteh WH. Novel strategies for the management of recurrent pregnancy loss. Semin Reprod Med. 2015;33:159–66.

Immunological Causes of Recurrent Pregnancy Loss

6

Ole Bjarne Christiansen, Astrid Marie Kolte, Elisabeth Clare Larsen, and Henriette Svarre Nielsen

Introduction

Recurrent pregnancy loss (RPL) is in Europe defined as three or more consecutive pregnancy losses prior to gestational week 22 [1] and affects approximately 2–3 % of all women aiming to get a child. In RPL women like in other women approximately half of the pregnancy losses are due to embryonal aneuploidy probably occurring by chance but with increased incidence with increased maternal age [2]. In the vast majority of couples no documented cause of pregnancy loss can be found, although a series of risk factors for pregnancy loss have been identified.

In this chapter we do not refer to "causes" of pregnancy loss since the only documented cause of pregnancy loss is severe embryonal malformation,

often caused by chromosomal aberration. Biomarkers associated with pregnancy loss or RPL will be entitled "risk factors" if they have been strongly associated with RPL or pregnancy outcome in case–control studies and/or in well-designed prospective studies. The main focus in RPL research has been on biomarkers relating to endocrinologic, thrombophilic, and immunological dysfunctions in the women suffering from RPL.

We provide an overview of the scientific evidence for immune aberrations being involved in the pathogenesis of RPL and we discuss which biomarkers related to immune function are candidates for further research or can already be used in clinical practice.

The feto-placental unit is often entitled the "feto-placental allograft" as it bears similarities to the transplantation of an organ such as a kidney from an allogenic donor. In this situation the allograft can only avoid being rejected when intensive immunosuppressive therapies are implemented. A priory, it must be presumed that the maternal immune system would make efforts to reject the feto-placental unit, which carries paternal alloantigens. The previous belief that rejection is avoided because alloantigens on the fetus or placenta are separated from the maternal immune-competent cells has now been abandoned; in contrast there is plenty of documentation that recognition of paternally derived antigens on the feto-placental unit is a normal feature in pregnancy. One such proof of immune recognition of paternal antigens is the observation

O.B. Christiansen, PhD, DMSc (✉)
Fertility Clinic 4071, Rigshospitalet, Copenhagen University Hospital, Blegdamsvej 9, 2100 Copenhagen, Denmark

Department of Obstetrics and Gynaecology, Aalborg University Hospital, Aalborg, Denmark
e-mail: obchr@post5.tele.dk

A.M. Kolte, MD
Recurrent Pregnancy Loss Unit, Fertility Clinic 4071, University Hospital Copenhagen, Rigshospitalet, Copenhagen, Denmark

E.C. Larsen, MD, PhD • H.S. Nielsen, MD, DMSci
Fertility Clinic 4071, Rigshospitalet, Copenhagen University Hospital, Blegdamsvej 9, 2100 Copenhagen, Denmark

that antipaternal human leukocyte antigen (HLA) antibodies develop in 10–30 % of all normal pregnancies [3]. However, in a meta-analysis of relevant studies their presence did not increase the risk of early pregnancy complications such as miscarriage [4].

The research in immunological biomarkers associated with RPL has focused on measurements of autoantibodies in the blood, natural killer (NK) cells in the blood or decidual tissue, and cytokines in the blood or decidual tissue and investigations of classical and nonclassical HLA polymorphisms in patients or couples with RPL and studies of HLA protein expression on trophoblast.

Autoantibodies

Much focus has been on investigation of autoantibodies in RPL since it was early recognized that women with specific autoimmune diseases, especially systemic lupus erythematosus (SLE), hypo- and hyperthyroidism, and inflammatory bowel disease had an increased risk of pregnancy loss in early and late gestation [5]. In SLE this increased risk was associated with the presence of antiphospholipid antibodies such as lupus anticoagulant (LAC) and anticardiolipin antibodies (ACA) and in thyroid disease the risk was associated with the presence of thyroid autoantibodies. LAC and probably also high-titer ACA are associated with an increased risk of venous and arterial thrombosis and are in many studies associated with a reduced chance of live birth in RPL patients [6]. The role of antiphospholipid antibodies will not be reviewed further here as it will be dealt with in another chapter in this book.

Thyroid autoantibodies can be found in 5–15 % of women of reproductive age but in the majority of cases they are not associated with thyroid dysfunction or reproductive problems. On the other hand almost all cases of clinical hyper- or hypothyroidism are associated with the presence of thyroid autoantibodies. The most prevalent thyroid autoantibody is thyroid peroxidase (TPO) antibody. A considerable number of studies have found thyroid autoantibodies with increased prevalence in RPL and a meta-analysis

including 8 case–control studies, most of them small, found that antithyroid antibodies are associated with RPL with odds ratio (OR) 2.3 (95 % CI 1.5–3.5) [7] . It remains to be elucidated whether the association between antithyroid antibodies and RPL reflects an increased risk of clinical hypothyroidism, which may lead to delayed embryonal development in pregnancy, or whether their presence is just a marker of a generally increased predisposition to an autoimmune response.

Another autoantibody, antinuclear antibody (ANA), has been extensively studied in RPL. In a review from 1996, Christiansen [8] reported that in 10 of 12 relevant case–control studies there was an increased ANA prevalence in RPL patients, though not always statistically significant. In the three relevant studies published subsequently, two found significant increased ANA prevalence in RPL compared with controls [9, 10] whereas one could not detect such an association [11]. In one study, the presence of ANA was associated with an increased risk of pregnancy loss in the next pregnancy [12].

A direct pathophysiologic link between the presence of autoantibodies in RPL and fetal death has not been convincingly documented. In our opinion, ACAs, antithyroid antibodies, ANA, and most other autoantibodies in RPL patients are most likely markers of a general breakage of autotolerance [5] or are epiphenomenons associated with carriage of specific HLA alleles such as HLA-DRB1*03. This HLA allele is associated with both production of ACA, antithyroid antibodies, and ANA and the risk of RPL [13, 14].

Cytokines

Cytokines are signaling molecules secreted from immune cells and usually bind to receptors on other immune cells resulting in stimulation or inhibition of function. One important division of cytokines is between the so-called T-helper type 1 cytokines, which promote T lymphocyte cytotoxicity and often inflammation and T-helper type 2 cytokines, which promote antibody production and anti-inflammation. Typical cytokines in the former group are interferon (IFN)-γ and interleukin (IL)-2 whereas IL-4 and IL-10 are characteristic T-helper type 2 cytokines. Tumor necrosis factor (TNF)-α is more difficult to classify but induces inflammation and apoptosis of target cells. Wegmann et al. [15] proposed the theory that normal pregnancy is characterized by a predominant production of T-helper type 2 cytokines, whereas adverse pregnancy outcomes such as RPL are characterized by a predominant T-helper type 1 cytokine production. This theory is probably too simplistic and has now been modified to include interactions between T-helper 17 cells secreting the pro-inflammatory cytokine IL-17 and T-regulatory cells [16]. It has been recognized that different cytokine profiles may be beneficial or harmful at different stages of pregnancy; for example IFN-γ, TNF-α, and other inflammatory cytokines seem to be crucial during the implantation process [17], whereas high levels of these cytokines may be harmful later in pregnancy. This fact makes research in the role of cytokines in RPL extremely difficult.

Since most cytokines display their effects at close range, interpretation of results from studies of cytokine secretion by peripheral blood lymphocytes or direct measurements of cytokines in the blood must be done with caution. Measurements of cytokines in endometrial biopsies or flushing or decidual tissue are subject to technical and methodological difficulties and will not be reviewed here.

TNF-α is one of the few cytokines with levels in the peripheral blood well above the detection limit of most assays, and since it is a typical pro-inflammatory cytokine it may be a good marker for the level of systemic inflammation. High plasma levels have been reported to increase the risk of pregnancy loss in RPL patients [18] and high TNF-α and TNF-α/IL10 ratios characterized women with euploid miscarriage compared with those with aneuploid miscarriage [19]. Kruse et al. [20] found that stimulated lymphocytes from RPL patients in very early pregnancy, who went on to miscarry, produced more TNF-α than those who gave birth. Lastly, it was reported that patients with RPL after a birth (secondary RPL) had significantly higher plasma levels of TNF-α

in very early pregnancy than RPL patients with exclusively early miscarriages (primary RPL) [21]. These observations suggest that a high systemic inflammatory stage in early pregnancy increases the risk of miscarriage and that in particular secondary RPL patients are in a pro-inflammatory stage from very early pregnancy.

Mannose-Binding Lectin

Mannose-binding lectin (MBL) is a plasma protein produced in the liver. After binding to oligosaccharides on the surface of microorganisms, it activates complement that can kill the microorganisms. Furthermore, MBL by enhancing phagocytosis can help in clearing apoptotic cells, cellular debris, and immune complexes, which would otherwise prompt inflammatory processes. The result of MBL deficiency may therefore be pro-inflammatory processes at the feto-maternal interface and MBL deficiency, which is genetically determined (see later), is therefore expected to increase the risk of pregnancy loss. In concordance with this assumption, MBL deficiency (<100 ng/ml) has been found to be associated with RPL in three case–control studies [22–24]. In the latter study, MBL deficiency was also associated with a significantly poorer prognosis in RPL patients.

Natural Killer Cells

In the search for immunological aberrations in RPL patients, there has been much focus on NK cells in the peripheral blood or decidual or endometrial tissue. NK cells are part of the innate immune system and in contrast to T lymphocytes they can recognize and react against target antigens typically on cells affected by intracellular infection or malignancy without prior sensitization. This reaction can result in killing of the cells (cytotoxicity) or secretion of an array of cytokines. The interest for NK cells in RPL and other pregnancy complications has been stimulated by three observations: (1) there is a unique composition of NK cells in the endometrium and decidual tissue. More than 90 % of lymphocytes in the endometrium in the luteal phase and in the decidual tissue in early pregnancy are low-cytotoxicity, high cytokine-producing NK cells, which carry a high density of the CD56 surface marker (CD56[bright]) by flow cytometry, but are negative for the CD16 marker [25]. In contrast, in peripheral blood, 90 % of the NK cells carry the CD56[dim]CD16 markers, which are associated with high cytotoxicity and low cytokine production; (2) the HLA molecules expressed on trophoblast subsets, HLA-G, HLA-C, and HLA-E, can all act as ligands for the three kinds of activating or inhibitory receptors found on NK cells and other cell types found in the uterus: the killer immunoglobulin-like receptors (KIRs), the CD94 receptors, and the immunoglobulin-like transcripts (ILTs) [26, 27]; (3) studies in NK- and T-cell-deficient transgenic mice with a high fetal loss rate show that restoration of NK cells by bone marrow transplantation results in a normal fetal resorption rate [28].

Investigations of NK cells in RPL can be divided into (1) studies of NK cell subsets by flow-cytometric analysis or tests of NK cytotoxicity of peripheral blood lymphocytes before or during pregnancy and (2) studies of NK cells in endometrial biopsies from before pregnancy or in decidual tissue collected from missed miscarriages and elective abortions.

Due to the easy availability, studies based on peripheral blood have been dominant. Excluding small studies (studies with <30 RPL patients), the majority of studies found that the percentage of CD56+ cells in peripheral blood taken prior to pregnancy is significantly higher in RPL women than controls [29–34]. Even so, some studies did not find any difference in percentage of CD56+,16+ cells or CD56+ cells [16, 35]. The fact that most of the investigated RPL women were nulliparous and most controls were multiparous is a methodological problem in this kind of studies [36] as a previous successful pregnancy can induce permanent changes in NK cell subsets [37]. The limitations of the immunological biomarkers tested in RPL and proposals for the research needed to clarify their clinical usefulness are listed in the table.

Cells from RPL patients collected before pregnancy have also been investigated in tests of NK cytotoxicity. In several studies in all RPL subsets [33, 38–40] or in primary RPL [37] a significantly increased NK cytotoxicity was found in patients compared with controls; however, Emmer et al. [41] in a large study did not find any difference between the two groups.

A series of studies have investigated the impact of high NK cytotoxicity on subsequent pregnancy outcome in RPL patients. Aoki et al. [42] first reported that RPL patients with high peripheral blood NK cytotoxicity before pregnancy had a significantly higher rate of pregnancy loss (71 %) in the next pregnancy than patients with lower NK cytotoxicity (20 %). Yamada et al. [43] found a significantly higher NK cytotoxicity in patients with a subsequent euploid miscarriage compared with those with live birth and Morikawa et al. [44] found a non-significant tendency for the same. In contrast Liang et al. [45] found similar NK cytotoxicity in RPL patients with subsequent pregnancy loss and live birth.

The strongest argument against a significant role for measurement of NK cytotoxicity in RPL patients came in a large prospective study by Katano et al. [46]. In a logistic regression analysis adjusting for recognized risk factors for miscarriage, high NK cytotoxicity before pregnancy had no impact on subsequent pregnancy loss rate.

The composition of endometrial lymphocytes fluctuates highly in the menstrual cycle with a six- to tenfold increase in the late luteal phase compared with the follicular phase [47] and as previously described the frequencies of the NK markers in the endometrium and peripheral blood vary as well. It has therefore rightly been questioned whether the endometrial NK cell subsets reflect those in the peripheral blood. A series of studies have investigated NK cells in endometrial biopsies taken in nonpregnant cycles in RPL patients and controls. Assessment of NK cell populations in these biopsies has been by immunohistochemistry or flow cytometry of homogenized tissue. The former technique is semiquantitative and subjective and the latter technique also has limitations, because the tissue undergoes enzymatic digestion, which influences marker expression. By flow cytometry, Lachapelle et al. found that the CD56[bright] subset was significantly lower in RPL patients than in controls [48]; using immunohistochemistry, Clifford et al. found that the frequency of CD56+ cells was significantly higher in RPL than controls [49]; Quenby et al. found that significantly more RPL patients than controls had NK cells >5 % [50]; and Tuckerman et al. reported that mean frequency of CD56+ cells was significantly higher in RPL than controls [51]. However, no relationship between CD56+ count in the endometrium and subsequent pregnancy outcome was found in the latter study: the patients who gave birth even tended to have higher NK cell numbers than those who miscarried again. Two quite small studies, using immunohistochemistry and flow cytometry, respectively, did not find any statistically significant difference in NK cell subsets in the endometrium between RPL patients and controls [52, 53].

Some studies have compared NK cell subsets in decidual tissue from missed miscarriages of RPL patients and fertile women having an elective termination and found differences in NK cell compositions between the two groups [54, 55]. Since the tissue in the former cases is often necrotic and inflamed due to the death of the fetus, whereas fresh and vital in the latter case, these kinds of studies provide limited valid information and they will not be reviewed further here.

T Regulatory Cells

T regulatory (Treg) lymphocytes have gained much attention in both general and reproductive immunology during the recent years. After being activated by tolerogenic antigen-presenting cells (APCs), Tregs can suppress the generation and the effector function of type 1 T-cell-mediated immune responses, which are considered harmful to pregnancy.

Studies in T-cell-deficient transgenic mice strains have clearly demonstrated that lymphocytes with the Treg phenotype CD4+, CD25+,Foxp3+

are important for implantation and successful pregnancy in allogenic matings [56]. The role in Tregs in human pregnancy and especially in RPL is still not clear, as relevant studies are small and sparse. Kwiatek et al. recently reported that the percentage of Tregs in the peripheral blood at the time of pregnancy loss was significantly lower in women with RPL than women with normal pregnancies at the same gestation age [57]. In women without a history of RPL, Jin et al. found that those who miscarried had significantly lower frequencies of CD4+,CD25[bright] cells in peripheral blood and deciduas than those with normal pregnancies [58].

A working hypothesis to guide future research that integrates the current knowledge from animal and human research of the role of Tregs in normal and adverse pregnancy has been proposed by Robertson et al. [59]: increasing plasma estrogen in the late follicular phase causes the Treg pool in the blood or regional lymph nodes to expand and causes increased uterine expression of chemokines resulting in the recruitment of T cells to the uterus. Male antigens and cytokines in seminal fluid in the vagina recruit tolerogenic APCs to the uterus and regional lymph nodes that activate local Tregs, which suppress pro-inflammatory T-helper type 1 immunity towards alloantigens on the embryo and trophoblast. The hypothesis is attractive as it introduces adaptive cellular immunity in the pathogenesis of adverse pregnancy outcomes such as RPL. In contrast to NK-cell-mediated immunity, an important feature of adaptive immunity is immunological memory, which is stored in memory T cells. Clinical observations such as the rare occurrence of preeclampsia in a second pregnancy with the same husband or the negative prognostic impact of the sex of the firstborn child in women with secondary RPL (see later) can most likely be explained by mechanisms, where tolerance or harmful immunity has developed in the first ongoing pregnancy and is remembered by memory T cells.

The current knowledge about Tregs in normal pregnancy and RPL illustrates the complexity of the research required in the future. It must take into account the very dynamic nature of the Tregs, which relocate between various compartments, proliferate, and activate according to cycle-specific endocrine factors and external antigen exposures provided, e.g., by coitus.

Immunogenetic Studies

All proteins which participate in immune interactions or are parts of immune cells are encoded by genes, which are often polymorphic due to single-nucleotide polymorphisms (SNPs) or copy number variations (CNVs) of DNA sequences. These polymorphisms may give rise to decreased or increased protein production and sometimes disturbances of immune functions.

By genome-wide screening, the polymorphisms suggested to affect gene function can be assigned to specific immunological or metabolic pathways modulated by the affected genes. In a recent study, CNVs that rearranged genes in pathways of "innate immune signaling," "complement cascade," or "interaction of Fc gamma receptors with antigen-bound IgG" were found highly significantly more often in RPL patients than in fertile controls [60].

In the following section we concentrate on studies of a single or a restricted series of candidate genes which a priori were considered likely to play a role in the immunological interactions being important for pregnancy.

Cytokine Genes

As discussed previously, it is generally believed that cytokines characterizing a T-helper type 1 or a pro-inflammatory immune response are involved in the pathogenesis of RPL. The plasma levels or the in vitro production of many cytokines are in part determined by polymorphisms in the genes coding for the cytokines. Many studies of cytokine gene polymorphisms have been undertaken in RPL patients. A review [61] concluded that some studies have reported altered prevalence of polymorphisms in genes coding for IFN-γ, IL-10, IL-6, and IL-1B, but the findings could not be confirmed in studies by other groups. The reasons for the lack of confirmed associations

may be that studies have been small, patient groups have been clinically heterogeneous, and the prevalence of the polymorphisms is very different between ethnic groups.

Mannose-Binding Lectin Genes

As previously discussed, two research groups have reported that MBL deficiency is associated with RPL and a poor prognosis in these patients. The plasma levels of MBL are determined by polymorphisms in the promoter region and exon 1 of the MBL-2 gene on chromosome 10. Specific combinations of genetic polymorphisms associated with low (<100 ng/ml) MBL levels have been reported with increased frequency in RPL patients and in particular in those with unexplained late fetal death [24, 62].

HLA

The HLA region located on the short arm of chromosome 6 contains the most polymorphic genes known in the human species. Dependent on the genetic distance between the various HLA loci, alleles in each locus display stronger or weaker linkage disequilibrium, which means that alleles in different loci are inherited together more often or less often than expected by chance. This is an important feature when studies of HLA polymorphisms in RPL and other disorders are evaluated.

The HLA molecules play an important role in both the adaptive and innate immune system. In the adaptive system, CD8+ lymphocytes can exert cytotoxic reactions against cells carrying class I HLA molecules, especially HLA-A and B, which play an important role in transplantation immunology. Class II HLA molecules (HLA-DR and -DQ) are carried primarily on APCs and present antigenic peptides to T-helper (CD4+) lymphocytes, which can initiate both humeral and cellular immune reactions. An individual's two sets of HLA class II alleles determine the repertoire of antigens that he/she can easily be immunized against, and which antigens will not give rise to an immune response. Due to this feature, HLA class II alleles are associated (sometimes strongly) with most autoimmune diseases, since these diseases are caused by an adverse reaction against one or several self-antigens.

NK cells, which belong to the innate immune system, were initially believed to react against all cells not carrying HLA molecules, but we now know that things are more complicated, as NK receptors can be inhibited or activated by HLA-C, HLA-G, and –E ligands, often dependent on the polymorphism of the HLA molecule.

Due to the different ways HLA can influence immune reactions, studies of HLA in RPL can be divided into three main categories: studies of HLA allele incompatibility (sharing) between partners with RPL; studies of HLA allele prevalences in women with RPL; and studies of HLA-C, -G, and -E alleles in couples with RPL.

All three kinds of studies have been addressed in a recent meta-analysis by Meuleman et al. [63], which provide a comprehensive review of the literature.

Increased HLA compatibility (sharing) was originally thought to decrease the probability that the mother would react immunologically adequate to the fetus and produce so-called blocking antibodies but the importance of these has never been documented. The vast majority of HLA-sharing studies is of older date, and used obsolete serological techniques for HLA determination, which can detect only broad antigen specificities of the HLA alleles. The meta-analysis [63] reported that allele sharing in the HLA-B, -DR, and -DQ loci was found with significantly higher frequency in RPL than control couples. However, these results should be interpreted with caution due to the obsolete methods used in most of these generally small studies.

Studies of HLA allele frequencies in RPL have focused on the HLA-DR or -DQ allele prevalences in RPL women and controls since these are the strongest immune response genes, as mentioned above. In the meta-analysis comprising eight case–control studies using modern polymerase chain reaction techniques, it was found that HLA-DRB1*04 and -DRB1*15 were significantly increased in RPL patients [63].

HLA-DRB1*03 was found with an OR of 1.32 (95 % CI: 0.89–1.97) in patients versus controls, which was not significant. However, we are convinced that HLA-DRB1*03 may be the strongest RPL susceptibility class II HLA allele in Caucasians. In a large case–control study [14] we found this allele to be highly significantly increased in RPL patients with increased prevalence with increased number of previous pregnancy losses. The reason why the HLA-DRB1*03 allele was not significantly increased in RPL in the meta-analysis may be due to several factors: Firstly, four of the included studies were Japanese. In Japan the HLA-DRB1*03 allele is very rare and the many Japanese patients and controls will dilute an association of HLA-DRB1*03 and RPL in the meta-analysis. Studies of associations between HLA polymorphisms and disease susceptibility should always be restricted to specific ethnic groups. Secondly, a large study with 234 patients and 360 controls [64] was excluded from the meta-analysis since the control group comprised normal blood donors rather than fertile women. This is an unjustified exclusion since individuals from an unselected population rather than individuals with no disease (fertile women) are fully accepted as controls in genetic case–control studies as long as the disease is rare (RPL prevalence 2–3 %). Third, in several of the included studies, patients (but not controls) with all kinds of autoantibodies were excluded. This will deplete the patient group for HLA-DRB1*03 positives since this allele is well known to be associated with autoantibody production [13].

In conclusion, taking the meta-analysis and our own full data set into consideration we conclude that HLA-DRB1*03, -DRB1*04, and -DRB1*15 may confer susceptibility to RPL in Caucasians. However, as all these alleles are quite frequent in a Caucasian population (combined frequency 80 %) this knowledge is not very useful in clinical practice.

Studies assessing the impact of maternal carriage of specific HLA class II alleles on future pregnancy outcome have provided information that can be more useful in clinical practice and in addition have highlighted the importance of a not previously recognized immune dysfunction in patients with RPL. Epidemiological studies have shown that among patients with RPL after a birth (secondary RPL), the birth of a boy in the pregnancy preceding the miscarriages is significantly more prevalent (61 % versus 39 %) and patients with a firstborn boy exhibit a significantly lower chance of live birth in their next pregnancy [65] and also after a period of 5 years [66]. Among RPL patients with a firstborn boy, maternal carriage of one of the three HLA-class II alleles, HLA-DRB1*15, -DQB1*0501/2, and -DRB3*0301, the chance of live birth was 22 % lower than in similar patients not carrying these alleles [67]. These alleles (HY-restricting class II HLA alleles) are known from in vitro models to present peptides derived from male-specific proteins (HY antigens) to T-helper cells and in transplantation immunology carriage of the alleles predisposes to graft-versus-host disease after sex-mismatched bone-marrow transplantation. Recently it has been reported that the HLA class II allele HLA-DRB1*07 also restricts immunity against HY antigens and in a new prospective study we confirmed that maternal carriage of this allele reduced the chance of live birth in patients with RPL after the birth of a boy [68]. Our hypothesis derived from the HLA studies and supported by a study of anti-HY antibodies in RPL patients [69] is that T-helper lymphocytes from some women carrying these HY-restricting class II HLA alleles recognize HY antigens on the placenta of their first ongoing pregnancy with a boy, which initiates a series of harmful immune reactions targeting the trophoblast in the subsequent pregnancies ultimately leading to RPL. More research confirming this mechanism of RPL is needed; in particular we need to isolate the suggested clones of HY-specific T lymphocytes that initiate or carry out the suggested immune reactions leading to RPL.

In the section about NK cells we were discussing the relationship between specific KIR receptor polymorphisms, HLA and RPL. It has been shown that feto-maternal mismatch for HLA-C alleles can induce Tregs that may promote tolerance to the pregnancy in the uterus [70]. HLA-C alleles can be divided into so-

called C1 and C2 groups according to a dimorphism at position 80 of the segment of HLA-C molecule that can bind KIRs. C1 allotypes are ligands for the inhibiting KIRDL2/3 and activating KIRDS2, whereas C2 allotypes are ligands for the inhibitory KIR2DL1 and activating KIR2DS1. Hiby et al. [71] published data suggesting a role for maternal KIR polymorphisms and parental HLA-C polymorphisms in RPL. It was found that situations where the woman carries a combination of KIR genes that is primarily inhibitory (so-called AA genotype) and where the father carries C2 allotypes are more frequent among RPL couples than couples with normal fertility. Hiby et al. suggested that this combination of mainly inactivating KIR genotypes in the woman and their ligands in the parents results in a predominant decidual NK cell inhibition that may lead to insufficient secretion of specific cytokines at the feto-maternal interface, resulting in defective trophoblast proliferation and invasion and subsequent RPL. Another large study [72] in contrast found that maternal carriage of the inhibitory KIR2DL1 in combination with C2 homozygosity in both partners was found significantly more often in controls than RPL women, whereas maternal carriage of the activating KIR2DS2 in conjunction med C1 homozygosity in both partners was found to be significantly increased in RPL patients. The conclusion from this study was the opposite of the above: that receptor-ligand combinations that promote inactivation of NK cells are beneficial for pregnancy and may prevent RPL. In the meta-analysis of HLA in RPL [63] no association between parental C2 allotypes and RPL could be detected.

Another set of studies have investigated HLA-G polymorphisms in RPL. HLA-G is a so-called nonclassical HLA gene, which exhibits much less polymorphism than classical HLA genes but has the interesting feature of being highly expressed in extravillous trophoblast cells in contrast to all other HLA genes except HLA-C and -E. No polymorphism in the coding part of the HLA-G gene has repeatedly been associated with RPL whereas many studies have been undertaken regarding a 14-base pair insertion/deletion dimorphism in exon 8 of the HLA-G gene, which may affect transcription of the gene. Several studies have showed an association between low levels of soluble HLA-G in plasma and homozygosity for the HLA-G 14-base pair insertion [73]. Low levels of soluble HLA-G may in itself result in reduced immunity against the trophoblast since soluble HLA-G can modulate NK cell function via inhibition of interactions between NK cells and specific antigen-presenting dendritic cells [74]. In the meta-analysis by Meuleman et al. combing results from seven studies, the HLA-G 14-base pair insertion was nonsignificantly increased in RPL compared with controls, OR 1.38 (95 % CI: 0.85–2.26) for the insertion/insertion genotype. However, two other recent meta-analyses including 17 studies [75] and 14 studies [76] found that the HLA-G 14-base pair insertion frequency was significantly increased in RPL with ORs 1.27 (95 % CI: 1.04–1.55) and OR = 1.47 (95 % CI: 1.13–1.91), respectively. In conclusion, the HLA-G 14-base pair insertion in exon 8 seems to predispose to RPL. Since the HLA-G 14-base pair insertion is in positive linkage disequilibrium with the HLA-DRB1*03 allele [77] the question remains whether the HLA-G gene insertion or HLA-DRB*03 is the main RPL susceptibility gene.

Conclusions

Overall, the three main arguments for immunological disturbances playing a role in RPL are the following:

1. The general knowledge that whenever allogenic tissue is introduced into an organism immune reactions develop and, if not abolished, rejection will occur
2. The observation that a series of autoimmune diseases and autoantibodies are found with increased prevalence in RPL
3. The observation that RPL women in the long term have an increased risk of atherosclerotic cardiovascular diseases attributable to a chronic pro-inflammatory state [78, 79]

Most of the non-genetic immunologic biomarkers (except autoantibody measurements) reviewed in this chapter have not been tested in assays with sufficient reproducibility or the reference values in normal women or during pregnancy have not been sufficiently established (Table 6.1). Regarding the genetic biomarkers, DNA-based tests are suggested to have high reproducibility, but in most cases their diagnostic values must be further studied in large studies of patients and controls, which are homogenous with regard to reproductive history and ethnicity.

The lack of tests with sufficient diagnostic value for detecting immunological causes of RPL has wide implications for the identification of patients for specific treatments or inclusion in randomized controlled trials. The failure to find significant beneficial effects of immunotherapeutic treatments such as prednisone [80] or intravenous immunoglobulin [81] in randomized controlled trials has by many researchers been attributed to the non-selection of patients for these trials due to the presence of immune biomarkers such as high NK cell cytotoxicity levels. We believe that as long as the diagnostic specificity of the immune tests is not well established, patients for treatment or participation in randomized trials must still be selected based on their reproductive history, e.g., a poor spontaneous prognosis evidenced by a high number of previous pregnancy losses.

In our view, not one but several disturbances or disruptions of pathways relating to immune interactions are probably causing many cases of RPL; the reproductive process is too important to be vulnerable to the disruption of only one immune pathway. We think that disturbances in several immune pathways (caused by SNPs or CNVs disrupting DNA sequences) in conjunction with immunizing events in previous pregnancies, such as a substantial transfer of fetal antigens (cells) into the maternal circulation [82], can promote pro-inflammatory reactions or breakage of autotolerance. This will predispose to RPL and other adverse pregnancy outcomes and ultimately lead to atherosclerotic or autoimmune disease.

Table 6.1 Immunological biomarkers investigated in recurrent pregnancy loss (RPL), their diagnostic value, and suggestions for further research

Biomarker		Associated to RPL	Prognostic value	Needed research
Autoantibodies	Antiphospholipid antibodies	+++	++	Standardization of assays and cutoff values Prognostic studies in untreated patients
	Thyroid antibodies Antinuclear antibodies	+++	?	Prognostic studies in untreated patients
Soluble immune biomarkes	Peripheral blood cytokines	?	?	More sensitive and reliable methods
	Mannose-binding lectin	++	+	More studies for further documentation
Immune cells	Peripheral blood NK cell subsets	+	?	Establishment of reference values in different phases of cycle or pregnancy
	Peripheral blood NK cytotoxicity	+	?	Establishment of reference values in different phases of cycle or pregnancy
	Endometrial NK cells	?/+	?	Establishment of reference values in different phases of cycle Standardization of methods Larger studies
	Decidual NK cells	?	-	Suitable control samples (aneuploid missed miscarriages?)
	Peripheral blood Treg cells	?	?	Establishment of reference values in different phases of cycle Standardization of methods Larger studies
Genetic biomarkers	Cytokine gene polymorphisms	?	–	More and larger studies Ethnic and diagnostic homogeneity of cases and controls
	Mannose lectin gene polymorphism	+	+	More studies
	HLA sharing	?	?	Studies using up-to-date techniques Clear definition of criteria for allele sharing
	HLA class II	++	+	Larger studies Studies homogeneous with regard to reproductive history and ethnicity
	HLA-C, HLA-G	+	?	Larger studies Studies homogeneous with regard to reproductive history and ethnicity

This suggested complexity of the pathogenesis of RPL will be a challenge for future research in the area, which is further complicated by the fact that almost half of all pregnancy losses in RPL women are due to embryonal aneuploidy with no immunological background. We find it important for researchers to acknowledge this complexity instead of narrow-sightedly dividing the patients into subgroups, each suggested to be caused by one specific (simple) immunological or non-immunological etiology.

Large epidemiological studies have now documented that RPL patients carry a substantial risk of developing later atherosclerotic disease [78, 79], which may be due to chronic activation of pro-inflammatory pathways. Research in the immunological abnormalities associated with RPL therefore both has the potential to disclose pathways leading to pregnancy loss that may be modified by specific therapies but it may also identify biomarkers, which can be used for identifying those patients who are in the greatest risk of contracting cardiovascular disease in order that preventive measures can be initiated.

References

1. Jauniaux E, Farquharson RG, Christiansen OB, Exalto N. Evidence-based guidelines for the investigation and medical treatment of recurrent miscarriage. Hum Reprod. 2006;21:2216–22.
2. Stephenson MD, Awartani KA, Robinson WP. Cytogenetic analysis of miscarriages from couples with recurrent miscarriage: a case-control study. Hum Reprod. 2002;17:446–51.
3. Van Kampen CA, Versteeg-van der Voort Maarschalk MF, Langerak-Langerak J van BE, Roelen BL, Claas FH. Pregnancy can induce long-persisting primed CTLs specific for inherited paternal HLA antigens. Hum Immunol. 2001;62:201–7.
4. Lashley EELO, Meuleman T, Claas EHJ. Beneficial or harmful effect of antipaternal human leukocyte antibodies on pregnancy outcome? A systematic review and meta-analysis. Am J Reprod Immunol. 2013;70:87–103.
5. Christiansen OB, Steffensen R, Nielsen HS, Varming K. Multifactorial etiology of recurrent miscarriage and its scientific and clinical implications. Gynecol Obstet Invest. 2008;66:257–67.
6. Robertson L, Wu O, Langhorne P, Twaddle S, Clark P, Lowe GD, Walker ID, et al. Thrombophilia in pregnancy: a systematic review. Br J Haematol. 2006;132:171–96.
7. Van den Boogaard E, Vissenberg R, Land JA, van Wely M, van der Post JAM, Goddijn M, et al. Significance of (sub)clinical thyroid dysfunction and thyroid autoimmunity before conception and in early pregnancy: a systematic review. Hum Reprod Update. 2011;17:605–19.
8. Christiansen OB. A fresh look at the causes and treatments of recurrent miscarriage, especially its immunological aspects. Hum Reprod Update. 1996;2:271–93.
9. Molazadeh M, Karimzadeh H, Azizi MR. Prevalence and clinical significance of antinuclear antibodies in Iranian women with unexplained recurrent miscarriage. Iran J Reprod Med. 2014;12:221–6.
10. Ticconi C, Rotondi F, Veglia M, Pietropolli A, Bernardini S, Ria F, et al. Antinuclear antibodies in women with recurrent pregnancy loss. Am J Reprod Immunol. 2010;64:384–92.
11. Bustos D, Moret A, Tambutti M, Gogorza S, Testa R, Ascione A, et al. Autoantibodies in Argentine women with recurrent pregnancy loss. Am J Reprod Immunol. 2006;55:201–7.
12. Cavalcante MB, da Silva Costa F, Junior EA, Barini R. Risk factor associated with a new pregnancy loss and perinatal outcomes in cases of recurrent miscarriage treated with lymphocyte immunotherapy. J Matern Fetal Med. Early Online: 1–5. 2014. doi:10.3109.
13. Christiansen OB, Ulcova-Gallova Z, Mohapeloa H, Krauz V. Studies on associations between human leukocyte antigen class II alleles and antiphospholipid antibodies in Danish and Czech women with recurrent miscarriage. Hum Reprod. 1998;12:3326–31.
14. Kruse C, Steffensen R, Varming K, Christiansen OB. A study of HLA-DR and -DQ alleles in 588 patients and 562 controls confirms that HLA-DRB1*03 is associated with recurrent miscarriage. Hum Reprod. 2004;19:1215–21.
15. Wegman TG, Lin H, Guilbert L, Mosmann TR. Birectional cytokine interactions in the maternal-fetal relationship: is successful pregnancy a Th2 phenomenon? Immunol Today. 1993;14:353–7.
16. Wang Q, Li T-C, Wu Y-P, Cocksedge KA, Fu Y-S, Kong Q-Y, et al. Reappraisal of peripheral NK cells in women with recurrent miscarriage. Reprod BioMed Online. 2008;17:814–9.
17. Haider S, Knöfler M. Human tumour necrosis factor: physiological and pathological roles in placenta and endometrium. Placenta. 2009;30:111–23.
18. Mueller-Eckhardt G, Mallmann P, Neppert J, Lattermann A, Melk A, Heine O. Immunogenetic and serological investigations in nonpregnant and in pregnant women with a history of recurrent spontaneous abortions. German RSA/IVIG Group. J Reprod Immunol. 1994;27:95–109.
19. Calleja-Agius J, Jauniaux E, Pizzey AR, Muttukrisna S. Investigation of systemic inflammatory response in first trimester pregnancy failure. Hum Reprod. 2012;27:349–57.
20. Kruse C, Varming K, Christiansen OB. Prospective, serial investigations of in-vitro lymphocyte cytokine production, CD62L expression and proliferative

response to microbial antigens in women with recurrent miscarriage. Hum Reprod. 2003;18:2465–72.

21. Piosek ZM, Goegebeur Y, Klitkou L, Steffensen R, Christiansen OB. Plasma TNF-α levels are higher in early pregnancy in patients with secondary compared with primary recurrent miscarriage. Am J Reprod Immunol. 2013;70:347–58.

22. Kilpatrick DC, Bevan BH, Liston WA. Association between mannan binding lectin deficiency and recurrent miscarriage. Hum Reprod. 1995;10:2501–5.

23. Christiansen OB, Klipatrick DC, Souter V, Varming K, Thiel S, Jensenius JC. Mannan-binding lectin deficiency is associated with unexplained recurrent miscarriage. Scand J Immunol. 1999;49:193–6.

24. Kruse C, Rosgaard A, Steffensen R, Varming K, Jensenius JC, Christiansen OB. Low serum level of mannan-binding lectin is a determinant for pregnancy outcome in women with recurrent spontaneous abortion. Am J Obstet Gynecol. 2002;187:1313–20.

25. Laird S, Mariee N, Wei L, Li TC. Measurements of CD56+ cells in peripheral blood and endometrium by flow cytometry and immunohistochemical staining in situ. Hum Reprod. 2011;26:1331–7.

26. Witt CS, Goodridge J, Gerbase-DeLima MG, Daher S, Christiansen FT. Maternal KIR repertoire is not associated with recurrent spontaneous abortion. Hum Reprod. 2004;111:2653–7.

27. Ponte M, Cantoni C, Biassoni R, Tradori-Cappai A, Bentivoglio G, Vitale C, Bertone S, Moretta A, Moretta L, Mingari MC. Inhibitory receptors sensing HLA-G1 molecules in pregnancy: decidua-associated natural killer cells express LIR-1 and CD94/NKG2A and acquire p49, an HLA-G1-specific receptor. Proc Natl Acad Sci U S A. 1999;96:5674–9.

28. Guimond M-J, Wang B, Croy BA. Engraftment of bone marrow from severe combined immunodeficient (SCID) mice reverses the reproductive deficits in natural killer-deficient tge mice. J Immunol. 2007;178:5949–56.

29. Kwak JYH, Beaman KD, Gilman-Sachs A, Ruiz JE, Schewitz D, Beer AE. Up-regulated expression of CD56+, CD56+/CD16+, and CD19+ cells in peripheral blood lymphocytes in pregnant women with recurrent pregnancy loss. Am J Reprod Immunol. 1995;34:93–9.

30. Beer AE, Kwak JYH, Ruiz JE. Immunophenotypic profiles of periferal blood lymphocytes in women with recurrent pregnancy losses and in infertile women with multiple failed in vitro fertilization cycles. Am J Reprod Immunol. 1996;35:376–82.

31. Perricone C, De Carolis C, Giacomelli R, Zaccari G, Cipriani P, Bizzi E, Perricone R. High levels of NK cells in the peripheral blood of patients affected with anti-phospholipid syndrome and recurrent spontaneous abortion: a potential new hypothesis. Rheumatology. 2007;46:1574–8.

32. King K, Smith S, Chapman M, Sacks G. Detailed analysis of peripheral blood natural killer (NK) cells in women with recurrent miscarriage. Hum Reprod. 2010;25:52–8.

33. Lee KL, Na BJ, Kim JY, Hur SE, Lee M, Gilman-Sachs A, Kwak-Kim J. Determination of clinical cellular

immune markers in women with recurrent pregnancy loss. Am J Reprod Immunol. 2013;70:398–411.

34. Ramos-Medina R, Garcia-Segovia A, Leon JA, Alonso B, Tejera-Alhambra M, Gil J, et al. New decision-tree model for defining the risk of reproductive failure. Am J Reprod Immunol. 2013;70:59–68.

35. Carbone J, Gellego A, Lanio N, Navarro J, Orera M, Aguaron A, et al. Quantitative abnormalities of peripheral blood distinct T, B, and natural killer cell subsets and clinical findings in obstetric antiphosphlipid syndrome. J Rheumatol. 2009;36:1217–25.

36. Christiansen OB. Research methodology in recurrent pregnancy loss. Obstet Gynecol Clin North Am. 2014;41:19–39.

37. Shakar K, Ben-Eliyahu S, Loewenthal R, Rosenne E, Carp H. Differences in number and activity of peripheral natural killer cell in primary versus secondary recurrent miscarriage. Fertil Steril. 2003;80:368–75.

38. Yoo JH, Kwak-Kim J, Han A-R, Ahn H, Cha S-H, Koong MK, et al. Peripheral blood NK cell cytotoxicities are negatively correlated with CD8+ T cells in fertile women but not in women with a history of recurrent pregnancy loss. Am J Reprod Immunol. 2012;68:38–46.

39. Karami N, Boroujerdnia MG, Nikbakht R, Khodadadi A. Enhancement of peripheral blood CD56^dim cell and NK cytotoxicity in women with recurrent spontaneous abortion or in vitro fertilization failure. J Reprod Immunol. 2012;95:87–92.

40. Hadinedoushan H, Mirahmadian M, Aflatounian A. Increased natural killer cell cytotoxicity and IL-2 production in recurrent spontaneous abortion. Am J Reprod Immunol. 2007;58:409–14.

41. Emmer PM, Veerhoek M, Nelen WLDM, Steegers EAP, Joosten I. Natural killer cell reactivity and HLA-G in recurrent spontaneous abortion. Transplant Proc. 1999;31:1838–40.

42. Aoki K, Kajiura S, Matsumoto Y, Ogasawara M, Okada S, Yagami Y, et al. Preconceptional natural-killer-cell activity as a predictor of miscarriage. Lancet. 1995;345:1340–2.

43. Yamada H, Morikawa M, Kato EH, Shimada S, Kobashi G, Minikami H. Pre-conceptional natural killer cell activity and percentage as predictors of biochemical pregnancy and spontaneous abortion with normal chromosome karyotype. Am J Reprod Immunol. 2003;50:351–4.

44. Morikawa M, Yamada H, Kato EH, Shimada S, Ebina Y, Yamada T, et al. NK cell activity and subsets in women with a history of spontaneous abortion. Gynecol Obstet Invest. 2001;52:163–7.

45. Liang P, Mo M, Li G-G, Yin B, Cai J, Wu T, et al. Comprehensive analysis of peripheral blood lymphocytes in 76 women with recurrent miscarriage before and after lymphocyte immunotherapy. Am J Reprod Immunol. 2012;68:164–74.

46. Katano K, Suzuki S, Ozaki Y, Suzumori N, Kitaori T, Sugiura-Ogasawara M. Peripheral natural killer cell

activity as a predictor of recurrent pregnancy loss: a large cohort study. Fertil Steril. 2013;100:1629–34.

47. Russell P, Sacks G, Tremeleln K, Gee A. The distribution of immune cells and macrophages in the endometrium of women with recurrent reproductive failure. III: further observations and reference ranges. Pathology. 2013;45:393–401.

48. Lachapelle M-H, Miron P, Hemmings R, Roy DC. Endometrial T, B and NK cells in patients with recurrent spontaneous abortion. Altered profile and pregnancy outcome. J Immunol. 1996;156:4027–34.

49. Clifford K, Flanagan AM, Regan L. Endometrial CD56+ natural killer cells in women with recurrent miscarriage: a histomorphometric study. Hum Reprod. 1999;14:2727–30.

50. Quenby S, Kalumbi C, Bates M, Farquharson R, Vince G. Prednisone reduces preconceptual endometrial natural killer cells in women with recurrent miscarriage. Fertil Steril. 2005;84:980–4.

51. Tuckerman E, Laird SM, Prakash A, Li TC. Prognostic value of the measurement of uterine natural killer cells in the endometrium of women with recurrent miscarriage. Hum Reprod. 2007;22:2208–13.

52. Michimata T, Ogasawara MS, Tsuda H, Suzumori K, Aoki K, Sasai M, et al. Distributions of endometrial NK cells, B cells, T cells, and Th2/Tc2 cells fail to predict pregnancy outcome following recurrent abortion. Am J Reprod Immunol. 2002;47:196–202.

53. Shimada S, Kato EH, Morikawa M, Iwabuchi K, Nishida R, Kishi R, et al. No difference in natural killer or natural killer T-cell population, but aberrant T-helper cell population in the endometrium of women with repeated miscarriage. Hum Reprod. 2004;19:1018–24.

54. Quack KC, Vassiliadou D, Pudney J, Anderson DJ, Hill JA. Leukocyte activation in the decidua of chromosomally normal and abnormal fetuses from women with recurrent abortion. Hum Reprod. 2001;16:949–55.

55. Yamamoto T, Takahashi Y, Kase N, Mori H. Role of decidual natural killer (NK) cells in patients with missed abortion: differences between cases with normal and abnormal chromosome. Clin Exp Immunol. 1999;116:449–52.

56. Aluvihare VR, Kallikourdis M, Betz AG. Regulatory T cells mediate maternal tolerance to the fetus. Nat Immunol. 2004;5:266–71.

57. Kwiatek M, Geca T, Krzyzanowski A, Malec A, Kwasniewska A. Peripheral dendritic cells and CD4 + CD25 + Foxp3+ regulatory T cells in the first trimester of normal pregnancy and in women with recurrent miscarriage. PLoS One. 2015;10, e0124747.

58. Jin LP, Chen QY, Zhang T, Guo PF, Li DJ. The CD4 + CD25 bright regulatory T cells and CTLA-4 expression in peripheral and decidual lymphocytes are down-regulated in human miscarriage. Clin Immunol. 2009;133:402–10.

59. Robertson SA, Prins JR, Sharkey DJ, Moldenhauser LM. Seminal fluid and the generation of regulatory T cells for embryo implantation. Am J Reprod Immunol. 2013;69:315–30.

60. Nagirnaja L, Palta P, Kasak L, Rull K, Christiansen OB, Nielsen HS, et al. Structural genomic variation as risk factor for idiopathic recurrent miscarriage. Hum Mutat. 2014;35:972–82.

61. Choi YK, Kwak-Kim J. Cytokine gene polymorphisms in recurrent spontaneous abortions: a comprehensive review. Am J Reprod Immunol. 2008;60:91–110.

62. Christiansen OB, Nielsen HS, Lund M, Steffensen R, Varming K. Mannose-binding lectin-2 genotypes and recurrent late pregnancy losses. Hum Reprod. 2009;24:291–9.

63. Meuleman T, Lashley LELO, Dekkers OM, van Lith JMM, Claas FHJ, Bloemenkamp KWH. HLA associations and HLA sharing in recurrent miscarriage: a systematic review and meta-analysis. Hum Immunol. 2015;76:362–73.

64. Christiansen OB, Rasmussen KL, Jersild C, Grunnet N. HLA class II alleles confer susceptibility to recurrent fetal losses in Danish women. Tissue Antigens. 1994;44:225–33.

65. Nielsen HS, Andersen ANM, Kolte AM, Christiansen OB. A firstborn boy is suggestive of a strong prognostic factor in secondary recurrent miscarriage: a confirmatory study. Fertil Steril. 2008;89:907–11.

66. Lund M, Kamper-Jørgensen M, Nielsen HS, Lidegaard O, Nybo Andersen AM, Christiansen OB. Prognosis for live birth in women with recurrent miscarriage. What is the best measure of success? Obstet Gynecol. 2012;119:37–43.

67. Nielsen HS, Steffensen R, Varming K, van Halteren AG, Spierings E, Ryder LP, Goulmy E, Christiansen OB. Association of HY-restricting HLA class II alleles with pregnancy outcome in patients with recurrent miscarriage subsequent to a firstborn boy. Hum Mol Genet. 2009;18:1684–91.

68. Kolte AM, Steffensen RN, Christiansen OB, Nielsen HS. The prognostic impact of HY restricting HLA class II alleles in secondary recurrent pregnancy loss. Reprod Sci. 2015;22 Suppl 1:321A (Meeting Abstract S-071).

69. Nielsen HS, Wu F, Aghai Z, Steffensen R, van Halteren AG, Spierings E, Christiansen OB, Miklos D, Goulmy E. H-Y antibody titers are increased in unexplained secondary recurrent miscarriage patients and associated with low male:female ratio in subsequent live births. Hum Reprod. 2010;25:2745–52.

70. Tilburgs T, Scherjon SA, van der Mast B, Haasnoot GW, Versteeg-van der Voort-Maarschalk M, Roelen DL, et al. Fetal-maternal HLA-C mismatch is associated with decidual T cell activation and induction of functional T regulatory cells. J Reprod Immunol. 2009;82:148–57.

71. Hiby SE, Regan L, Lo W, Farrell L, Carrington M, Moffett A. Association of maternal killer-cell immunoglobulin-like receptors and parental HLA-C genotypes with recurrent miscarriage. Hum Reprod. 2008;23:972–6.

72. Faridi RM, Agrawal S. Killer immunoglobulin-like receptors (KIR) and HLA-C allorecognition patterns implicative of dominant activation of natural killer

cells contribute to recurrent miscarriage. Hum Reprod. 2011;20:491–7.

73. Hviid TV, Rizzo R, Christiansen OB, Melchiorri L, Lindhard A, Baricordi OR. HLA-G and IL-10 in serum in relation to HLA-G genotype and polymorphisms. Immunogenetics. 2004;56:135–41.

74. Gros F, Cabillic F, Toutirais O, Maux AL, Sebti Y, Amiot L, et al. Soluble HLA-G molecules impair natural killer/dendritic cell crosstalk via inhibition of dendritic cells. Eur J Immunol. 2008;38:742–9.

75. Fan W, Li S, Huang Z, Chen Q. Relationship between HLA-G polymorphism and susceptibility to recurrent miscarriage: a meta-analysis of non-familly based studies. J Assist Reprod Genet. 2014;31:173–84.

76. Wang X, Jiang W, Zhang D. Association of 14-bp insertion/deletion polymorphism in couples with recurrent spontaneous abortions. Tissue Antigens. 2013;81:108–15.

77. Hviid TVF, Christiansen OB. Linkage disequlibrium between human leucocyte antigen (HLA) class II and HLA-G – possible implications for human reproduction and autoimmune disease. Hum Immunol. 2005;66:688–99.

78. Ranthe MF, Andersen EAW, Wohlfarht J, Bundgaard H, Melbye M, Boyd HA. Pregnancy loss and later risk of atherosclerotic disease. Circulation. 2013;127:1775–82.

79. Kessous R, Shoham-Vardi I, Pariente G, Sergienko R, Holcberg G, Sheiner E. Recurrent pregnancy loss: a risk factor for long-term maternal atherosclerotic morbidity? Am J Obstet Gynecol. 2014;211:414e1–11.

80. Laskin CA, Bombardier C, Hannah C, Mandel ME, Ritchie JW, Farewell V, et al. Prednisone and aspirin in women with autoantibodies and unexplained recurrent fetal loss. N Eng J Med. 1997;337:148–53.

81. Christiansen OB, Larsen EC, Egerup P, Lunoee L, Egestad L, Nielsen HS. Intravenous immunoglobullin treatment for secondary recurrent miscarriage: a randomised, double-blind, placebo-controlled trial. BJOG. 2015;122:500–8.

82. Nielsen HS, Steffensen R, Lund M, Egestad L, Mortensen LH, Andersen AM, Lidegaard Ø, Christiansen OB. Frequency and impact of obstetric complications prior and subsequent to unexplained secondary recurrent miscarriage. Hum Reprod. 2010;25:1543–52.

Anatomical Aspects in Recurrent Pregnancy Loss

Asher Bashiri, David Gilad, David Yohai, and Tullio Ghi

Introduction

The overall incidence of uterine malformations in the general population is hard to determine with accuracy due to a wide range of epidemiologic data reported in the literature. It is reasonable to estimate that uterine malformations are found in approximately 0.1–4 % of the general population and in approximately 15 % of patients with RPL [1]. Some reports describe a prevalence as high as 25 % of the general population [2]. As for the incidence of the specific types of anomalies, it appears that septate and arcuate uterus represent 55 % of congenital uterine malformations [1] with the former being the most

A. Bashiri, MD (✉)
Director Maternity C and Recurrent Pregnancy Loss Clinic, Department of Obstetrics and Gynecology, Soroka University Medical Center, Faculty of Health Sciences, Ben-Gurion University of the Negev, Be'er Sheva, Israel
e-mail: abashiri@bgu.ac.il

D. Gilad, MMedSc
Department of Physiology and cell Biology, Joyce and Irwing Goldman Medical school, Ben-Gurion University, Be'er Sheva, Israel

D. Yohai, MD
Department of Obstetrics and Gynecology, Soroka Medical Center, Ben-Gurion University of the Negev, Be'er Sheva, Israel

T. Ghi, PhD
Department of Obstetrics and Gynecology, University of Parma, Parma, Italy

common congenital uterine anomaly encountered in clinical practice [2]. Women suffering from Müllerian anomalies (congenital malformations of the uterus and Fallopian tube) face reproductive challenges in pregnancy maintenance as well as in conception. The associated clinical implications of uterine anomalies include an increased risk of spontaneous abortion, malpresentation, placental abruption, intrauterine growth restriction, prematurity, operative delivery, retained placenta, and fetal mortality [2].

Embryology

During embryogenesis, between 5 and 8 weeks of gestation, the development of the male and female genital systems is sex indifferent, with the presence of both the mesonephric (Wolffian) and paramesonephric (Müllerian) ducts. In a normal female fetus the absence of a Y chromosome does not allow for the expression of the testis-determining factor (TDF) gene, also known as sex determining region Y (SRY), located in the Y chromosome of a male fetus. Therefore, in a female fetus a developing testis does not form and will not liberate anti-Müllerian hormone (AMH), also known as Müllerian inhibitory factor (MIF), as occurs in the male fetus. This process promotes the degeneration of the mesonephric ducts, and bidirectional development of the Müllerian ducts along the lateral aspects of the gonads into the uterus, uterine cervix, fallopian tubes, and upper

© Springer International Publishing Switzerland 2016
A. Bashiri et al. (eds.), *Recurrent Pregnancy Loss*, DOI 10.1007/978-3-319-27452-2_7

two thirds of the vagina forming the anatomy of a female reproductive system.

Between 8 and 20 weeks gestation, the Müllerian duct will progressively undergo elongation, fusion, canalization, and septal resorption in a cephalic direction. Fusion of the paramesonephric ducts occurs primarily in their caudal portions forming the uterovaginal primordium. Their non-fused cranial directions will give rise to the developing Fallopian tubes with most cranial ends forming the ostium. Once fusion is complete a median septum is formed from the now apposed walls of the two fused paramesonephric ducts. In order to form single uterine and vaginal cavities, this septum must degenerate. Abnormalities of the formation of the cranial paramesonephric ducts will give rise to anomalies of the uterine tubes, and malformation of the caudal portions may result in a myriad of possible congenital uterine anomalies collectively referred to as Müllerian anomalies, ranging from complete absence or formation of a rudimentary uterus (e.g., complete agenesis of the uterus, Müllerian aplasia, uterine hypoplasia), unilateral aplasia of the paramesonephric ducts (e.g., uterus unicornis, uterus bicornis unicollis), and partial to complete retention of the apposed walls (forming a uterus subseptus unicollis and uterus bicornis septus, respectively), with complete failure of unification forming a double uterus (uterus didelphys) that may be associated with a single or correspondingly double vagina. Defective fusion is considered to be the most common cause of congenital uterine anomalies.

The Bcl-2 gene mediates the regression of the uterine septum caused by apoptosis, and persistence of the septum has been suggested to be a result of impaired Bcl-2 gene activity. There are two suggested theories regarding the process of this regression; the classic theory suggests a unidirectional regression of the septum, from the caudal to the cranial aspect of the uterovaginal canal; the second theory suggests a bidirectional regression in which the regression occurs simultaneously in the caudal and cranial directions [3, 4].

The urinary and genital systems both arise from a common ridge of mesoderm developing along the dorsal body wall, and both rely on normal development of the mesonephric system.

Hence, abnormal differentiation of the mesonephric or paramesonephric ducts may also be associated with anomalies of the kidneys including renal agenesis and renal ectopy [2, 5]. In their original study, Buttram and Gibbons [6] reported that 31 % of patients with Müllerian anomalies had coincident urinary anomalies. Moreover, unilateral abnormalities of the paramesonephric ducts are more frequently associated with renal defects. In a study specifically looking at urinary tract anomalies associated with unicornuate uterus, 40.5 % had an accompanying renal anomaly; of them, the most frequent was renal agenesis contralateral to the unicornuate uterus [7]. Thus, imaging study of the kidneys should be undertaken when a Müllerian anomaly is found, specifically an obstructive Müllerian anomaly.

Paramesonephric duct abnormalities may also rarely alter the normal anatomical location of the ovaries [8]. In patients with a unilateral rudimentary horn uterus or in patients with complete Müllerian agenesis, an ectopic location or a complete absence of the gonad on the affected side may also be found. Such occurrences may be observed in women with a normal uterus. The reported frequency of altered gonad location is as high as 20 % when the uterus is absent and 42 % in cases of unicornuate uterus. The ovaries in those patients may be found in the upper abdomen, at the level of the pelvic brim or in the inguinal canal [9, 10].

Prevalence and Inheritance

Estimating the exact incidence of Müllerian anomalies in the general population is challenging, as most of these women may not have an adverse reproductive outcome and will escape clinical detection. Overall congenital anomalies are estimated to occur in about 0.1–4 % of the general female population [2]. In a study of 679 women with normal reproductive outcomes evaluated with laparoscopy or laparotomy prior to tubal ligation, the incidence of congenital uterine anomalies was 3.2 % [11].

Interestingly, among women with adverse reproductive outcomes, the prevalence of uterine anomalies is higher. Congenital uterine anomalies were present in 12.6 % of patients with RPL. The prevalence of uterine anomalies among women with recurrent first trimester miscarriage ranged from 5 to 10 %, and reached 25 % in patients with recurrent second trimester pregnancy loss [2].

Congenital uterine malformations were found to be 21 times more frequent among infertile women than among those with normal fertility [12].

In a meta-analysis of 22 studies including unselected fertile patients referred for uterine morphologic assessment at the time of hysteroscopic tubal occlusion, or abdominal sterilization, or cesarean delivery, the prevalence of a Müllerian malformation was 1 in 594 [12]. These data clearly demonstrate a significant variation in the reported prevalence of congenital uterine anomalies amongst women with and without adverse reproductive outcomes.

A large case–control study conducted by Sugiura-Ogasawara et al. included 1676 patients with two or more consecutive pregnancy losses found major uterine anomalies in 3.2 % of the study population by hysterosalpingography and laparotomy/laparoscopy [13].

Jaslow and Kutteh [14] studied the effect of prior birth or miscarriage on the prevalence of both acquired and congenital uterine anomalies in women with RPL. The study population consisted of 875 women who suffered from two or more consecutive pregnancy losses. Uterine anomalies (both congenital and acquired) were diagnosed in 169 of the women (19.3 %). Women with primary RPL were more likely to have a structural uterine anomaly compared to women with secondary RPL. Congenital anomalies were more prevalent in the primary RPL group (9 % vs. 4.6 %) with septate uterus being significantly more common in the primary RPL group compared to the secondary RPL group (6.5 % vs. 3.2 %). Interestingly, no significant difference in the prevalence of acquired anomalies was found between the primary and secondary RPL groups. The prevalence of uterine anomalies among the 169 women was as follows: septate uterus had the highest occurrence rate (4.9 %), followed by bicornuate uterus with 0.8 %, unicornuate uterus 0.7 %, T-shaped uterus 0.3 %, and didelphic uterus 0.2 %. In summary, this important study

suggests that uterine anomalies are more prevalent in cases of primary RPL compared to secondary RPL. Furthermore, not only is septate uterus the most common congenital uterine anomaly, it is also the most common uterine anomaly associated with primary RPL.

Although the incidence of the various subtypes of uterine anomalies varies across the studies, the septate uterus is consistently reported as the most common uterine anomaly encountered, while Mayer-Rokitansky-Küster-Hauser syndrome (MRKH), also known as Müllerian Agenesis, seems the rarest [15].

Familial cohorts of these disorders are uncommonly reported and the inheritance of congenital uterine anomalies remains unclear [16]. Among the genetic conditions characterized by Müllerian malformations, the hand-foot-genital syndrome presenting with bilateral great toe, thumb hypoplasia, and various grades of incomplete fusion of the Müllerian duct must be acknowledged. Additionally, 7.7 % of women with congenital uterine anomalies were found to have abnormal karyotypes. Müllerian anomalies are considered to be multifactorial and polygenic, and since many women with Müllerian anomalies do not present clinical signs, familial studies involving Müllerian defects are challenging [2].

Classification of Uterine Anomalies

Several classifications of uterine malformation were suggested over the years. In 1979, Buttram and Gibbons [6] were the first to propose a classification that was based on the failure of normal degree of development. In 1988, the American Fertility Society [17] introduced a modified version of this classification that remains the most widely accepted classification. More recently, in 2004 and 2005, two classification systems were proposed by different research groups—the embryological clinical classification system of genito-urinary malformations, by Acién et al. [18]; and the vagina, cervix, uterus, adnexae, and associated malformations system based on the tumor, nodes, metastases (TNM) system in oncology, by Oppelt et al. [19]. Both systems had limitations regarding effective categorization, clinical usefulness, and simplicity, leading some experts to strive for a comprehensive updated classification system. Finally, in 2013, a new classification by the ESHRE/ESGE (European Society of Human Reproduction and Embryology/ European Society of Gynaecological Endoscopy) was introduced [20] (Table 7.1). The new classification system is based on four major leading concepts:

1. The basis for the categorization of the anomalies is the anatomy.
2. The main classes are based on the type of uterine anomalies derived from the same embryological origin.
3. Subclasses are defined as anatomical variations of the main classes expressing different degrees of uterine deformity.
4. Cervical and vaginal anomalies are classified separately, from the less severe variants to the most severe in the order they appear in the classification system. In a recent study, Di Spiezio Sardo concluded that the comprehensiveness of the ESHRE/ESGE classification adds objective scientific validity [21]. This may, therefore, promote its further dissemination and acceptance, with a probable positive outcome in clinical care and research.

Uterine Anomalies Diagnostic Modalities and Techniques

Several diagnostic modalities including both invasive and noninvasive techniques are available for the diagnosis of anatomical anomalies of the uterus. In RPL patients, imaging studies play an important role during the initial work-up.

3D Ultrasonography

A noninvasive method, currently available in most clinics and considered to be the preferred diagnostic modality. It is a relatively quick imaging method that allows the evaluation of the external contours of the uterus (Fig. 7.1) with

MRI comparable results. Examples of TVS findings in various congenital uterine anomalies are presented in Figs. 7.2, 7.3, 7.4, and 7.5. The ability of 3D ultrasonography to visualize both the uterine cavity and the myometrium, as well its ability to differentiate subseptate from bicornuate uteri, makes it an accurate modality for the detection of uterine anomalies [22]. Szkodziak et al. [23] compared the performance of hysterosalpingography (HSG) and 3D transvaginal sonography (TVS) in diagnosing uterine anomalies. In 22 cases out of 155 the diagnosis of arcuate, septate, and bicornuate uterus was possible only after the use of 3D TVS. Importantly, in five patients the HSG exam could not be completed due to severe pain and lack of cooperation; a 3D TVS was performed and found all five cases to have normal uterus. The authors concluded that 3D TVS can accurately demonstrate uterine anomalies. Salim et al. [24] examined the reproducibility of the diagnosis of congenital uterine anomalies and the repeatability of the measurements of uterine cavity dimensions using 3D TVS. Two independent observers evaluated the data. Eighty-three 3D TVS volumes were examined and both investigators diagnosed 27 uteri as normal, 33 as arcuate, 19 as subseptate, and 3 as unicornuate; only a single uterine anomaly was classified by one as arcuate and by the other as subseptate (kappa 0.97). They concluded that 3D TVS is a reproducible method in diagnosing congenital uterine anomalies (Fig. 7.1).

Ghi et al. [25] studied the accuracy of 3D ultrasound in the diagnosis of congenital uterine anomalies among a group of women with RPL.

Ultrasound scan was performed using a machine equipped with a multi-frequency volume endovaginal probe. The insonation technique was standardized according to the following criteria: probe frequency set at 9 mHz, a midsagittal view of the uterus filling 75 % of the screen, three-dimensional (3D) box size including the uterus from fundus to the cervix, sweep angle of 90°, and sweep velocity adjusted to maximum quality. As shown in Fig. 7.1, the volume reconstruction technique was standardized according to the following criteria: the volume rendering box was as narrow as possible in the sagittal

Table 7.1 ESHRE 2013 Müllerian anomaly classification system

Class	Subclass	Main characteristics	Image
Class U0 = normal uterus		Straight curved line but with an internal indentation at the fundal midline not exceeding 50 % of the uterine wall thickness	
Class U1 = dysmorphic uterus		Uterine deformity defined by the proportion of the uterine anomaly landmarks Normal uterine outline but with an abnormal shape of the uterine cavity excluding septa	
	Class U1a/T-shaped uterus	Narrow uterine cavity due to thickened lateral walls with a correlation 2/3 uterine corpus and 1/3 cervix	
	Class U1b/uterus infantilis	Narrow uterine cavity without lateral wall thickening and an inverse correlation of 1/3 uterine body and 2/3 cervix	
	Class U1c or others	All minor deformities of the uterine cavity including those with an inner indentation at the fundal midline level of <50 % of the uterine wall thickness	
Class U2 = septate uterus		Normal fusion and abnormal absorption of the midline septum	
	Class U2a/partial septate uterus	Existence of a septum dividing partly the uterine cavity above the level of the internal cervical os	
	Class U2b/complete septate uterus	Existence of a septum fully dividing the uterine cavity up to the level of the internal cervical os. These patients could have or not cervical (e.g., bicervical septate uterus) and/or vaginal defects	
Class U3 = bicorporeal uterus		All cases of fusion defects—an abnormal fundal outline Characterized by the presence of an external indentation at the fundal midline exceeding 50 % of the uterine wall thickness. This indentation could divide partly or completely the uterine corpus including in some cases the cervix and/or vagina. It is also associated with an inner indentation at the midline level that divides the cavity as happens also in the case of septate uterus	
	Class U3a/partial bicorporeal uterus	External fundal indentation partly dividing the uterine corpus above the level of the cervix	
	Class U3b/complete bicorporeal uterus	External fundal indentation completely dividing the uterine corpus up to the level of the cervix	
	Class U3c/bicorporeal septate uterus	Presence of an absorption defect in addition to the main fusion defect. The width of the midline fundal indentation exceeds by 150 % the uterine wall thickness. Could have or not co-existent cervical (e.g., double cervix/formerly didelphys uterus) and/or vaginal defects (e.g., obstructing or not vaginal septum)	

(continued)

Table 7.1 (continued)

Class	Subclass	Main characteristics	Image
Class U4 = hemi-uterus		All cases of unilateral formed uterus, defined as the unilateral uterine development; the contralateral part could be either incompletely formed or absent. It is a formation defect	
	Class U4a/hemi-uterus with a rudimentary (functional) cavity	The presence of a communicating or non-communicating functional contralateral horn	
	Class U4b/hemi-uterus without rudimentary (functional) cavity	Characterized either by the presence of non-functional contralateral uterine horn or by aplasia of the contralateral part. The presence of a functional cavity in the contralateral part is the only clinically important factor for complications, such as hemato-cavity or ectopic pregnancy in the rudimentary horn or hemato-cavity	
Class U5 = aplastic uterus		All cases of uterine aplasia. Absence of any fully or unilaterally developed uterine cavity. In some cases there could be bi- or unilateral rudimentary horns with cavity, while in others there could be uterine remnants without cavity	
	Class U5a/aplastic uterus with rudimentary cavity	Presence of bi- or unilateral functional horn	
	Class U5b/aplastic uterus without rudimentary (functional) cavity	Presence of uterine remnants or by full uterine aplasia. The presence of a horn with cavity is clinically important and it is used as a criterion for subclassification because it is combined with health problems (cyclic pain and/or hemato-cavity) necessitating treatment	
Class U6		Incorporates unclassified cases. Cases of infrequent anomalies, subtle changes, or combined pathologies that could not be allocated correctly to one of the six groups	

plane and adjusted on the uterine corpus in the coronal plane, cut plane scrolled in anterior-posterior fashion with slice thickness set at 1 cm, transparency low (<50 %), and volume rendering by a mix of surface and maximum mode. The analysis of uterine morphology was performed in a standardized reformatted section with the uterus in the coronal view using the interstitial portions of fallopian tubes as reference points. Specific

ultrasound diagnosis of uterine anomalies was based on the classification system originally proposed by the American Fertility Society and subsequently modified according to 3D ultrasound landmarks [10] (Table 7.2).

Women with negative ultrasound findings subsequently underwent office hysteroscopy; a combined laparoscopic-hysteroscopic assessment was performed in cases of suspected Müllerian

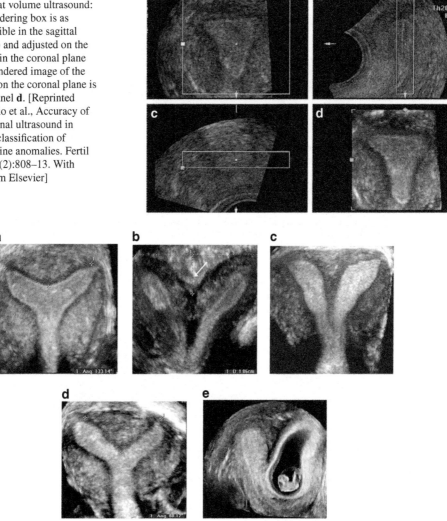

Fig. 7.1 Multiplanar imaging of a normal uterus at volume ultrasound: the volume rendering box is as narrow as possible in the sagittal plane (panel **b**) and adjusted on the uterine corpus in the coronal plane (panel **a**). A rendered image of the normal uterus on the coronal plane is displayed in panel **d**. [Reprinted from Ghi, Tullio et al., Accuracy of three-dimensional ultrasound in diagnosis and classification of congenital uterine anomalies. Fertil Steril. 2009;92(2):808–13. With permission from Elsevier]

Fig. 7.2 Examples of three-dimensional transvaginal sonography findings in congenital anomalies of the uterus. (**a**) Arcuate uterus, (**b**) Bicornuate uterus, (**c**) Septate uterus, (**d**) Subseptate uterus, (**e**) Pregnancy in septate uterus. (**a–d**) [Reprinted from Ghi, Tullio et al., Accuracy of three-dimensional ultrasound in diagnosis and classification of congenital uterine anomalies. Fertil Steril. 2009;92(2):808–13. With permission from Elsevier]. (**e**) [Courtesy of Tullio Ghi, MD, PhD]

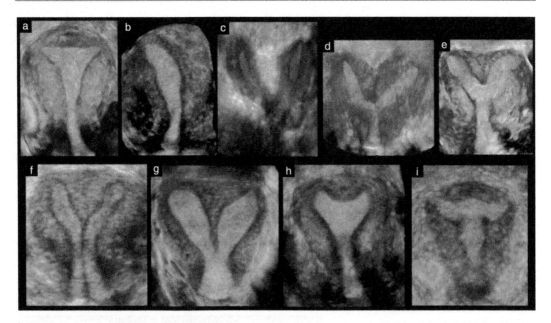

Fig. 7.3 Three-dimensional surface-rendered ultrasound images showing different types of uterine malformation using the American Fertility Society classification: (**a**) normal uterus; (**b**) unicornuate uterus; (**c**) didelphic uterus; (**d**) complete bicornuate uterus; (**e**) partial bicornuate uterus; (**f**) septate uterus with two cervices; (**g**) partial septate/subseptate uterus; (**h**) arcuate uterus; (**i**) uterus with DES drug-related malformations. [Reprinted from Bermejo, C., Martinez Ten, P., Cantarero, R., Diaz, D., Perez Pedregosa, J., Barron, E. Ruiz Lopez, L. Three-dimensional ultrasound in the diagnosis of Mullerian duct anomalies and concordance with magnetic resonance imaging. Ultrasound Obstet Gynecol, 2010;35(5), 593–601. With permission from John Wiley & Sons, Inc.]

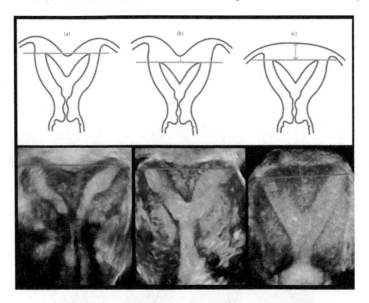

Fig. 7.4 To distinguish bicornuate uteri from septate uteri with three-dimensional ultrasound we used the formula proposed by Troiano and McCarthy: a line was traced joining both horns of the uterine cavity. If this line crossed the fundus or was ≤5 mm from it, the uterus was considered bicornuate (**a** and **b**); if it was >5 mm from the fundus it was considered septate, regardless of whether the fundus was dome-shaped (**c**), smooth or discretely notched. [Reprinted from Bermejo, C., Martinez Ten, P., Cantarero, R., Diaz, D., Perez Pedregosa, J., Barron, E. Ruiz Lopez, L. Three-dimensional ultrasound in the diagnosis of Mullerian duct anomalies and concordance with magnetic resonance imaging. Ultrasound Obstet Gynecol, 2010;35(5), 593–601. With permission from John Wiley & Sons, Inc.]

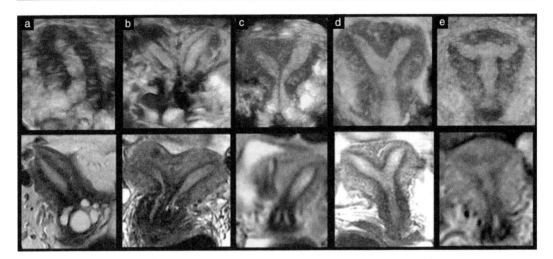

Fig. 7.5 Comparison of three-dimensional ultrasound and magnetic resonance imaging in cases of uterine malformation; the two imaging modalities are extremely similar. Images, according to the American Fertility Society classification, show: (**a**) unicornuate uterus (Type IId); (**b**) bicornuate bicollis uterus (Type IVb); (**c**) septate uterus with two cervices (Type Va); (**d**) partial septate uterus (Type Vb); (**e**) uterus with diethylstilbestrol (DES) drug-related malformations (Type VII). [Reprinted from Bermejo, C., Martinez Ten, P., Cantarero, R., Diaz, D., Perez Pedregosa, J., Barron, E. Ruiz Lopez, L. Three-dimensional ultrasound in the diagnosis of Mullerian duct anomalies and concordance with magnetic resonance imaging. Ultrasound Obstet Gynecol, 2010;35(5), 593–601. With permission from John Wiley & Sons, Inc.]

anomaly. A specific Müllerian malformation was sonographically diagnosed in 54 of the 284 women (19 %) included in the study group. All negative ultrasound findings were confirmed at office hysteroscopy. Among the women with abnormal ultrasound findings, the presence of a Müllerian anomaly was endoscopically confirmed in all. Concordance between ultrasound and endoscopy around the type of anomaly was verified in 52 of the 54 (96.3 %) cases, including all cases with a septate uterus and two out of three with bicornuate uterus. This important study concluded that volume TVS appears to be extremely accurate for the diagnosis and classification of congenital uterine anomalies and should conveniently become the first recommended step in the assessment of the uterine cavity in patients with a history of recurrent miscarriage. Three-dimensional ultrasound enables the clinician to comprehensively assess uterine morphology, thus alleviating the need for invasive tests.

Hysterosalpingography (HSG) is a radiographic procedure performed in order to mainly examine the patency of the Fallopian tubes and the morphology of the uterine cavity. It is usually indicated in the early stages of an infertility work-up [26]. The radio-opaque contrast medium fills the cavity, allowing the accurate identification of filling defects due to Müllerian malformations. However, this technique cannot accurately differentiate a septate uterus from a bicornuate uterus [22]. It is also unable to determine the myometrial thickness above the defect or the size of the defect itself. Therefore, the major limitation of this exam lies in its inability to evaluate the external uterine contour [5]. Another disadvantage is the exposure to ionizing radiation in typically young women.

Magnetic Resonance Imaging (MRI)

An expensive, powerful but noninvasive and accurate technique. It has displayed promising results in the diagnosis and categorization of uterine malformations with an accuracy of up to 100 % in the evaluation of Müllerian anomalies [5]. In a study by Bermejo et al. [27], a high degree of concordance between 3D TVS and MRI was reported for the diagnosis of uterine malformations. The structural relationship between the uterine cavity and fundus was equally well visualized with both techniques. Currently MRI is indicated as a complementary

Table 7.2 Classification of congenital uterine anomalies according to volume transvaginal ultrasound

Uterine morphology	Fundal contour	External contour
Normal	Straight or convex	Uniformly convex or with indentation <10 mm
Arcuate	Concave fundal indentation with central point of indentation at obtuse angle	Uniformly convex or with indentation <10 mm
Subseptate	Presence of septum, which does not extend to cervix, with central point of septum at an acute angle	Uniformly convex or with indentation <10 mm
Septate	Presence of uterine septum that completely divides cavity from fundus to cervix	Uniformly convex or with indentation <10 mm
Bicornuate	Two well-formed uterine cornua	Fundal indentation >10 mm dividing the two cornua
Unicornuate with or without rudimentary horn	Single well-formed uterine cavity with a single interstitial portion of Fallopian tube and concave fundal contour	–

Reprinted from Ghi, Tullio et al., Accuracy of three-dimensional ultrasound in diagnosis and classification of congenital uterine anomalies. Fertil Steril. 2009;92(2):808–13. With permission from Elsevier

imaging modality to 3D ultrasound only in cases of complex abnormalities that involve in addition to the uterus both the cervix and the vagina [22].

Diagnostic Hysteroscopy

Hysteroscopy has become the gold standard for the evaluation of the uterine cavity and is a reliable and safe method in an office setting [22]. This tech-nique allows visualization of the inner part of the cervix and uterus, offering direct vision of the uter-ine cavity and its internal structures and allows guided biopsies to be obtained if necessary [28]. However, it is also an invasive method that may cause patient discomfort. Hysteroscopy alone is unable to differentiate a septate uterus from a bicor-nuate uterus [22]. In a retrospective analysis per-formed by Valli et al. [29], 344 women with RPL and 922 controls were referred for diagnostic hys-teroscopy. There was a significantly higher rate of major and minor uterine anomalies (septate and unicornuate uterus) in the RPL group compared to the control group (32 % vs. 6 %, $p < 0.001$). There was no significant difference in uterine adhesions between the two groups. Another retrospective analysis by Weiss et al. [30] compared the preva-lence of uterine anomalies between women referred to hysteroscopy for RPL after two or more consec-utive miscarriages. There was no significant differ-ence in uterine abnormality rates between the 67 patients with 2 RPLs and the 98 patients with 3 or more RPLs (32 % vs. 28 %, respectively).

Diagnostic Laparoscopy

This modality gives the surgeon the ability to assess the outer surface of the uterus as well as other pelvic structures. Nonetheless, it is more expensive and invasive [5] compared to the previ-ously reviewed modalities. Currently, diagnostic laparoscopy is generally reserved for women in whom interventional therapy is likely to be under-taken and rarely used for uterine anatomic evalua-tion purposes [22]. As shown by some, the high accuracy of 3D TVS or MRI allows a noninvasive diagnosis and characterization of uterine anomalies without the need for diagnostic laparoscopy [28].

Sonohysterography

A transvaginal sonogram used in combination with a saline contrast medium injected into the uterine cavity. This is a simple and quick proce-dure with minimal discomfort to the patient and is now being increasingly used for a routine evaluation of the uterine cavity [22]. Goldberg et al. [26] performed transvaginal sonohysterography on 40 consecutive patients with infertility or RPL previously diagnosed with uterine abnormalities by HSG. The study found that sonohysterography was more accurate than HSG and provided more information about uterine abnormalities. It also provides additional information on the relative proportion of the intracavitary and intramyometrial components of submucous myomas, as well as extracavitary myomas and adhesions [26].

RPL in Different Types of Müllerian Duct Anomalies and Treatment Options

Uterine anomalies have been associated with adverse pregnancy outcomes including spontaneous abortion, recurrent miscarriage, malpresentation, placental abruption, IUGR, prematurity, operative delivery, retained placenta, and fetal mortality [2, 31]. However, it is difficult to assess reproductive outcome precisely, because the majority of studies do not have a control group. In the following section we discuss the treatment of the uterine malformations among women with RPL.

Septated Uterus (ESHRE Classification Class U2)

Septated uterus is the most common Müllerian anomaly, accounting for about 55 % of all Müllerian duct anomalies [5]. It is also the most common major uterine anomaly in women with RPL [32], with a reported prevalence of 15–26 %.

The etiology of RPL in a septated uterus was originally attributed to the fibrous and vascular nature of the septum, despite the lack of histologic data [33, 34]. However, thanks to the use of MRI and histology it is now clear that the septum is composed primarily of smooth muscle and not fibrous tissue [5].

The increased risk of pregnancy loss is most probably related to the decreased connective tissue of the septum that may result in poor decidualization and reduced implantation rate, while increased muscular tissue may result in increased contractility of the tissue. In addition to the inherent deficiencies of the composition of the septum, the overlying endometrium has been shown to be defective [35]. Studies employing electron microscopy reported that the septal endometrium was found to be irregular in morphology, with a decreased sensitivity to preovulatory hormonal changes [36]. Morphologic narrowing of the cavity by the septum, causing a reduction in endometrial capacity, is also believed to play a role in the pathophysiology of adverse reproductive outcome [37].

Finally, inadequate vascularization within the septum and altered relationships between the endometrial, myometrial vessels and myometrial nerves are also considered to be associated with RPL [33, 34]. If this is true, the likelihood of miscarriage caused by septal implantation should increase with the severity of the disruption of uterine morphology [24].

Adverse pregnancy outcome seems to be increased in women with septate uterus as shown in several studies with fetal survival between 6 and 28 % [2]. Ghi et al. [38] reported on pregnancy outcome in women with incidental diagnosis of septate uterus at first trimester scan. They found that in 24 patients diagnosed at a median gestational age of 8.2 weeks, the cumulative pregnancy progression rate was 33.35 % due to the occurrence of early (≤13 weeks) or late (14–22 weeks) miscarriages in 13 and 2 cases, respectively.

Septate uterus is amenable to surgical correction. Hysteroscopic septectomy is the treatment of choice [22]. This procedure is considered to be simple and safe and is reported to increase the live birth rate in patients affected by RPL. It is important to emphasize that although hysteroscopic septectomy is easy and safe to perform, it is critical to demonstrate the external uterine contour by 3D ultrasound before the procedure to rule out a bicornuate uterus for which a different therapeutic approach should be considered (see below).

In addition to some reports on the improvement of infertility and fecundity (38.6 % vs. 20.4 %) after septectomy treatment [39], other studies suggested that the treatment improved birth rate in RPL patients [1, 39].

Fedele et al. [40] reported good results after septectomy in 102 patients with RPL and infertility who had a complete or partial septum. The cumulative pregnancy rate and birth rate after 36 months were 89 and 75 %, respectively, in the septated uterus and 80 and 67 % in the subseptated group.

Homer et al. [32] published a meta-analysis on pregnancy outcomes before and after septectomy and showed a marked improvement after surgery. However, this meta-analysis includes nonrandomized observational methodology. Grimbizis et al. [1] published a nonrandomized study that included patients with previous delivery and live birth rate of only 5 %. After septectomy, the subsequent term delivery rate was around 75 % and the live birth rate was around 85 %.

On the other hand, some authors claim that surgical therapy for septate uterus is not necessary. For example, Homer et al. [32] in their review state that septated uterus is not an indication for surgical intervention. Heinonen [41] reported on 67 patients with a uterine septum and a longitudinal vaginal septum in whom pregnancy outcome was favorable without surgical intervention.

In our opinion, resection of the septum is highly recommended for those with infertility or with RPL to optimize the uterine cavity and minimize adverse obstetrical outcomes once pregnancy is achieved [2].

The procedure includes several methods for removal of the uterine septum using a hysteroscope or resectoscope, including mechanical scissors, electrosurgery with knife electrode or vaporization by bipolar electrodes, yag laser, and mechanical morcellators. The most acceptable procedure is the use of a hysteroscope with mechanical scissors. The septum should be cut from its middle portion where its vasculature is usually most scarce. The preferable timing for the procedure is during the follicular period of the menstrual cycle and should be performed by an experienced surgeon. Complications of the procedure include bleeding, fluid overload, uterine perforation, formation of intrauterine adhesions, and uterine rupture in a subsequent pregnancy. Future deliveries following the procedure do not mandate a cesarean section [42].

It remains uncertain if prophylactic removal of incidentally discovered uterine septa detected prior to childbearing would be indicated in order to improve fertility and pregnancy outcomes [43].

In cases with a cervical septum, the resection of the septum is controversial in regard to the risk of cervical os incompetence once pregnancy has been achieved. At present, a cervical septum should be resected when surgically feasible since inadequate evidence exists for the risk of cervical os incompetence [2].

Unicornis Uterus (ESHRE Classification Class U4, Hemi-uterus)

Unicornis uterus is associated with the worst reproductive outcome, with 30 % of pregnancies resulting in miscarriage [22]. Furthermore this malformation is also associated with intrauterine growth restriction (IUGR), malpresentation, preterm labor, cesarean section, and cervical incompetence [44]. In one recent review of 175 patients and 468 pregnancies, 24.3 % ended in first trimester miscarriage and 9.75 % in second trimester miscarriage with an overall live birth rate of 49.9 % [45].

The presence of a rudimentary uterine horn containing functional endometrium is associated with endometriosis, hematometra, hematosalpinx, pelvic pain, and acute abdomen secondary to ruptured rudimentary horn containing ectopic pregnancy. In those cases, the data support laparoscopic removal in order to prevent these complications [46, 47].

Uterus Arcuatus (ESHRE Classification Class U1c)

Classification of arcuate uterus has been challenging, because it remains unclear whether this variant should be classified as a true anomaly or as an anatomic variant of normal [5]. By definition, this uterus has an intrauterine indentation less than 1 cm [22]. It has an estimated prevalence of 20 % in the general population [1]. Data regarding the reproductive outcomes of patients with an arcuate uterus are extremely limited and widely disparate. In small studies, both poor and good obstetric outcomes have been reported, although an arcuate configuration is generally thought to be compatible with normal term gestation, with a quoted live birth rate of 85 %. In a study of 38 fertile women with live newborns and a history of RPL, uterine malformations were observed in 7.5 % of the cases. The frequency of arcuate uterus was higher than the 4.6 % found in 131 fertile women with live newborns and no history of RPL [48]. However, after excluding all possible extrauterine factors for infertility, surgical hysteroscopy may be considered in selected patients with RPL, particularly those with a prominent or broad configuration of the fundal myometrium. This type of uterine malformation must be considered as part of the differential diagnosis of a partial septate uterus. Some experts consider arcuate uterus as a subtype of a partial septate uterus, even though the natural history and clinical manifestations of arcuate uterus malformation are relatively benign [1]. Even though the pathophysiology of pregnancy loss in women with this malformation remains uncertain, one can view arcuate uterus as a minor alteration of the uterine cavity shape but with no major external change of the contour. This is supported by a long-term study that found a term delivery rate of almost 80 % with a live birth rate of 82.7 % and no adverse impact on reproduction [49].

Uterine Didelphi (ESHRE Classification Class U3c)

This type of uterus, also referred to as a double uterus, may result from complete failure of the fusion of the two Müllerian ducts. This results in a separate and narrower uterus developing from each duct. Each uterus may have its own cervix or both uteri may share a single one. This type of uterus is associated with a double vagina (each referred to as "hemivagina") in 67 % of cases, separated by a thin wall [22]. However, this anomaly is relatively rare. Nahum [12] found uterine didelphi in 11 % of all congenital uterine anomalies. Heinonen [50] studied the clinical implications and long-term follow-up of 49 cases

of didelphic uterus. Complications such as an obstructed hemivagina and renal agenesis were found, as well as ovarian neoplasm [9 %]. As for pregnancies, 94 % of the women had at least one pregnancy and the miscarriage rate was 21 %. Ectopic pregnancy occurred in 2 % of the cases, prenatal mortality in 5.3 %, and prematurity in 24 %. The study concluded that women with this type of uterus do not have a notably impaired fertility. Grimbizis et al. [1] instead reported a term delivery rate of approximately 45 % in women with didelphic uteri.

While the nonobstructive type is usually asymptomatic, the didelphic uterus with a hemivaginal obstruction could become symptomatic at the time of menarche and present with dysmenorrhea. Other complications that may be associated are endometriosis and pelvic adhesions, possibly secondary to retrograde menstrual flow in patients with an obstruction [5].

Bicornuate Uterus (ESHRE Classification Classes U3a and U3b)

A bicornuate uterus results from a partial fusion of the Müllerian ducts. Bicornuate uteri may be classified into two subtypes, depending on the level of the caudal extension of the fundal indentation: bicornuate unicollis if at the level of the internal cervical os, bicornuate bicollis if at the level of the external cervical os. The horns of this uterus are not fully developed and are thus smaller than those of a didelphic uterus [22]. In a series of 67 pregnancies among 261 patients with untreated bicornuate uterus, Grimbizis et al. [1] found poor pregnancy outcomes, with a mean miscarriage rate of 36 %. The mean preterm delivery rate was 23 % and the mean live birth rate was 55.2 %. They concluded that the pregnancy outcome was significantly poorer ($p < 0.001$) than that of women with a normal uterus. Usually this type of malformation is not a candidate for surgical correction, but a Strassman metroplasty with a wedge resection of the medial aspect of each uterine horn followed by the unification of the two cavities may be considered in women with RPL [2].

Diethylstilbestrol Exposure

Diethylstilbestrol (DES) is an orally active synthetic estrogen that was used between 1948 and 1971 in the prevention of pregnancy loss in women suffering from RPL. When administered to pregnant women, it has been shown to increase the risk of malformations and tumors in the genitalia of the offspring. The use of this medication in pregnancy was discontinued due to its teratologic effects. When hysterosalpingography was performed on 267 DES-exposed women, 69 % of them presented a congenital malformation of the uterus. The most common abnormality was a T-shaped uterine cavity (ESHRE classification class U1a). How DES affects the uterine development is not clear. A)relationship between in utero DES exposure and the occurrence of cervical incompetence was also noted.

Treatment of Uterine Malformations

Raga et al. [49], in their review, summarized the current management of the different types of uterine malformations. For septate and arcuate uterus, hysteroscopic metroplasty is the treatment of choice. The other anomalies, which are less frequently encountered, may require more complicated abdominal or combined procedures or may even not have a surgical solution. The strategy of management must be based either on the obstetric history of the patient or on the prognosis of the malformation itself. Most clinicians do not recommend the Strassman procedure, which was associated with a high percentage of complications. The main concept in the treatment of uterine malformations is close monitoring and follow-up in high-risk pregnancy clinic, bed rest, and progesterone treatment for the prevention of preterm delivery.

Cerclage is indicated in cases with cervical os incompetence diagnosed by medical history or shortened cervical length by ultrasound. Cervical os incompetence is difficult to diagnose and is not a common cause of RPL even in patients with profound structural uterine abnormality. However, cerclage has recently been offered as a treatment for women with RPL and a uterine anomaly other than a septate uterus. Seidman et al. [51] compared the survival rate of fetuses in 86 women with congenital uterine anomalies and 106 women with normal anatomy. The incidence of cervical os incompetence proven by HSG was 23 % in the two groups. Sixty-seven out of 86 and 29 out of 106 were managed with cervical cerclage. The obstetric outcome was stratified by cervical incompetence and obstetric history. The viable live birth rate was significantly higher in the malformed group with cerclage (88 %) compared with the malformed group without cerclage (47 %). No statistically significant differences in live birth rate were found in the normal uterus with cerclage even when only those women with a history of RPL were considered. The indications for cerclage are still controversial. The CIPRACT study found that therapeutic cerclage with bed rest reduced neonatal morbidity and preterm delivery rates in women with risk factors (including DES exposure and uterine anomaly) and/or cervical os incompetence and cervical length of <27 mm before 27 weeks gestational age [52].

Yassaee and Mostafaee [53] studied 40 patients with uterine anomalies, 26 were treated with cerclage and 14 without cerclage. In patients with bicornuate uterus and cervical cerclage, term delivery rate was 76.2 % compared to 27.35 % in the group without cerclage ($p < 0.05$). Among patients with uterus arcuatus, preterm delivery rate was not statistically different between those with or without cerclage.

Cervical os incompetence is still considered an infrequent cause of pregnancy loss in patients with major structural anomalies of the uterus. We recommend to consider prophylactic cerclage for those patients with uterine anomalies such as bicornuate uterus and unicornis uterus with a history of RPL or preterm delivery.

Acquired Uterine Structural Malformations

Myomas

A uterine myoma, also known as fibroid, is a benign solid tumor made of fibrous tissue of the uterus. The myomas' size and number may vary;

they are usually slow-growing and asymptomatic. Myomas are associated with abnormal uterine bleeding including heavy menstrual bleeding, infertility, RPL, and complaints related to the effect of an enlarged uterus on the adjacent structures in the pelvis [54]. RPL is usually the result of lesions that distort the endometrial cavity, being close to the endometrium. The presence of submucous myomas may deform the uterine cavity; the overlying endometrium is usually thin and therefore inadequate for normal implantation. Myomas are common in woman of reproductive age with a prevalence as high as 70–80 % in woman aged 50 years [55]. The location of the myomas may affect the reproductive outcome and function in women, and the removal of the myoma prior to conception may have a positive influence on pregnancy rate [56]. In a meta-analysis by Pritts et al. [56] women with submucous myomas had significantly higher spontaneous miscarriage rates (RR 1.68, 95 % CI 1.37–2.05, $p = 0.022$). The mechanism by which submucous myomas affect pregnancy outcomes is unknown. Histologic testing did show glandular atrophy of the endometrium overlying the myomas and opposite to the myomas. The atrophy has been suggested to impair the implantation and nourishment of the developing embryo [57, 58]. Other suggested mechanisms are impaired transport of gametes, altered uterine contractility, and other negative effects such as enlarging or deforming the endometrial cavity and obstructing tubal ostia [59, 60]. Myomas may also cause implantation failure by physically altering the uterine shape, preventing discharge of intrauterine blood or clots, and by altering the normal endometrial development [60]. Due to the increasing use of US, there has been a rise in the diagnosis of uterine leiomyomas in women with unexplained infertility [61].

Regarding the recommended treatment, another interesting finding of the study performed by Casini et al. [62] was that there is an important role for the removal of fibroids before conception and pregnancy. However, it is still undetermined who are the patients that may benefit the most from the invasive surgical approach. In a study by Pritts et al. [56] the relative risk of spontaneous

pregnancy following submucous myomectomy was 0.77, compared to the control subjects who did not undergo myomectomy. This confirms the important role of uterine fibroids in infertility as well as the importance of fibroid removal before conception, to improve both the chances of fertilization and pregnancy maintenance. Patients who had submucous fibroids larger than 2 cm distorting their uterine cavities had a higher pregnancy rate following hysteroscopic resection [22]. It seems that subserosal myomas have little, if any, effect on reproductive outcome, especially if they are up to 5–7 cm in diameter. Intramural myomas that do not invade the endometrium may be considered as well to be relatively harmless to reproduction, as long as they are smaller than 4–5 cm in diameter [60]. Submucosal as well as some intramural myomas that compress the uterine cavity significantly reduce pregnancy rates, and surgical removal should be considered before assisted reproductive techniques are used [63].

The association between submucous myomectomy and pregnancy loss is less evident as there is insufficient data regarding this association. Moreover, an inherited bias exists due to the increased risk of first trimester loss. The available evidence is suggestive of benefit. Clearly more data are required, but this evidence suggests that, at least in selected patients, submucous myomectomy may reduce the risk of spontaneous miscarriage [61]. Therefore, one can conclude that the two parameters influencing better outcomes of a future pregnancy are the location and size of the myomas. Hysteroscopic myomectomy is the gold standard for the treatment of submucous myomas. For other myomas, abdominal or laparoscopic myomectomy by a trained surgeon is the best alternative [60]. It is now recommended that most of the intramural and subserosal uterine myomas should be treated with laparoscopic myomectomy in women who desire to preserve their uterus. The post-laparoscopy pregnancy rates are estimated to be 50–60 % [64]. Another less invasive surgical approach is laparoscopic-assisted myomectomy (LAM), which became a safe and efficient alternative to both laparoscopic myomectomy and myomectomy by laparotomy for patients with numerous large or deep intramural myomas [22].

Uterine Polyps

Polyps are growths, endometrial masses attached to the inner lining of the uterus. They can be differentiated from fibroids by the fact that while fibroids are mainly composed of muscle tissue, polyps are made of endometrial tissue. Polyps consist of benign hyperplastic endometrial growth. It is suggested that polyps with intracavity extensions may act like foreign bodies within the uterine cavity [22]. Another suggestion is that they play a role in inducing chronic inflammatory changes in the endometrium, causing the area to be less receptive for pregnancy implantation and support. However, the association between endometrial polyps and RPL is yet to be proven. Several more hypotheses have arisen more recently. A case–control study by Rackow et al. [65] evaluated the effect of hysteroscopically identified endometrial polyps on the endometrium using known molecular markers of endometrial receptivity. Marked decrease in the mRNA levels of the HOXA10 and HOXA11 was observed in a uterus with endometrial polyps. These molecular markers are thought to impair implantation. These findings offer a possible molecular mechanism to support the clinical findings of lower pregnancy rates in women with endometrial polyps.

Even though the association between endometrial polyps and pregnancy loss is yet to be proven, polyps are more common in patients with recurrent spontaneous miscarriage [29]. The current treatment approach to infertile women, particularly those undergoing in vitro fertilization and embryo transfer, is to perform hysteroscopic polypectomy when intrauterine filling defects are diagnosed [66]. Perez-Medina et al. [67] attempted to determine whether hysteroscopic polypectomy before intrauterine insemination (IUI) resulted in better pregnancy outcomes. Two hundred and fifteen infertile women scheduled to undergo IUI participated in the study and it was reported that, compared to women who did not undergo the procedure, hysteroscopic polypectomy improved the likelihood of conception, with a relative risk of 2.1 (95 % CI 1.5–2.9).

It seems that hysteroscopic polypectomy enhances fertility [68]. Therefore, one should consider performing polypectomy in women with uterine polyps and RPL, especially when no other etiology has been found.

Intrauterine Adhesions

Intrauterine adhesions, also known as Asherman syndrome, occur most often due to exaggerated postpartum or postmiscarriage dilatation and curettage. Other causes include genital tuberculosis, previous uterine surgery [69], and endometritis [22]. The adhesions may result in infertility and/or RPL [70]; although this is not a common cause it may lead to secondary infertility in these patients. These intrauterine scars can interfere with the normal implantation process, therefore being responsible for pregnancy loss. The type and extent of intrauterine adhesions vary. They are expected to be found more often in women with RPL since vacuum aspiration, which is one of the leading causes of uterine adhesions, is a common procedure in cases of early pregnancy loss. In a study performed by Ventolini et al. [71], among 23 patients with an otherwise unexplained history of three or more first or second trimester miscarriages and no live births, hysteroscopy showed that 5 (21.8 %) of the women had intrauterine adhesions. Classifying the adhesions can be done according to the amount of the involved uterine cavity. Minimal adhesions are defined by the involvement of less than one-fourth of the uterine cavity with thin and filmy adhesions. If affecting one-fourth of the uterine cavity with no agglutination of the walls, ostial areas and partial occlusion of the upper fundus, it is defined as moderate adhesions. Severe adhesions involve more than three-fourths of the uterine cavity, with agglutination of the walls or thick bands and occlusion of the ostial areas and upper uterine cavity [69].

It is agreed that adhesions should be hysteroscopically resected. In a retrospective case report series published by Pabuccu et al. [69], 40 women with RPL or infertility underwent hysteroscopic adhesiolysis. The majority of women included in the study had a history of vigorous curettage and two had a history of genital tuberculosis. Women with previous uterine surgery were excluded from the study. All women with RPL conceived after surgery and 71 % of pregnancies resulted in term or viable preterm infants. Out of eight patients with mild adhesions, seven conceived after surgery, as did three out of four patients with moderate adhesions.

Hysteroscopic synechiae resection seems to be indicated when the adhesions are classified as moderate to severe or the access to the tubal ostia is blocked [69]. When no other cause for RPL is found, and mild adhesions are present, one should consider performing adhesiolysis as well. It should be noted that uterine adhesions caused by genital tuberculosis are usually cohesive and have a tendency to recur, therefore conferring a poor prognosis. The reproductive outcome correlates with the severity of the initially diagnosed adhesions.

Summary

Congenital Müllerian and acquired uterine structural abnormalities are important in the pathophysiology, diagnosis, and therapy of RPL. Therefore, an anatomical work-up is recommended for RPL patients according to ASRM guidelines. The initial diagnostic modality is 2D followed by 3D transvaginal ultrasonography. These modalities will provide the diagnosis in more than 95 % of the cases. The findings should be classified using the newer and simplified ESHRE classification. Following diagnosis, appropriate interventions should be considered when indicated, like septectomy for a septate uterus or adhesiolysis for intrauterine adhesions. Other (non-septate) Müllerian anomalies require close monitoring and a few of them may benefit if cervical cerclage is performed. For acquired malformation, adhesiolysis as well as synechiae and resection of uterine myomas are recommended in the setting of RPL.

References

1. Grimbizis GF, Camus M, Tarlatzis BC, Bontis JN, Devroey P. Clinical implications of uterine malformations and hysteroscopic treatment results. Hum Reprod Update. 2001;7(2):161–74.
2. Reichman DE, Laufer MR. Congenital uterine anomalies affecting reproduction Best practice and research clinical obstetrics and gynaecology, volume 24. Amsterdam: Elsevier; 2010. p. 193–208.
3. Muller P, Musset R, Netter A, Solal R, Vinourd JC, Gillet JY. State of the upper urinary tract in patients with uterine malformations. Study of 133 cases. Presse Med. 1967;75(26):1331–6.
4. Lee DM, Osathanondh R, Yeh J. Localization of Bcl-2 in the human fetal müllerian tract. Fertil Steril. 1998;70(1):135–40.
5. Troiano RN, McCarthy SM. Mullerian duct anomalies: imaging and clinical issues. Radiology. 2004;233:19–34.
6. Buttram VC, Gibbons WE. Müllerian anomalies: a proposed classification. (An analysis of 144 cases). Fertil Steril. 1979;32(1):40–6.
7. Fedele L, Bianchi S, Agnoli B, Tozzi L, Vignali M. Urinary tract anomalies associated with unicornuate uterus. J Urol. 1996;155(3):847–8.
8. Narang HK, Warke HS, Mayadeo NM. Mullerian anomaly with ovary at deep inguinal ring: a rare case finding. J Obstet Gynaecol. 2013;33(3):317–8.
9. Ombelet W, Verswijvel G, de Jonge E. Ectopic ovary and unicornuate uterus. N Engl J Med. 2003;348(7):667–8.
10. Dabirashrafi H, Mohammad K, Moghadami-Tabrizi N. Ovarian malposition in women with uterine anomalies. Obstet Gynecol. 1994;83(2):293–4.
11. Simón C, Martinez L, Pardo F, Tortajada M, Pellicer A. Müllerian defects in women with normal reproductive outcome. Fertil Steril. 1991;56(6):1192–3.
12. Nahum GG. Uterine anomalies. How common are they, and what is their distribution among subtypes? J Reprod Med. 1998;43(10):877–87.
13. Sugiura-Ogasawara M, Ozaki Y, Kitaori T, Kumagai K, Suzuki S. Midline uterine defect size is correlated with miscarriage of euploid embryos in recurrent cases. Fertil Steril. 2010;93(6):1983–8.
14. Jaslow CR, Kutteh WH. Effect of prior birth and miscarriage frequency on the prevalence of acquired and congenital uterine anomalies in women with recurrent miscarriage: a cross-sectional study. Fertil Steril. 2013;99(7):1916–22. e1.
15. Shulman LP. Müllerian anomalies. Clin Obstet Gynecol. 2008;51(2):214–22.
16. Battin J, Lacombe D, Leng JJ. Familial occurrence of hereditary renal adysplasia with müllerian anomalies. Clin Genet. 1993;43(1):23–4.
17. The American Fertility Society classifications of adnexal adhesions, distal tubal occlusion, tubal occlusion secondary to tubal ligation, tubal pregnancies, mullerian anomalies and intrauterine adhesions. Fertil Steril. 1988;49(6):944–55.

18. Acién P, Acién M, Sánchez-Ferrer M. Complex malformations of the female genital tract. New types and revision of classification. Hum Reprod. 2004;19(10):2377–84.

19. Oppelt P, Renner SP, Brucker S, Strissel PL, Strick R, Oppelt PG, et al. The VCUAM (Vagina Cervix Uterus Adnex-associated Malformation) classification: a new classification for genital malformations. Fertil Steril. 2005;84(5):1493–7.

20. Grimbizis GF, Gordts S, Di Spiezio Sardo A, Brucker S, De Angelis C, Gergolet M, et al. The ESHRE-ESGE consensus on the classification of female genital tract congenital anomalies. Gynecol Surg. 2013;10(3):199–212.

21. Di Spiezio Sardo A, Campo R, Gordts S, Spinelli M, Cosimato C, Tanos V, et al. The comprehensiveness of the ESHRE/ESGE classification of female genital tract congenital anomalies: a systematic review of cases not classified by the AFS system. Hum Reprod. 2015;30(5):1046–58.

22. Carp HJ. Recurrent pregnancy loss- causes, controversies and treatment. 1st ed. London: Informa UK Ltd, Taylor & Francis e-Library; 2008. 305.

23. Szkodziak P, Wozniak S, Czuczwar P, Paszkowski T, Milart P, Wozniakowska E, et al. Usefulness of three dimensional transvaginal ultrasonography and hysterosalpingography in diagnosing uterine anomalies. Ginekol Pol. 2014;85(5):354–9.

24. Salim R, Regan L, Woelfer B, Backos M, Jurkovic D. A comparative study of the morphology of congenital uterine anomalies in women with and without a history of recurrent first trimester miscarriage. Hum Reprod. 2003;18(1):162–6.

25. Ghi T, Casadio P, Kuleva M, Perrone AM, Savelli L, Giunchi S, et al. Accuracy of three-dimensional ultrasound in diagnosis and classification of congenital uterine anomalies. Fertil Steril. 2009;92(2):808–13.

26. Goldberg JM, Falcone T, Attaran M. Sonohysterographic evaluation of uterine abnormalities noted on hysterosalpingography. Hum Reprod. 1997;12(10):2151–3.

27. Bermejo C, Ten Martinez P, Cantarero R, Diaz D, Perez Pedregosa J, Barron E, et al. Three-dimensional ultrasound in the diagnosis of Mullerian duct anomalies and concordance with magnetic resonance imaging. Ultrasound Obstet Gynecol. 2010;35(5):593–601.

28. Dueholm M, Lundorf E, Hansen ES, Ledertoug S, Olesen F. Evaluation of the uterine cavity with magnetic resonance imaging, transvaginal sonography, hysterosonographic examination, and diagnostic hysteroscopy. Fertil Steril. 2001;76:350–7.

29. Valli E, Zupi E, Marconi D, Vaquero E, Giovannini P, Lazzarin N, et al. Hysteroscopic findings in 344 women with recurrent spontaneous abortion. J Am Assoc Gynecol Laparosc. 2001;8(3):398–401.

30. Weiss A, Shalev E, Romano S. Hysteroscopy may be justified after two miscarriages. Hum Reprod. 2005;20:2628–31.

31. Hua M, Odibo AO, Longman RE, Macones GA, Roehl KA, Cahill AG. Congenital uterine anomalies and adverse pregnancy outcomes. Am J Obstet Gynecol. 2011;205(6):558.e1–5.

32. Homer HA, Li TC, Cooke ID. The septate uterus: a review of management and reproductive outcome. Fertil Steril. 2000;73(1):1–14.

33. Fayez JA. Comparison between abdominal and hysteroscopic metroplasty. Obstet Gynecol. 1986;68(3):399–403.

34. Fedele L, Bianchi S. Hysteroscopic metroplasty for septate uterus. Obstet Gynecol Clin North Am. 1995;22(3):473–89.

35. Candiani GB, Fedele L, Zamberletti D, De Virgiliis D, Carinelli S. Endometrial patterns in malformed uteri. Acta Eur Fertil. 1983;14(5):311–8.

36. Fedele L, Bianchi S, Marchini M, Franchi D, Tozzi L, Dorta M. Ultrastructural aspects of endometrium in infertile women with septate uterus. Fertil Steril. 1996;65(4):750–2.

37. Patton PE, Novy MJ. Reproductive potential of the anomalous uterus. In: Seminars in reproductive endocrinology, Vol. 6, No. 2, 1988. p. 217–33. http://ohsu.pure.elsevier.com/en/publications/reproductive-potential-of-the-anomalous-uterus(55ded2b8-5dba-45ef-99b9-a3bed82fc108).html.

38. Ghi T, De Musso F, Maroni E, Youssef A, Savelli L, Farina A, et al. The pregnancy outcome in women with incidental diagnosis of septate uterus at first trimester scan. Hum Reprod. 2012;27(9):2671–5.

39. Mollo A, De Franciscis P, Colacurci N, Cobellis L, Perino A, Venezia R, et al. Hysteroscopic resection of the septum improves the pregnancy rate of women with unexplained infertility: a prospective controlled trial. Fertil Steril. 2009;91:2628–31.

40. Fedele L, Arcaini L, Parazzini F, Vercellini P, Di Nola G. Reproductive prognosis after hysteroscopic metroplasty in 102 women: life-table analysis. Fertil Steril. 1993;59(4):768–72.

41. Heinonen PK. Complete septate uterus with longitudinal vaginal septum. Fertil Steril. 2006;85(3):700–5.

42. Valle RF, Ekpo GE. Hysteroscopic metroplasty for the septate uterus: review and meta-analysis. J Minim Invasive Gynecol. 2013;20(1):22–42.

43. Pabuçcu R, Gomel V. Reproductive outcome after hysteroscopic metroplasty in women with septate uterus and otherwise unexplained infertility. Fertil Steril. 2004;81(6):1675–8.

44. Cohen AW, Chhibber G. Obstetric complications of congenital anomalies of the paramesonephric ducts.

45. Reichman D, Laufer MR, Robinson BK. Pregnancy outcomes in unicornuate uteri: a review. Fertil Steril. 2009;91(5):1886–94.

46. Canis M, Wattiez A, Pouly JL, Mage G, Manhes H, Bruhat MA. Laparoscopic management of unicornuate uterus with rudimentary horn and unilateral extensive endometriosis: case report. Hum Reprod. 1990;5(7):819–20.

47. Nezhat F, Nezhat C, Bess O, Nezhat CH. Laparoscopic amputation of a noncommunicating rudimentary horn after a hysteroscopic diagnosis: a case study. Surg Laparosc Endosc. 1994;4(2):155–6.

48. Acien P. Incidence of Mullerian defects in fertile and infertile women. Hum Reprod. 1997;12(7):1372–6.

49. Raga F, Bauset C, Remohi J, Bonilla-Musoles F, Simon C, Pellicer A. Reproductive impact of congenital Mullerian anomalies. Hum Reprod. 1997;12(10): 2277–81.
50. Heinonen PK. Clinical implications of the didelphic uterus: long-term follow-up of 49 cases. Eur J Obstetr Gynecol Reprod Biol. 2000;91:183–90.
51. Seidman DS, Ben-Rafael Z, Bider D, Recabi K, Mashiach S. The role of cervical cerclage in the management of uterine anomalies. Surg Gynecol Obstet. 1991;173(5):384–6.
52. Althuisius S, Dekker G, Hummel P, Bekedam D, Kuik D, van Geijn H. Cervical Incompetence Prevention Randomized Cerclage Trial (CIPRACT): effect of therapeutic cerclage with bed rest vs. bed rest only on cervical length. Ultrasound Obstet Gynecol. 2002;20(2):163–7.
53. Yassaee F, Mostafaee L. The role of cervical cerclage in pregnancy outcome in women with uterine anomaly. J Reprod Infertil. 2011;12(4):277–9.
54. AAGL practice report: practice guidelines for the diagnosis and management of submucous leiomyomas. J Minim Invasive Gynecol 2012;19:152–71.
55. Baird DD, Dunson DB, Hill MC, Cousins D, Schectman JM. High cumulative incidence of uterine leiomyoma in black and white women: ultrasound evidence. Am J Obstet Gynecol. 2003;188(1):100–7.
56. Pritts EA, Parker WH, Olive DL. Fibroids and infertility: an updated systematic review of the evidence. Fertil Steril. 2009;91(4):1215–23.
57. Deligdish L, Loewenthal M. Endometrial changes associated with myomata of the uterus. J Clin Pathol. 1970;23(8):676–80.
58. Maguire M, Segars JH. Benign uterine disease: leiomyomata and benign polyps. The endometrium: molecular, cellular and clinical perspectives. 2nd ed. London: Informa Health Care; 2008.
59. Farhi J, Ashkenazi J, Feldberg D, Dicker D, Orvieto R, Ben Rafael Z. Effect of uterine leiomyomata on the results of in-vitro fertilization treatment. Hum Reprod. 1995;10(10):2576–8.
60. Kolankaya A, Arici A. Myomas and assisted reproductive technologies: when and how to act? Obstet Gynecol Clin North Am. 2006;33(1):145–52.
61. Klatsky PC, Tran ND, Caughey AB, Fujimoto VY. Fibroids and reproductive outcomes: a systematic literature review from conception to delivery. Am J Obstet Gynecol. 2008;198(4):357–66.
62. Casini ML, Rossi F, Agostini R, Unfer V. Effects of the position of fibroids on fertility. Gynecol Endocrinol. 2006;22:106–9.
63. Carranza-Mamane B, Havelock J, Hemmings R, Reproductive E, Infertility C, Cheung A, et al. The management of uterine fibroids in women with otherwise unexplained infertility. J Obstetr Gynecol. 2015;37(3):277–88.
64. Goldberg J, Pereira L. Pregnancy outcomes following treatment for fibroids: uterine fibroid embolization versus laparoscopic myomectomy. Curr Opin Obstet Gynecol. 2006;18(4):402–6.
65. Rackow BW, Jorgensen E, Taylor HS. Endometrial polyps affect uterine receptivity. Fertil Steril. 2011;95(8):2690–2.
66. Silberstein T, Saphier O, van Voorhis BJ, Plosker SM. Endometrial polyps in reproductive-age fertile and infertile women. Isr Med Assoc J. 2006;8(3): 192–5.
67. Pérez-Medina T, Bajo-Arenas J, Salazar F, Redondo T, Sanfrutos L, Alvarez P, et al. Endometrial polyps and their implication in the pregnancy rates of patients undergoing intrauterine insemination: a prospective, randomized study. Hum Reprod. 2005; 20(6):1632–5.
68. Varasteh NN, Neuwirth RS, Levin B, Keltz MD. Pregnancy rates after hysteroscopic polypectomy and myomectomy in infertile women. Obstet Gynecol. 1999;94(2):168–71.
69. Pabuçcu R, Atay V, Orhon E, Urman B, Ergün A. Hysteroscopic treatment of intrauterine adhesions is safe and effective in the restoration of normal menstruation and fertility. Fertil Steril. 1997;68(6): 1141–3.
70. ASHERMAN JG. Traumatic intra-uterine adhesions. J Obstet Gynaecol Br Emp. 1950;57(6):892–6.
71. Ventolini G, Zhang M, Gruber J. Hysteroscopy in the evaluation of patients with recurrent pregnancy loss: a cohort study in a primary care population. Surg Endosc. 2004;18(12):1782–4.

Male Factors in Recurrent Pregnancy Loss

8

Luna Samanta, Gayatri Mohanty, and Ashok Agarwal

Introduction

In the process of human reproduction, germ cells become distinct early in life and undergo a process of differentiation with an objective of generating progenitor cells for perpetuation of the species. Shaping of the sperm nucleus occurs in late spermiogenesis with remarkable condensation of sperm chromatin that enables the spermatozoa to thrive in hostile environments. This includes the passage of the spermatozoa in acidic environment of the vaginal tract, and encountering certain inhospitable conditions, such as the opposing motion of cilia within the uterus and fallopian tubes. Within this setting, the male germ cells fulfill their final task of delivering the paternal genome after meeting the oocyte. Remarkable modulation of gene expression must underlie the rapid and dramatic changes in the morphology and biochemistry of the germ cell during spermatogenesis. Some elements of this newly established genomic organization in relation to spermatozoa

have been known for a long time including the DNA-packaging proteins, histone variants, transition proteins, and protamines which are expressed and act in a sequence-specific manner [1]. However, critical information on specific factors managing these elements is still missing. Although a growing number of studies investigate functional genome organization in somatic cell nuclei, it is largely unknown how mammalian genome organization is established during embryogenesis. This is utterly important in the context of recurrent pregnancy loss (RPL) as even after a successful fertilization, 30–50 % of the conceptions are lost before the end of first trimester while 15–20 % of clinical pregnancies end through spontaneous abortions [2–5]. In modern times, RPL has been defined as two or more consecutive pregnancy loss in less than or equal to 20 weeks of gestation [6] and is usually studied from the women's perspective due to the close association between the mother and the developing embryo. Moreover, the significance of the unique features of gene expression in spermatogenic cells is controversial. Some workers believe that these features have special functions in meiosis and differentiation of spermatozoa while others, suggest that they are a symptom of leaky, inappropriate, or promiscuous transcription [7]. Last few years have seen dramatic changes with a plethora of publications that sheds light on how a nucleosome-based genome of a spermatozoon loses its fundamental organizing structural unit and adopts a new packaging principle, which is apt to be recognized and taken

L. Samanta, PhD • G. Mohanty, MPhil
Redox Biology Laboratory, Department of Zoology, Ravenshaw University, College Square, Cuttack, Odisha 753003, India

A. Agarwal (✉)
American Center for Reproductive Medicine, Cleveland Clinic, 10681 Carnegie Avenue, Desk X11, Cleveland, OH 44195, USA
e-mail: agarwaa@ccf.org

© Springer International Publishing Switzerland 2016
A. Bashiri et al. (eds.), *Recurrent Pregnancy Loss*, DOI 10.1007/978-3-319-27452-2_8

in charge by the maternal genome reprogramming factors in the egg. These new findings in the context of RPL will be discussed with emphasis concomitant with the currently available working models for the molecular basis of histone-to-protamine transition.

Sperm Chromatin

A key feature of mammalian spermatozoa is its unique chromatin structure. Male germ cells undergo unique and extensive chromatin remodeling soon after their specification (determination to become a spermatocyte) and during the differentiation process to become a mature spermatozoon [8]. Haploid male germ cells package their DNA into a volume that is typically 10 % or less than that of a somatic cell nucleus. To achieve this remarkable level of compaction, spermatozoa replace most of their histones with smaller, highly basic arginine- and (in eutherians) cysteine-rich protamines. In other words, testis-specific nuclear proteins, the transition proteins, and the protamines, are responsible for this chromatin condensation. In early spermatids, DNA is compacted around nucleosomes containing histones, the universal organization units of the genome [9]. The first step of the process of compaction occurs in round spermatids which involves displacement of the histones with the transition nuclear proteins (TP1 and TP2). Subsequently, in elongating spermatids, two isoforms of protamine proteins, protamine 1 (P1) and 2 (P2), take the place of transition proteins in the sperm chromatin. The ratio of incorporated P1 and P2 is tightly regulated at ~1:1 in the mature sperm [10–13]. With the aforementioned transition, a high degree of chromatin compaction is achieved that results in trancriptionally silent paternal DNA, thus, effectively protected against DNA damage (Fig. 8.1) [14]. In effect, protamination is responsible for the removal of core epigenetic layer from the paternal chromatin that leads to the belief that spermatozoa are incompetent to drive epigenetic changes in the embryo and their utility lies only in the delivery of an undamaged DNA blueprint to the embryo.

However, recent evidence challenges this dogma that demonstrates how highly specialized and unique modifications retained in sperm chromatin may actually provide significant influence in the early embryo [15]. However, even after the replacement, there still remain a small portion of histones which include testes-specific histone variants and canonical histones. Intriguingly, the retention of these histones could be either a result of inefficient replacement machinery or some regulatory mechanism. Interestingly, recent studies have found that this histone retention to be programmatic in nature [16]. Thus, the mammalian sperm chromatin can be categorized into three domains: (a) the large majority of DNA is packaged by protamines, (b) a smaller amount (~15 %) retains histone-bound chromatin and (c) the nuclear matrix attachment region (MARs) for the attachment of DNA (Fig. 8.1). However, the mechanisms underlying the replacement of these histones remain largely unknown [17]. Current evidence suggests that the larger structural domain (i.e., DNA packaged with protamines) plays a pivotal role in gene silencing during spermatogenesis but have no role post-fertilization and embryo development rather is protective in nature [7, 18, 19]. While, latter two structural domains, mentioned earlier are transferred to the paternal pronucleus and play a pivotal role during fertilization and embryonic development. The nuclear matrix organization is essential for DNA replication, and the histone-bound chromatin identifies genes that are important for embryonic development. Accordingly, well programmed chromatin packaging in sperm could potentially deliver epigenetic information to the oocyte and the zygote, post-fertilization. However, the contention that sperm protamines have no discrete role in early embryogenesis and they are mainly protective in function during and post-fertilization has been supported by three lines of evidence. Firstly, the replacement of protamines by histones in the first 2–4 h post-fertilization enables the paternal chromatin to be accessible to the chromatin of the oocyte [20, 21]. Secondly, the high resistive nature of sperm chromatin to mechanical disruption as compared to somatic cell supports the fact that protamines have a role

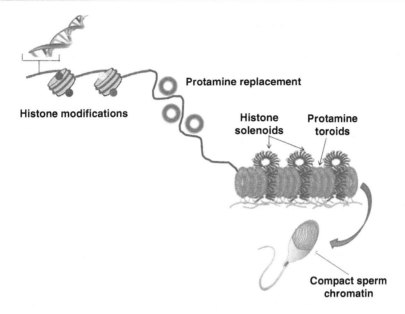

Fig. 8.1 Schematic representation of organization and compaction of sperm chromatin

in DNA protection. Finally, injection of round spermatids into mouse oocytes resulted in normal development of pups, thus concluding that protamines are not the prerequisite for normal embryogenesis [22]. Various hypotheses explain why sperm exhibit unique chromatin structure. First, condensation of sperm chromatin may help to generate a compact hydrodynamic shape. Second, the compaction of chromatin may protect the paternal genome from physical and chemical damage. And third, protamines could be involved in epigenetic regulation [23]. Thus, packaging of sperm chromatin have been categorized into four different levels of organization which includes (1) chromosomal anchorage-attachment of the DNA to the nuclear annulus; (2) formation of DNA loop domains (3) chromatin condensation which refers to the replacement of somatic cell-like histones by sperm-specific protamines for condensation of DNA into compact doughnuts; and (4) chromosomal positioning [24]. However, the retention of nearly 10–15 % of the histone-based nucleosomal structure has raised several questions with regard to the utility of paternal epigenome in embryonic development. Furthermore, it has been demonstrated that histones with specific modifications in the sperm cell are also present in the paternal pronucleus, thus reflecting on the fact that they were never replaced [25, 26]. In theory, this selective retention in sperm could allow for targeted gene activation or silencing in the embryo. An additional feature in the organization of sperm chromatin is the MAR as mentioned earlier [27]. The sperm chromatin is organized into loop domains and attached to a proteinaceous nuclear matrix. These MARs are no larger than 1000 base pairs and located between each protamine toroid by anchoring the toroids into place and thereby often termed as toroid linkers. Several pieces of evidence support a functional role for the sperm nuclear matrix in the function of the paternal genome during early embryogenesis [7]. These toroid linkers are enriched with histone and thereby extremely sensitive to nuclease activity. In addition to providing association between the DNA and the nuclear matrix, these MARs also function as a checkpoint for sperm DNA integrity after fertilization. Thus, the transmission of sperm histones and associated chromatin structures, suggests the possibility of the newly fertilized oocytes inheriting histone-based chromatin structural organization from the spermatozoa. This series of nucleoprotein exchanges during spermiogenesis provides an excellent model for the sequential gene expression and therefore, is a matter of general interest.

Nuclear Proteome of the Spermatozoa and Its Role in DNA Stability

The first sign of sperm chromatin packaging is a massive increase in the level of acetylation of core histones as revealed by immunocytochemistry and western blot analysis. This results in the incorporation of noncanonical, replication-independent testis-specific histone variants into the nucleosomes of developing spermatocytes and implies that histones are displaced prior to global replacement [28]. It is therefore, imperative to understand the attributes of the core histones of the nucleosome-bound DNA of the sperm chromatin that assist in the formation of the nucleoprotein make up of the spermatozoa. In early spermatids, DNA is compacted around nucleosomes, the universal organization units of the genome. A nucleosome is comprised of DNA coiled around an octamere of canonical histones (i.e., H2A, H2B, H3, and H4) [16]. These are a subset of histones found in somatic chromatin and are more susceptible to covalent modifications such as methylation, acetylation, ubiquitination, and phosphorylation. Each of these chemical modifications to histones works alone or in concert, under the name of the "histone code" to influence gene repression and/or activation [23]. These subsets of histones include histone H2 that takes the form of two minor variants, called H2A.X and H2A.Z, and the histones H3 and H4 and are extensively acetylated. As a prelude to removal of the histones, the stable nucleosome structure is relaxed by processes linked with acetylation of histone H4 [29]. Within the amino-terminal tail of histone H4, four lysines can be acetylated: lysine 5, lysine 8, lysine 12, and lysine 16 (H4K5, H4K8, H4K12, H4K16). In humans, however, H4K8 and H4K16 acetylations occur in elongating spermatids. In addition, acetylation of histone H3 (H3K9) can be detected in elongating spermatids

of humans [1, 15]. It has been reported that these modified histones are responsible for the formation of slightly smaller nucleosomes that apparently lack either H3 or H4 and repackage at least some of the pericentric/chromocentric DNA, providing evidence for novel nucleosome-like complexes in spermnuclei that are delivered to the egg at fertilization (Fig. 8.2). The establishment and removal of acetylation is accomplished by histone acetyl transferases (HATs) and deacetylases (HDACs), respectively. Histone acetylation relaxes chromatin and makes it accessible to transcription factors, whereas deacetylation is associated with gene silencing [23]. It has been hypothesized that H4 hyperacetylation in mammalian spermatids leads to an open chromatin structure that facilitates and induces histone displacement. Further evidences suggest that sperm H4Ac being species-specific is either not lost from the sperm during pericentric condensation or is present as a separate, nonpericentric compartment, possibly located in the posterior of the sperm [30] or peripheral nuclear regions [31]. It is a matter of concern as to whether these paternally derived histones contribute to and persist in zygotic chromatin is currently unresolved. However, both H2AL1/2 rapidly disappear after fertilization in the mouse [32] while H3.1/H3.2 persists in human and mouse zygotes prior to DNA replication which could be an effect of the heterologous system used [26]. Apart from acetylation, histone methylation signals have been observed in elongating spermatids, such as strong H3K4 mono-, di-, and tri-methylation. These modifications in concert with acetylation might assist in achieving a more-open chromatin configuration. It has been seen that H3K4methylation is generally associated with gene expression whereas H3K9 and H3K27 methylation is linked to gene silencing and heterochromatin. Nevertheless, methylation pattern associated with repressed chromatin are observed in elongating spermatids which includes H3K9 mono-, di-, and tri-methylation as well as H3K27 di- and tri-methylation [19, 33]. However, the timing of establishment and removal of methylation markers is critical to spermatogenesis. It has been often observed that the methylation level of H3K4 peaks in spermatogonial stem cells which signals the stem cells to begin differentiation and to

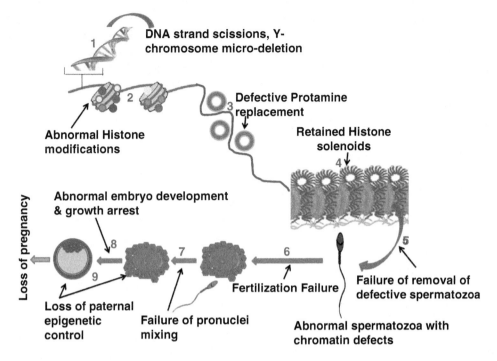

Fig. 8.2 Schematic representation of proposed mechanism(s) for defective packaging of sperm chromatin leading to early pregnancy loss

go on to become spermatocytes and is removed during meiosis. In contrast, the methylation level of H3K9 and H3K27 increases during meiosis, but the removal of H3K9me at the end of meiosis is essential to the onset of spermiogenesis [23, 34]. Expression of different histone methyltransferases and demethylases has been observed during spermatid elongation. This coexistence of both types of enzymes might be crucial to balance regions of "opened" and "closed" chromatin. However, it has been demonstrated in human spermatozoa that histone enrichment were not randomly distributed but were rather enriched at loci important for embryo development which are transmitted to the oocyte during fertilization. These loci included imprinted gene clusters, miRNA, HOX gene clusters, developmental promoters, and signaling factors [35]. Similarly, Arpanahi et al. found that histone-bound DNA regions of human spermatozoa were associated with regulatory regions of the genome [36]. An epigenetic marking of these retained histones was observed showing key developmental genes bivalently marked with H3K4me3 and H3K27me3, as observed in embryonic stem cells. Additionally,

H3K4me2 was preferentially located at promoters of developmental gene and H3K4me3 at HOX regions, noncoding RNAs, and paternally imprinted loci [35]. This radical change in chromatin configuration is expected to involve mechanism that facilitates the eviction of nucleosomes in favor of incorporation of transition proteins, followed by a subsequent exchange of transition proteins for protamines. The functional activity of each transition protein is still debatable. Some reports suggest that TP1 decreases the melting temperature of DNA, relaxes the DNA in nucleosomal core particles, and stimulates the DNA-relaxing activity of topoisomerase I which indicates that TPs could help chromatin remodeling by making the DNA more flexible. However, others have reported that neither TP1 nor TP2 is able to cause topological changes in supercoiled DNA. Rather, TP1 has been found to stimulate repair of single-strand DNA breaks [37]. Whatever the case might be, data from knockout mouse model suggests that TP1 and TP2 might not be required for histone removal and protamine loading, yet are important for proper regulation of chromatin structure. Subsequently these transition proteins are replaced by the protamines. Protamines are the major class of sperm nuclear proteins. They are of two types, namely, protamine1 (P1) encoded by a single-copy gene and the family of protamine 2 (P2) proteins (P2, P3, and P4), all encoded by a single gene that is transcribed and translated into a precursor protein [38]. The question then arises as to how the DNA binding proteins (such as protamines) of the mammalian spermatozoa fit themselves into the sperm nucleus? Balhorn proposed a model for protamine–DNA binding that accounts for such discrepancy in sperm volume [39]. He stated that the protamines bind to DNA by lying lengthwise inside the minor groove. He opined that positively charged arginine-rich protamines can completely neutralize the negatively charged phosphate groups of DNA and protamine-DNA complex of one strand would fit into the major groove of a neighboring DNA strand so that the DNA strands of sperm nucleus would be packaged side by side in a linear array. Furthermore, the sperm chromatin is stabilized by inter- and intramolecular disulfide bridges between protamines which enable the whole DNA to be tightly packaged in a small volume. An additional process that occurs during chromatin reorganization in elongating spermatids of mammals is the transient appearance of DNA strand breaks [16, 37]. Presumably, the elimination of nucleosomes during spermiogenesis leaves a great number of unconstrained DNA supercoils in the male germ cell that needs to be removed. This elimination is performed in particular by the introduction of single- or double-strand breaks in DNA that relieves the helical tension. Subsequently, upon elimination of strand breaks, effective mechanisms are employed to seal or repair the DNA backbone.

DNA Damage and Male Infertility

Mammalian spermatogenesis entails a major biochemical and morphological restructuring of the germ cell DNA into the condensed spermatid nucleus. In association with the chromatin restructuring, other well documented nuclear events includes an increase in histone acetylation, an increase in the activity of ubiquitin system,

SUMOylation as well as a change in DNA topology resulting from the elimination of the negative supercoiling induced by the removal of DNA-bound nucleosomes. It has been hypothesized that incomplete protamination could render spermatozoa DNA more vulnerable to damage by endogenous or exogenous agents such as nucleases, free radicals, and mutagens. Thus, progressive oxidation of free sulfhydryl or thiol (SH) groups of protamines to disulfides (SS) groups in the epididymis further stabilizes the compacted sperm DNA [40]. Abnormality in the deposition of sperm protamines during spermiogenesis or incomplete oxidation of sperm protamine SH groups during epididymal transit can lead to enhanced susceptibility of sperm DNA to injury. This results in sperm DNA fragmentation and impaired sperm decondensation during fertilization. Spermatozoa with fragmented DNA may initiate apoptosis and interfere with transmission of paternal genetic information to the developing embryo [41]. Several independent investigators have demonstrated the importance of DNA integrity in predicting male reproductive potential. In fact, sperm DNA damage is an objective marker of sperm function, with a lower coefficient of variation than conventional semen parameters. Besides, the several exogenous sources of sperm DNA damage, it is pertinent to focus on the inherent nature of spermatozoa and its maturation process that may cause for sperm DNA damage. In this regard reactive oxygen species (ROS) which are produced by both exogenous and endogenous factors warrants special mention. In general, a mature spermatozoon is accomplished with a small amount of cytoplasm and hence with a limited supply of cytoplasmic antioxidants. Concomitantly, the plasma membrane of the spermatozoa is rich in unsaturated fatty acids that maintain the fluidity of the membrane. Such property leaves the spermatozoa particularly vulnerable to oxidative stress brought upon by increased generation of ROS [42].

Role of Reactive Oxygen Species in Sperm DNA Damage

The sperm genome is encoded with information that needs to be accurately transmitted to the oocyte—a feature vital for the pre- and postnatal development of the offspring. Under normal physiological conditions, germ cells produce physiological amounts of ROS that modulate gene and protein activities required for maturation, capacitation, acrosome reaction, and oocyte fusion. The pathogenic effect of ROS occurs when an imbalance between pro- and anti-oxidants is disturbed leading to oxidative stress as onserved during sperm maturation in epididymis or in the seminal plasma [43]. ROS are short-lived, highly reactive, autocatalytic, and nonspecific reactive intermediates of metabolism that oxidize lipids, amino acids, and carbohydrates as well as are responsible for DNA strand breaks and mutations. ROS includes hydroxyl ion, superoxide ion, nitric oxide, peroxyl, lipid peroxyl, and Thiyl and nonradical molecules singlet oxygen, hydrogen peroxide, hypochloric acid, lipid peroxides, and ozone [41]. Spermatozoa are constantly exposed to the interphase between oxidation through high amounts of ROS produced by themselves as during metabolism and by leukocytes present in semen; and reduction by means of scavengers and antioxidants. Generation of ROS involves two mechanisms which includes the nicotinamide adenine dinucleotide phosphate oxidase system at the level of the sperm plasma membrane and/or the nicotinamide adenine dinucleotide-dependent oxido-reductase reaction at the mitochondrial level. Mitochondrial respiration is the main biological source of ROS under physiological conditions [44]. Normally, oxygen is tetravalent reduced to water by the mitochondrial cytochrome c oxidase while incomplete reduction leads to leakage of these radicals [45]. Spermatozoa are densely populated with mitochondria since a constant supply of energy is required for their motility. The lipid composition of plasma membrane of mammalian spermatozoa are rich in polyunsaturated fatty acids (PUFA), thus, render them susceptible to ROS attack. These lipids contain unconjugated double bonds separated by methylene groups that, weakens the methyl carbon hydrogen bond making hydrogen extremely susceptible to abstraction and oxidative damage. When the level of ROS escapes the antioxidant defense, they primarily attack PUFA, to initiate chain reactions resulting in lipid peroxidation (LPO). Superoxide ($O_2^{\cdot-}$) is the major

ROS generated in human spermatozoa. This electron-deficient product of O_2 generates H_2O_2 via dismutation. These in turn undergo Fenton reaction to form $\cdot OH$ that is a potent initiator of chain reaction leading to LPO of membrane lipids. Therefore, may lead to sperm dysfunction due to loss of membrane fluidity [40]. Biopositive effect of ROS is seen at low considerations and is known to act selectively on the metabolism of prostanoids, in gene regulation or in the regulation of cellular growth, intracellular signaling, and in other types of signal transduction while excessive generation leads to cell death [44]. As described in the previous section, sperm chromatin is prone to oxidative damage leading to base modifications and DNA fragmentation. Damaged DNA has been observed in testicular, epididymal, and ejaculated human spermatozoa. Single-strand breaks are a direct result of oxidative damage on sperm DNA, while double-strand breaks may arise from exposure to 4-hydroxyl-2-nonenal a major product of LPO. Two types of DNA adducts, namely, 8-hydroxy-2-deoxyguanosine and two ethenonucleosides (1, N6-ethenoadenosine and 1, N6-ethenoguanosine) are found in human spermatozoa, both of which have been considered key biomarkers of DNA damage caused by oxidative stress [45].

Most of the DNA damages incurred to germ cell during spermatogenesis are taken care of by DNA repair systems. Any insult to such machinery may result in production of spermatozoa with damaged DNA which when fertilizes the ovum may impair embryo development.

DNA Repair Systems in Spermatozoa

An intriguing feature of chromatin remodeling is the introduction of DNA strand breaks concomitant with the general progression for the removal of nucleosomes that leaves the DNA with unconstrained supercoils. To reduce the torsional stress induced by an alteration in DNA topology, there occurs the transient appearance of DNA strand breaks to provide the swivel effect [36, 45]. It has been surmised that the integrity of the DNA condensing process plays a key role in the elimination of DNA strand breaks since the breaks are transient and are no longer detected at later steps of the spermiogenesis process where the nuclear protein transition is completed. Due to haploid nature of post-meiotic spermatids, DNA repair relies mostly on nonhomologous end joining. The basic nuclear proteins, i.e. the transition proteins and protamines would therefore act as "alignment factors" in nonhomologous end joining of the free ends of the DNA [36]. With the absence of DNA ligating activity in the DNA binding proteins it has been proposed that in elongating spermatids, topoisomerase II is responsible for generating as well as ligating DNA strand breaks that overlaps with the appearance of histone variant H2AX foci, a marker of DNA double-strand breaks [46]. H2AX in response to DSBs, acts by recruiting DNA repair factors to sites of DNA damage where it is rapidly phosphorylated resulting in formation of H2AX foci. Also, evidence suggests that ubiquitination and SUMOylation are involved in DNA repair pathways in elongating spermatids thus facilitating appropriate level of histone–protamine exchange [47]. However, a mature spermatozoon being transcriptionally and translationally inactive, the termination of DNA repair process occurs during its transit through the epididymis and post-ejaculation. Ultimately, the breaks in the DNA that may have escaped repair prior to compaction or damage occurring after the completion of chromatin remodeling are delivered to the oocyte. Oxidative stress impairs sperm DNA by introducing adducts such as ethenonucleosides that impair nucleotide excision repair in oocyte [48, 49]. Oocytes and early embryos have been shown to repair sperm DNA damage to some extent, so the biological effect of sperm DNA damage depends cumulatively on the magnitude of sperm chromatin damage and the capacity of the oocyte to repair it after fertilization.

From the above-mentioned facts, it is important to understand that proteins involved in chromatin remodeling and condensation are important for the repair of DNA in vivo. Under such circumstances, it is expected that targeted deletion of these respective genes or any alteration in their sequences would lead to the persistence of strand breaks up to much later stages of spermiogenesis

or even in a matured spermatozoa. In this context, targeted deletion of mouse TP1 or TP2 gene have been compensated with a marked increase in the expression of other genes so that their function is apparently reduced. As a consequence of these mutations, it did not result in major sperm head abnormalities although alterations in the condensation state of the nuclei were nevertheless observed in both cases [50].

Gene Deletion and Sperm DNA Integrity

Y-Chromosome harbors several genes critical for spermatogenesis and development of gonads. Extensive research has been performed on the association of Y-chromosome deletions with male infertility. The Y-chromosome locus is divided into three regions; the proximal, middle, and distal of Yq11 and is labeled as AZF-a, b, and c after the azoospermia factor AZF. Patients with microdeletions in the AZFa region have been reported with congenital oligozoospermia or partial spermatogenic arrest, whereas patients with AZFb and AZFc are usually reported with azoospermia or oligozoospermia [51]. However, microdeletions in the overlapping area between the latter two regions may present with range of sperm counts (azoospermia to normal sperm count) [52].

Apoptosis

As the male germ cell development progress, apoptosis orchestrates the production and function of these cells from the early stages of gonadal differentiation to the moment of fertilization. It has been suggested that an early apoptotic pathway is initiated in spermatogonia and spermatocytes which express Fas. On the other hand, Sertoli cells express Fas ligand which upon binding to Fas on germ cells leads to death of the later. This mechanism enables Sertoli cells to limit the population of germ cells that adhere to it for support. Infact, apoptosis plays a significant role in the regulation of germ cell development by removing damaged cell in the seminiferous tubules and thus, safeguarding the genome integrity [42]. However, absence of timely repair or DNA damage if tolerated, the cells that harbor the damage are removed by the apoptosis pathway. Sperm DNA damage and impaired fertilization has often been correlated with unsuccessful apoptosis in the germ cell. The presence of apoptosis in ejaculated spermatozoa could be the result of various types of injuries. Testicular causes including hormonal depletion, irradiation, toxic agents, chemicals, and heat have been shown to induce apoptosis, while those in the epididymis are signals released by abnormal or defective spermatozoa or leukocytes, such as ROS and other mediators of inflammation/infection [53]. Irrespective of source or origin, the fertilization capacity of apoptotic sperm has been observed at the same rate as intact spermatozoa. However, the in vitro embryo development to the blastocyst stage is closely related to the integrity of the DNA. As a result of oxidative stress, the human ejaculate expresses various apoptotic markers that initiate apoptosis, some of which include Fas, phosphatidylserine (PS), Bcl-Xl, and p53. This apoptotic pathway in turn induces release of cytochrome c from mitochondrial membranes that triggers caspases, such as caspases 3 and 9, and annexin-V binding (Annexins are calcium-dependent phospholipid-binding proteins, which bind to PS). This pathway eventually leads to sperm apoptosis [54, 55]. It has been observed that mature spermatozoa from infertile patients with increased ROS levels had significantly higher levels of apoptosis than mature spermatozoa from the control group [40]. More dramatically, they may pose the risk of carrying a damaged genome into the egg, resulting in poor embryo development, miscarriage, or birth defects.

Ubiquitination

In response to DNA damage, cells activate a highly conserved signaling network, commonly referred to as the DNA damage response (DDR), to safeguard genomic integrity. It is well understood that chromatin reorganization not only facilitates the compaction of the paternal genome into the sperm head but also protect the DNA from damaging agents. The DDR consists of a set of tightly regulated events, including detection of DNA damage, accumulation of DNA repair factors at the site of damage, and finally physical repair of the lesion. One of the process by which DNA damage is detected is histone ubiquitination. H2A and H2B ubiquitination are known to be enriched at sites of DNA damage albeit the primary function of histone ubiquitination is suggested to be sex chromosome inactivation during meiotic prophase and nucleosome removal at post meiotic stages [56–58]. RNF8 is a 485-residue nuclear polypeptide that is known to have ubiquitin E3 ligase activity. Upon DNA damage, RNF8 has been shown to be rapidly recruited to sites of DNA damage via its interaction with γH2AX. At sites of DNA damage, RNF8 ubiquitinates histones—H2A and H2B, promoting the recruitment of downstream DNA damage response factors such as 53BP1, BRCA1, and Rad51 [59]. However, more recently it has been reported that H4K8 acetylation and H4K16 acetylation are not affected in elongating spermatids of RNF8-deficient mice leaving this issue unresolved [60]. Ubiquitin is one of the 200 major proteins secreted in apocrine fashion by the epididymal epithelium which has the property of binding covalently to other proteins, via an isopeptide bond between the C-terminal glycine of ubiquitin and the E-amino group of a lysine, in substrate proteins [61]. Upon overwhelming damage, the DDR provokes detrimental cellular actions by involving the apoptotic machinery and inducing a coordinated demise of the damaged cells. Moreover, recent observations highlighted the role of ubiquitination in orchestrating the DDR, providing a dynamic cellular regulatory circuit helping to guarantee genomic stability and cellular homeostasis. Abnormal spermatozoa produced as a result of endogenous or exogenous insult become ubiquitinated and subsequently phagocytised by epididymal epithelial cells [62]. Despite this safety mechanism available during the epidiymal transit of the spermatozoa, some of the ubiquitinated spermatozoa are believed to escape phagocytosis and find their way into ejaculate [62, 63] and cause defects in head and axoneme. Protein ubiquitination typically occurs in the cell cytosol or nucleus and it has been postulated that sperm-acrosomal ubiquitin C-terminal hydrolases are involved in sperm-ZP interactions and antipolyspermy defense. In the studies of Sutovsky et al. in bovine semen, ubiquitination have been associated with DNA fragmentation. It is suggested that sperm ubiquitination is associated with poor-quality sperm parameters in men. In contradiction to the above, studies have revealed that ubiquitination is involved in the fertilization process, and once the process of ubiquitin–proteasome is inhibited, the percentage of fertilization is reduced [64]. Apart from DDR, protein ubiquitination has also been detected in several regions of human sperm and is initially inversely related to semen quality [63] while other studies have suggested that ubiquitination also plays a role in normal sperm function [63, 65–67]. During spermatogenesis, ubiquitination is a crucial process that is responsible for the replacement of the spermatid's nuclear histones by transition proteins, followed by permanent substitution with protamines [53]. Ubiquitination also has a principal role in the dramatic reduction of human sperm centrosome that occurs during spermatid elongation. Thus, ubiquitination, principally a death signal for proteins is involved in maintaining the protein homeostasis in the spermatozoa, however, beyond threshold level is associated with anomalies is sperm structure and function.

SUMOylation

One of the critical phenomena for preserving genome integrity is the sheltering of chromosomal ends from unwanted DNA repair reactions and maintenance of telomere length homeostasis. A growing body of evidence suggests that covalent protein modification (SUMOylation) by SUMO (small ubiquitin-like modifier) to be critical in the regulation of numerous DNA transactions, including DNA repair and transcription, as well as heterochromatin formation and maintenance. These SUMO proteins exist in three isoforms: 1, 2, and 3. Of the three isoforms, SUMO2 and 3 are 95 % identical and are often referred to as SUMO2/3 [68–70]. Amongst the many targeted PTMs, SUMOylation have not been identified as a

potential target although such targets are critical for understanding the role of SUMO in normal and impaired sperm function. SUMO proteins have been localized to different subcompartments of mouse and human testicular cells [71–73] while SUMO1 is localized mostly to the heads of human sperm [74]. A recent study by Vigodner et al. demonstrated the localization and identification of SUMOylated proteins in the defective spermatozoa by immunofluorescence and electron microscopy. They revealed that SUMO proteins were highly expressed in the neck area of human sperm and were also detectable in the flagella and head regions. High levels of SUMOylation were detected in defective spermatozoa in the neck and tail region relative to normal spermatozoa [75]. The study concluded that numerous proteins are modified by SUMOylation in human spermatozoa; wherein excessive SUMOylation is a marker of defective spermatozoa.

Sperm DNA and Recurrent Pregnancy Loss

Past research have focused on the contributions of the fertilizing spermatozoon to the oocyte and have limited their observation to spermatozoon by being a carrier or vector that transfers the DNA to the egg. DNA in the male germ cell is tightly compacted and is considered evolutionarily as a highly conserved process. Owing, to this silent state of the compacted nucleus, it was long thought spermatozoon transcripts did not play a role in embryo development and that only maternal transcripts were involved. It is now well established that apart from being a mere cargo for the delivery of DNA, spermatozoa transmit information to the next generation via the genome as well as the epigenome. Several recent studies however suggest that this tight packaging of the sperm chromatin conveys important epigenetic message to the embryo. The possible mechanism underlying this phenomenon is the extensive cross-talk between the fertilizing spermatozoa and the oocyte which leads to activation of the egg on one hand and sperm head decondensation on the other. This is extremely important to understand in the light of RPL, as here the problem is not the inability to impregnate or conceive but rather the limitation in carrying the conceptus to a live birth. The male gamete confers 50 % of the genomic material on the embryo, and also contributes to placental and embryonic development [76]. Genetic and epigenetic alterations of sperm may therefore have dire consequences in early pregnancy loss. In this context, it is noteworthy to state that while genetic inheritance is based on the DNA code, epigenetic information comprises modifications occurring directly on DNA or on the chromatin. The major type of DNA modification is methylation, whereas on the chromatin various modifications occur on specific residues of histones, including methylation, phosphorylation, acetylation, and ubiquitination. The mammalian genome undergoes two major phases of epigenetic reprogramming, once in the primordial germ cells and once in the preimplantation embryos. After the crucial process of fertilization, protamines in sperm chromatin are rapidly replaced with histones which are hyperacetylated, while the male pronucleus DNA undergoes demethylation in the absence of DNA replication. Therefore, it is speculated that any alteration of chromatin structure is an important mechanism for regulating DNA transcription.

DNA Damage and Sperm Function

As the paternal genome is inactive transcriptionally till 2 days after fertilization, a damaged sperm DNA does not impair fertilization or cleavage [77]. However, activation of paternal genome with modifications at the level of the DNA nucleotides and/or DNA strand breaks that are beyond the oocyte repair capacity after fertilization are not compatible with normal embryo and fetal development. This raises the question as to whether the retention of paternal gene sequences having some potentially important embryological function in a more relaxed chromatin configuration is more susceptible to DNA damage than the bulk, protamine-packaged DNA [53]. Since, abnormal paternal genome modifications lead to poor blastocyst

development, unequal cleavage, implantation failure, or early fetal loss. As mentioned earlier, small DNA damages in spermatozoa as result of endo-or exogenous insults are repaired by pre- and postreplication repair mechanisms, but large DNA damages cannot be repaired. Decreased elimination and subsequent accumulation of the DNA-damaged spermatozoa results in poor-quality sperm. This is due largely to inefficient apoptotic machinery and poor DNA integrity and abnormal chromatin packaging [78]. Sperm chromatin packaging anomalies are closely associated with poor fertility outcomes and higher levels of DNA damage are an accompanying feature of dysfunctional sperm [37]. Thus, men who are partners of couples with recurrent pregnancy loss may have sperms with normal morphology, whose, germ cells may harbor damaged DNA. This causes an alteration in sperm quality and function, sperm-oocyte interaction, implantation, and early embryo development all of which are good indicators of successful pregnancy.

Aneuploidy

As a subpopulation, men with normal semen parameters who are partners in a couple with RPL or unexplained recurrent IVF failure are commonly overlooked [79]. Elevated levels of sperm aneuploidies are known to be associated with RPL. Sperm aneuploidy has been defined as the abnormality in the number of chromosome resulting from defective meiosis during spermatogenesis. As a result, a spermatozoon that is disomic or nullisomic for a particular chromosome will develop. Arguably, delivery of an intact chromosome by the spermatozoon to the ovum is the most important function of sperm. Fertilization with such type of abnormal sperm cell results in monosomic or trisomic embryos, the majority of which are incompatible with a viable birth. It is unfortunate, that, with the available technologies we can have a gross identification of sperm with abnormal morphology than detecting the underlying genetic abnormality such as aneuploidy [79]. Carrell and his colleagues reported a significant increase in sperm chromosome aneuploidy, apoptosis, and abnormal sperm morphology in some patients with recurrent loss of pregnancy [80]. The incidence of aneuploidy increases as the standard semen parameters worsen. Even though men within fertility exhibit high rates of sperm aneuploidy genetic testing in clinics for men with infertility is restricted to detection of chromosomal abnormalities using a karyotype and Y-chromosome microdeletion analysis. It is important to realize that sperm aneuploidy rates can be high even in men with normal sperm morphology. Cytogenetic analysis of sperm using fluorescence in situ hybridization (FISH) provides a method to test for sperm chromosomal aneuploidy and can help evaluate potential causes of RPL or recurrent IVF failure [79] which has been detailed below. Recently, a study was undertaken in order to bring about an association between sperm aneuploidies and normal semen parameters in men who are partners of RPL using the cytogenetic technique FISH. The study showed that nearly was 40 % of men with RPL and normal sperm density/motility had abnormal sperm aneuploidy while no association was found between sperm DNA fragmentation and sperm aneuploidy [79].

DNA Fragmentation

Recent advances in the understanding of mammalian sperm chromatin and function have changed our perception of spermatozoa as a silent carrier of paternal DNA. However, there are several theories with relation to DNA strand breakage and subsequent DNA fragmentation that needs to be resolved. The question of whether DNA strand break occurs exclusively during spermiogenic compaction of chromatin and is not repaired in the seminiferous tubules, or rather is a result of aggressors acting on the male genital tract, is still unresolved [78]. To explain the origin of sperm DNA damage, several hypotheses have been proposed. DNA strand separation is a physiological process that accompanies the recombination step that occurs at the time of protamine-ordained compaction. DNA fragmentation is often a result of double or single-strand breaks which have been induced in the DNA prior to, or post, ejaculation of the spermatozoa. The causes of sperm DNA fragmentation are still unclear, even if apoptosis, oxidative assault, and defects in chromatin maturation are hypothesized. Several studies have reported a significant negative association between the percentage of sperm with DNA fragmentation and fertilization rate in the context of RPL. A recent meta-analysis including 16 studies found a highly significant increase in miscarriage rate in couples where the male partner had elevated levels of sperm DNA damage compared to those where the male partner had low levels of sperm DNA damage (risk ratio = 2.16, $P < 0.00001$) [81]. In another study comparing fertile sperm donors with couples who have unexplained recurrent miscarriage, showed that 85 % of the couples affected with recurrent miscarriage had a profile with high values of double-stranded DNA damage compared to only 33 % among fertile sperm donors, suggesting a specific paternal explanation in these otherwise unexplained cases [82]. Several mechanisms have been proposed in explanation to the genesis of sperm DNA fragmentation but none have completely clarified the causes and site of origin of sperm DNA fragmentation and our knowledge is still limited to hypothesis and theories. Amongst the many proposed mechanism, one theory states that DNA nicks, as a part of the remodeling process of sperm chromatin are produced which are not completely repaired due to an impairment of sperm maturation process. Abortive apoptosis can be associated with DNA cleavage and can also be provoked by the attack of free radicals including ROS, acting both in testis and in post-testicular sites. The major DNA adducts found 8-hydroxy-2-deoxyguanosine and two ethenonucleosides (1, N6-ethenoadenosine and 1, N6-ethenoguanosine) are found in human sperm DNA which have been considered key biomarkers of DNA damage caused by OS [40]. Many direct and indirect studies prove the aforementioned hypothesis by stating that increased levels of sperm DNA fragmentation show high degree of cell immaturity, apoptosis, or oxidative stress. Whatever the case may be, it is important to understand that a damaged DNA does not inhibit fertilization or prevent the formation of a zygote rather prohibits further development of the embryo beyond the two-celled stage. It is therefore, pertinent to understand other underlying causes such as alterations in the epigenetic programming of the sperm chromatin that may have a profound effect on sperm DNA.

DNA Methylation

DNA compaction in male germ cells is a fundamental biologic process and a prerequisite for transmission of the male genome to the next generation. Several studies suggest that this sperm-specific genome packaging structure conveys an important epigenetic message to the embryo [22]. Epigenetic programming in the spermatozoa is unique with as erasure of epigenetic marks occurs in primordial germ followed by its establishment during post-meiotic maturation. Therefore, understanding the epigenetic processes in the male germ cells may contribute to understanding paternal effects on early embryonic development. DNA methylation as one of the most studied epigenetic markers of male germ cells refers to the addition of a methyl group from S-adenosyl-methionine to the fifth position of the cytosine ring (5meC) in CpG dinucleotides. Nearly, 3–5 % of the cytosine residues in mammalian genomic DNA appear in the form of 5meC [83]. The process of methylation in germ cells is unique and necessary for proper spermatogenesis and sperm production. Three structurally distinct chromatin configurations may occur as follows: histone-packaged hypomethylated DNA, histone-packaged methylated DNA, and protamine-packaged hypomethylated DNA [27, 84]. It is observed that only four imprinted loci are methylated in the male germ line which includes Igf2/H19, Rasgrf1, Dlk1-Gtl2, and Zdbf2. A specific family of methyltansferases (DNMTs) is also involved in DNA methylation. DNMT1 ensures methylation maintenance while DNMT3A, 3B, and 3L specifically allow the methylation process in germ cells. DNMT3A and 3B have a catalytic activity, whereas DNMT3L lacks this catalytic activity and acts as a cofactor to DNMT3A [85, 86]. After fertilization, the decondensation of the male pronucleus follows an epigenetic reprogramming with DNA demethylation along with protamine-to-histone transition, and histone modifications that contributes to genome activation in the embryo and subsequent embryonic development. But, there still remain many facts unclear with regard to mechanism and function of paternal genome. Post-fertilization, histones incorporated into the male pronucleus are highly acetylated, however, immediately upon histone incorporation; H3K4me1, H3K9me1, and H3K27me1 are detectable which is at a time when DNA methylation is still present in the male pronucleus. Although these findings raise the question that whether any of these epigenetic marks in the paternal pronucleus protect specific regions such as the centromeres from demethylation remains known. These suggest that the sperm genome may be packaged and poised for two programs: first is a reminiscent gametogenesis program (active chromatin marks), and second is a future embryonic program (bivalent domains) [34]. Nevertheless, the progressive histone modification and concomitant demethylation in the paternal pronucleus presumably leads to a chromatin state easily accessible by the maternal genome. However, this does not devoid the paternal genome from acquiring unique epigenetic marks early on in development which are important for imprinting and X chromosome inactivation [87]. Furthermore, the dynamics of DNA methylation and histone modifications during epigenetic reprogramming raise several questions about additional mechanistic links. For example, specific sequences in the male pronucleus escape demethylation which generates special interest. Secondly, is there sequence preference for demethylation or are there regions in the sperm genome that contain histones rather than protamines, perhaps carrying particular modifications? Are the stepwise histone modifications of the paternal genome marks for later de novo methylation events? In an answer to these mechanistic links, it is possible that during reprogramming these appear to be developmentally regulated and may depend on the precise developmental stage, cell type, and genomic region. This may account for developmental plasticity and regulation, which is typical of pluripotent cell types. The fact that there are so many open questions means that this is an area with exciting discoveries ahead of us.

Errors in Imprinting

Implications of genomic imprinting in embryo/fetal growth are fairly a recent event. Several studies have evaluated the sperm DNA methylation status of the differentially methylated regions (DMRs) of a number of imprinted genes. Genomic imprinting refers to the monoallelic regulation of gene expression according to the parent of origin of the gene. It is mediated by the establishment of sex-specific epigenetic marks on DNA called "imprints" in the form of DNA methylation at imprinting control regions (ICRs) in the genomic DNA [88]. Houshdaran et al. reported significant associations between sperm concentration, motility, and morphology and the methylation status of four genes: NTF3, MT1A, PAX8, and PLAGL1 [89]. Studies conducted by Nanassy et al. reported abnormal sperm DNA hypermethylation at several CpGs in CREM associated with abnormal P1/P2 ratio which was subsequently confirmed in a larger cohort of patients and controls [90, 91]. Considerably, the evaluation of sperm DNA methylation status has been focused primarily either to a few genes or to global methylation levels by evaluation of repetitive elements or immunostaining of 5-methylcytosine. Hence, a clear indication of all the spermatozoa within a population are affected with aberrant DNA methylation is not obtained. In order to better characterize the involvement of sperm DNA methylation in male infertility, an array-based using the Illumina Infinium Human Methylation 27 Beadchip assay, which measures genome-wide sperm DNA methylation was done. More than 27,000 CpG sites was assessed in the genome of men with abnormal P1/P2 ratios and in men who have undergone IVF/intracytoplasmic sperm injection (ICSI) cycles that resulted in poor embryo quality in the absence of female factors. The study identified three individuals displaying broad spectrum of aberrant sperm DNA methylation profiles. As these findings were limited to small

sample set the results may be an important signature in some infertile men. Functional studies will be necessary to characterize the developmental consequences of such epigenetic disruption [92]. Although majority of the focus has been on the methylation status of imprinted genes, methylation of nonimprinted genes has been evaluated to a lesser extent. DAZL methylation seems to be normal in infertile men however differential methylation of the DAZL promoter was observed in the sperm of OAT men [93]. Elucidation of the exact mechanism leading to such aberrant methylation may lead to development of appropriate therapeutic strategies. Understanding the fact that epigenetic programming is crucial for the proper functioning of the male genome and any alteration may have an impact on embryonic development have also been studied in the light of RPL. Significant reduction in the H19 ICR methylation without significant difference in the sperm parameters demonstrated aberrant imprinting in patients affected with idiopathic recurrent spontaneous miscarriage [94]. In another setting, methylation aberrations in spermatozoa at developmentally important imprinted regions and its role in early embryo loss in idiopathic recurrent spontaneous miscarriages (RSM) was ascertained by the same group. The study confirmed that the conventional notion of DLK1-GTL2, PEG1, and ZAC (PLAGL1) promoter being essential during later stages of gestation and suggest that the methylation of these loci may not be indispensable for early development. The study also concluded that these sites may not be good epigenetic markers unlike the H-19 imprinting control region for diagnosis of idiopathic RSM [88]. Although all the aforementioned studies support the hypothesis that sperm DNA methylation patterns of imprinted as well as nonimprinted genes are essential for normal sperm function, fertility, and embryo development, still there are many unanswered questions that need to be defined. Amongst them the most relevant are whether these methylation errors acquired during fetal or early postnatal development? Are they linked to abnormal methylation maintenance during spermatogenesis? Along with the causes the timing of their occurrence remains largely unknown. Under such circumstances, it is commented that in the absence of the guidance of global spermatozoa epigenome, developmental progression is likely to be a haphazard affair, prone to many epigenetic errors that lead to nonviable embryos [27]. This fact has its relevance in the light of RPL, as mentioned earlier, that the problem here is not to impregnate or conceive rather carrying a conceptus to a live birth. If this assistance rendered by the paternal chromatin is lost once pluripotent ES cells become committed to establishing the earliest cell lineages, then successful totipotent reprogramming of a somatic cell nucleus would be very difficult to achieve as revealed through several cloning experiments [95]. Functional studies will therefore be necessary to characterize the developmental consequences of such epigenetic disruption [92].

Methods to Detect Sperm DNA Damage

The unique packaging of the sperm chromatin has important implications for both the development of male infertility screening tests and understanding of sperm chromatin characteristics. Over the years sperm DNA integrity tests have gained importance and have been proposed as a means to assess male gamete competence. Although sperm DNA integrity assays are more often used as a supplement to traditional semen analysis, the point at which DNA damage occurs during spermiogenesis, and to what degree, remains to be elucidated [78]. Sperm DNA damage has also been shown to have the lowest variability of all semen parameters and rapid advance of molecular biology has resulted in numerous techniques to assess DNA and chromatin quality [96].

Microscopic Analysis of DNA Damage

Fluorescent In Situ Hybridization (FISH)

The basis for FISH lies in the analysis of the hybridization of chromosome-specific DNA probes labeled with different fluorochromes to complementary DNA sequences on target chromosomes. This is followed by the detection by means of an optical microscope equipped with fluorescence apparatus and filters for the dyes that is to be used. Advantage of the technique relies on the centromeric or locus-specific probes that can enumerate chromosomes in interphase nuclei and their use allows for the study of thousands of spermatozoa in a limited period of time [97]. It should be noted that FISH is an indirect method of assessing chromosomal anomalies as only the fluorescent signals, rather than chromosomes, are scored. An important limitation to FISH analysis is its inefficiency to obtain a complete karyotype as the analysis only considers the chromosomes investigated and does not allow for the detection of structural chromosomal anomalies [97].

Alkaline Comet Assay

The comet assay, also known as single-cell gel electrophoresis is a direct assessment of DNA damage in an individual cell. The damage is quantified by measuring the displacement between the genetic material of the nucleus "comet head" and the resulting tail [98]. This method is a multistep process which involves embedding of cells in agarose, lysis of cell in neutral or alkaline condition, electrophoresis of lysed cells followed by DNA staining and microscopic image analysis. The tail lengths are used as an index for damage as damaged cells appear as a "comet" with a brightly fluorescent head and tail, whose length and fluorescence intensity depend on the number of DNA strand breaks. The Comet assay is a rapid and sensitive method that allows the evaluation of DNA fragmentation on a few sperm; thus, it can be employed in cases of severe oligozoospermia. The tail moment can be more precisely defined as being equivalent to the torsional moment of the tail. The comet is a well-standardized assay that correlates significantly with other tests for the measurement of DNA damage. It is simple to perform, has a low intra-assay coefficient of variation, and a low performance cost. The disadvantages of the Comet assay are the lack of standardized protocols and the need for software to conduct image analysis. Moreover, the presence of residual RNA can bring about an overestimation of DNA damage as it creates background analysis, or can be underestimated because of proteins which hamper the movement of fragments during electrophoresis. Incomplete chromatin decondensation may not allow breaks to be revealed [99].

TUNEL Assay

Terminal deoxynucleotidyl transferase-mediated fluorescein-dUTP nick-end labeling (TUNEL) is also a direct measure for the assessment of sperm DNA damage. The assay quantifies the amount of cellular DNA breakage by incorporating fluorescent dNTPs at single- and double-stranded DNA ends breaks in a reaction catalyzed by the template-independent enzyme terminal deoxynucleotidyl transferase (TdT). This aforementioned enzyme incorporates biotinlyated deoxyuridine to 3′-OH of DNA to create a signal, which increases with the number of DNA breaks. These incorporated labeled nucleotides can be detected in spermatozoa by flow cytometry, flourecence microscope, or light microscope [54]. On detection by fluorescence microscopy, spermatozoa with normal DNA having capped telomeres at the 3′OH end have only background staining/fluoresce while those with fragmented DNA (multiple 3′OH ends) stain/fluoresce brightly. The clinical utility of TUNEL assay lies in the fact that it can simultaneously detect single- and double-strand breaks unlike comet assay which requires different protocols for studying both types of strand breakages. But it too has many limitations. By the use of TUNEL the degree of damage within a cell is not quantified wherein the data reveals DNA damage within a population. Moreover due to lack of thresholds and lack of nonvalidated data, the assay is still not being used in routine clinical tests.

Flow Cytometric Chromatin Evaluation (FCCE)

The relative degree of sperm DNA fragmentation can be revealed by flow cytometry and/or fluorescence microscopy depending on the method used. However, whereas flow cytometry has the capacity to analyze hundreds of thousands of cells, fluorescence microscopy is usually limited to several hundred cells. The sperm chromatin structure Assay (SCSA) is a flow cytometric assay that relies on the fact that abnormal sperm chromatin is highly susceptible to physical induction of partial DNA denaturation in situ. The SCSA method measures the susceptibility of sperm DNA to acid denaturation by measuring the metachromatic shift of acridine orange from green (indicative of intercalation into double-stranded DNA) to red fluorescence (indicative of association with single-stranded DNA) [78]. The assay has the ability to analyze many thousands of spermatozoa at one time. The most important parameter of the SCSA is the DNA fragmentation index (%DFI), which represents the population of cells with DNA damage.

Choosing the Assay and Evaluating Consequences

Sperm DNA is an independent measure of sperm quality that provides better diagnostic and prognostic capabilities than standard sperm parameters for male fertility potential. The clinical utility of sperm DNA testing remains controversial. A metaanalysis was conducted which included 13 studies involving 2161 in vitro fertilization/ICSI treatments revealed high levels of DNA damage significantly increases the risk of pregnancy failure. But concluded that testing was not clinically useful in discriminating couples who would conceive [99]. It is worth noting that the establishment of a cut-off point between normal levels in the average fertile population and the minimal levels of sperm DNA integrity required to achieve pregnancy using these different assays is still lacking. This lack in the predictive power of sperm DNA testing as well as the diagnostic ignorance frustrates both the patient and physician because without pathophysiological understanding, specific treatment is unlikely. The clinician also has a duty to inform the couple, wherever possible, of the reason for the male's disability and identify treatable disorders. Until that time, a handful of DNA assessment assays are available with different level of efficacy that hints at general damage riddling the male genome. Based upon the limited available test clinicians need to counsel their patients accordingly. For couples planning their first pregnancy, test for sperm DNA damage especially SCSA are good predictors of negative pregnancy outcome. When high levels of sperm DNA damage is detected in the male partner, IVF or ICSI is the recommended choice as these tests are only fair predictors of negative or positive pregnancy outcomes [100]. A more precise, noninvasive technique is the need of the hour that will elucidate the entire story of male genome and indicate poorly scripted passages that will warn the technician from inserting that sperm into a similarly interrogated ovum.

Future Directions: Potential of Omics Studies

It is evident from mammalian sperm chromatin research that nonrandomly located nucleosomal domains in spermatozoal nuclei are conserved throughout the spermatogenic process, all supporting the hypothesis that the spermatozoon delivers a novel epigenetic signature to the egg that may be crucial for normal development. This certainly provides insights on why this signature may be required in early embryogenesis. It seems more and more evident that various epigenetic alterations associated with male factor deformity are linked together. Abnormal methylation levels are in fact associated with histone/protamine disequilibrium as well as to RNA retention. Clearly, the sum of these epigenetic alterations has dire consequences not only on male reproductive potential but also on the formation and development of the embryo. As a subpopulation, men with grossly normal semen parameters and repeated pregnancy failure are usually not counseled on any particular causes and are not encouraged to undergo any further testing. If epigenetic profiles of the mature spermatozoa are critical, then any alterations in the epigenetic patterns can provide a logic for the

increased risk for preterm birth or repeated miscarriage. Histone retention and DNA demethylation contribute to a poised state that ensures transcriptional competence and activation of developmental regulators in the early embryo. Albeit, this continuous process of epigenetic reprogramming enables the spermatozoa to be susceptible to several impediments, ramifications of the altered chromatin states in the germ-line are not entirely known. It is therefore, hoped that no sooner with the advancement of technology a noninvasive technique will be developed that has the ability to read the genetic book contained within the single male gamete. Future studies are needed to establish the cause and effect of paternally retained modified nucleosomes in the early embryo, and their potential effects if abnormally retained. In light of this, proteomics is considered as one of the burgeoning field of research in reproductive medicine in the postgenomic era. It is a natural consequence of the huge advances in genome sequencing, bioinformatics and the development of robust, sensitive, reliable, and reproducible analytical techniques. Documenting specific changes in the spermatozoa proteins may aid in the better understanding of the functional changes associated with men who are partners in couples affected with RPL. Furthermore, the candidate proteins of interest may be utilized as potential markers and help in understanding the cause of implantation failure with no female factor abnormality. Mature sperm are almost transcriptionally and translationally silent, thus posttranslational modifications are critical for the functionality of the spermatozoa during its epididymal transit and post-ejaculation. A variety of PTMs are observed in spermatozoa that are remnants of testicular spermatogenesis. Recent identifications suggest that histones, a core group proteins present in the sperm chromatin can undergo 67 novel modifications [101]. This indicates that we have just scratched the surface in trying to unravel the histone code, and in understanding how histone modifications could regulate the histone-to-protamine transition. Proteomics can help recognize these modifications and facilitate to understand the downstream events with altered chromatin structure. The most-studied histone modifications include acetylation, methylation, phosphorylation, ubiquitination, and SUMOylation. Proteomics forms a basis for the identification of protein substrates and the site for PTMs fundamental to the biochemical dissection of PTM pathways. Studies on differentially expressed proteins between fertile and men affected with recurrent pregnancy may demonstrate several modifications in candidate genes as well as identify biomarkers that can, in turn, help clinicians determine certain peptides or metabolites that may be linked to male factor deformity. Furthermore, the alteration of chromatin-associated proteins such as the protamines contributes to decreased fertility and poor embryonic growth. Most of the techniques used to detect sperm chromatin defects only detect gross defects in DNA integrity, while the roles of the associated proteins remain a mystery. Therefore, it is suggested that the use of such noninvasive technique will not only allow for a better understanding of posttranslational modifications and offer an opportunity to identify proteins that are differentially expressed in the spermatozoa that may lead to early embryo loss. Minimun set of test with maximum functional coverage is the need of the hour in order to establish a practical and cost effective service. Such endeavors are long overdue.

References

1. Brunner AM, Nanni P, Mansuy IM. Epigenetic marking of sperm by post-translational modification of histones and protamines. Epigenetics Chromatin. 2014;7(1):2.
2. Rai R, Regan L. Recurrent miscarriage. Lancet. 2006;368(9535):601–11.
3. Gupta S, Agarwal A, Banerjee J, Alvarez JG. The role of oxidative stress in spontaneous abortion and recurrentpregnancy loss: a systematic review. Obstet Gynecol Surv. 2007;62(5):335–47.
4. P K, Malini SS. Positive association of sperm dysfunction in the pathogenesis of recurrent pregnancy loss. J Clin Diagn Res. 2014;8(11):7–10.
5. Nabi A, Khalili MA, Halvaei I, Ghasemzadeh J, Zare E. Seminal bacterial contaminations: probable factor in unexplained recurrentpregnancy loss. Iran J Reprod Med. 2013;11(11):925–32.
6. ASRM 2013.
7. Ward WS. Function of sperm chromatin structural elements in fertilization and development. Mol Hum Reprod. 2010;16(1):30–6.
8. Seki Y, Hayashi K, Itoh K, Mizugaki M, Saitou M, Matsui Y. Extensive and orderly reprogramming of genome-wide chromatin modifications associated with specification and early development of germ cells in mice. Dev Biol. 2005;278(2):440–58.
9. Campos EI. Reinberg D histones: annotating chromatin. Annu Rev Genet. 2009;43:559–99.
10. Balhorn R, Reed S, Tanphaichitr N. Aberrant protamine 1/protamine 2 ratios in sperm of infertile human males. Experientia. 1988;44(1):52–5.
11. Hecht NB. Regulation of 'haploid expressed genes' in male germ cells. J Reprod Fertil. 1990;88(2):679–93.
12. Oliva R, Dixon GH. Vertebrate protamine gene evolution I. Sequence alignments and gene structure. J Mol Evol. 1990;30(4):333–46.
13. Dadoune JP. The nuclear status of human sperm cells. Micron. 1995;26(4):323–45.
14. Deal RB, Henikoff JG, Henikoff S. Genome-wide kinetics of nucleosome turnover determined by metabolic labeling of histones. Science. 2010;328(5982):1161–4.
15. Jenkins TG, Carrell DT. The sperm epigenome and potential implications for the developing embryo. Reproduction. 2012;143(6):727–34.
16. Rathke C, Baarends WM, Awe S, Renkawitz-Pohl R. Chromatin dynamics during spermiogenesis. Biochim Biophys Acta. 2014;1839(3):155–68.
17. Chen YS, Qiu XB. Transcription-coupled replacement of histones: degradation or recycling? J Genet Genomics. 2012;39(11):575–80.
18. Carrell DT, Emery BR, Hammoud S. Altered protamine expression and diminished spermatogenesis: what is the link? Hum Reprod Update. 2007;13(3):313–27.
19. Rathke C, Baarends WM, Jayaramaiah-Raja S, Bartkuhn M, Renkawitz R, Renkawitz-Pohl R. Transition from a nucleosome-based to a protamine-based chromatin configuration during spermiogenesis in Drosophila. J Cell Sci. 2007;120(Pt 9):1689–700.
20. van der Heijden GW, Dieker JW, Derijck AA, Muller S, Berden JH, Braat DD, van der Vlag J, de Boer P. Asymmetry in histone H3 variants and lysine methylation between paternal and maternal chromatin of the early mouse zygote. Mech Dev. 2005;122(9):1008–22.
21. Ajduk A, Yamauchi Y, Ward MA. Sperm chromatin remodeling after intracytoplasmic sperm injection differs from that of in vitro fertilization. Biol Reprod. 2006;75(3):442–51.
22. Ogura A, Matsuda J, Yanagimachi R. Birth of normal young after electrofusion of mouse oocytes with round spermatids. Proc Natl Acad Sci U S A. 1994;91:7460–2.
23. Boissonnas CC, Jouannet P, Jammes H. Epigenetic disorders and male subfertility. Fertil Steril. 2013;99(3):624–31.
24. Ward WS, Coffey DS. DNA packaging and organization in mammalian spermatozoa: comparison with somatic cells. Biol Reprod. 1991;44(4):569–74.

25. van der Heijden GW, Derijck AA, Ramos L, Giele M, van der Vlag J, de Boer P. Transmission of modified nucleosomes from the mouse male germline to the zygote and subsequent remodeling of paternal chromatin. Dev Biol. 2006;298(2):458–69.

26. van der Heijden GW, Ramos L, Baart EB, van den Berg IM, Derijck AA, van der Vlag J, Martini E, de Boer P. Sperm-derived histones contribute to zygotic chromatin in humans. BMC Dev Biol. 2008;8;34.

27. Kumar K, Thilagavathi J, Deka D, Dada R. Unexplained early pregnancy loss: role of paternal DNA. Indian J Med Res. 2012;136(2):296–8.

28. Miller D, Brinkworth M, Iles D. Paternal DNA packaging in spermatozoa: more than the sum of its parts? DNA, histones, protamines and epigenetics. Reproduction. 2010;139(2):287–301.

29. Meistrich ML, Trostle-Weige PK, Lin R, Bhatnagar YM, Allis CD. Highly acetylated H4 is associated with histone displacement in rat spermatids. Mol Reprod Dev. 1992;31(3):170–81.

30. Li Y, Lalancette C, Miller D, Krawetz SA. Characterization of nucleohistone and nucleoprotamine components in the mature human sperm nucleus. Asian J Androl. 2008;10(4):535–41.

31. Pittoggi C, Renzi L, Zaccagnini G, Cimini D, Degrassi F, Giordano R, Magnano AR, Lorenzini R, Lavia P, Spadafora C. A fraction of mouse sperm chromatin is organized in nucleosomal hypersensitive domains enriched in retroposon DNA. J Cell Sci. 1999;112(Pt 20):3537–48.

32. Wu F, Caron C, De Robertis C, Khochbin S, Rousseaux S. Testis-specific histone variants H2AL1/2 rapidly disappear from paternal heterochromatin after fertilization. J Reprod Dev. 2008;54(6):413–7.

33. De Vries M, Ramos L, Housein Z, De Boer P. Chromatin remodelling initiation during human spermiogenesis. Biol Open. 2012;1(5):446–57.

34. Godmann M, Auger V, Ferraroni-Aguiar V, Di Sauro A, Sette C, Behr R, Kimmins S. Dynamic regulation of histone H3 methylation at lysine 4 in mammalian spermatogenesis. Biol Reprod. 2007;77(5):754–64.

35. Hammoud S, Liu L, Carrell DT. Protamine ratio and the level of histone retention in sperm selected from a density gradient preparation. Andrologia. 2009;41(2):88–94.

36. Arpanahi A, Brinkworth M, Iles D, Krawetz SA, Paradowska A, Platts AE, Saida M, Steger K, Tedder P, Miller D. Endonuclease-sensitive regions of human spermatozoal chromatin are highly enriched in promoter and CTCF binding sequences. Genome Res. 2009;19(8):1338–49.

37. Boissonneault G. Chromatin remodeling during spermiogenesis: a possible role for the transition proteins in DNA strand break repair. FEBS Lett. 2002;514(2-3):111–4.

38. Aoki VW, Moskovtsev SI, Willis J, Liu L, Mullen JB, Carrell DT. DNA integrity is compromised in protamine-deficient human sperm. J Androl. 2005;26(6):741–8.

39. Balhorn R. A model for the structure of chromatin in mammalian sperm. J Cell Biol. 1982;93(2):298–305.

40. Zini A, Kamal KM, Phang D. Free thiols in human spermatozoa: correlation with sperm DNA integrity. Urology. 2001;58(1):80–4.

41. Agarwal A, Mulgund A, Alshahrani S, Assidi M, Abuzenadah AM, Sharma R, Sabanegh E. Reactive oxygen species and sperm DNA damage in infertile men presenting with low level leukocytospermia. Reprod Biol Endocrinol. 2014;12:126.

42. Agarwal A, Prabakaran SA. Mechanism, measurement, and prevention of oxidative stress in male reproductive physiology. Indian J Exp Biol. 2005;43(11):963–74.

43. Agarwal A, Said TM. Role of sperm chromatin abnormalities and DNA damage in male infertility. Hum Reprod Update. 2003;9(4):331–45.

44. Henkel RR. Leukocytes and oxidative stress: dilemma for sperm function and male fertility. Asian J Androl. 2011;13(1):43–52.

45. Sanocka D, Kurpisz M. Reactive oxygen species and sperm cells. Reprod Biol Endocrinol. 2004;2:12.

46. González-Marín C, Gosálvez J, Roy R. Types, causes, detection and repair of DNA fragmentation in animal and human sperm cells. Int J Mol Sci. 2012;13(11):14026–52.

47. Leduc F, Nkoma GB, Boissonneault G. Spermiogenesis and DNA repair: a possible etiology of human infertility and genetic disorders. Syst Biol Reprod Med. 2008;54(1):3–10.

48. Bergink S, Jentsch S. Principles of ubiquitin and SUMO modifications in DNA repair. Nature. 2009;458(7237):461–7.

49. Ahmadi A, Ng SC. Fertilizing ability of DNA-damaged spermatozoa. J Exp Zool. 1999;284(6):696–704.

50. Steger K, Cavalcanti MC, Schuppe HC. Prognostic markers for competent human spermatozoa: fertilizing capacity and contribution to the embryo. Int J Androl. 2011;34(6 Pt 1):513–27.

51. Adham IM, Nayernia K, Burkhardt-Göttges E, Topaloglu O, Dixkens C, Holstein AF, Engel W. Teratozoospermia in mice lacking the transition protein 2 (Tnp2). Mol Hum Reprod. 2001;7(6):513–20.

52. Tahmasbpour E, Balasubramanian D, Agarwal A. A multi-faceted approach to understanding male infertility: gene mutations, molecular defects and assisted reproductive techniques (ART). J Assist Reprod Genet. 2014;31(9):1115–37.

53. Foresta C, Moro E, Ferlin A. Y chromosome microdeletions and alterations of spermatogenesis. Endocr Rev. 2001;22(2):226–39.

54. Barroso G, Valdespin C, Vega E, Kershenovich R, Avila R, Avendaño C, Oehninger S. Developmental sperm contributions: fertilization and beyond. Fertil Steril. 2009;92(3):835–48.

55. Agarwal A, Saleh RA, Bedaiwy MA. Role of reactive oxygen species in the pathophysiology of human reproduction. Fertil Steril. 2003;79(4):829–43.

56. Aitken RJ, Baker MA. Causes and consequences of apoptosis in spermatozoa; contributions to infertility and impacts on development. Int J Dev Biol. 2013;57(2-4):265–72.

57. Bergink S, Salomons FA, Hoogstraten D, Groothuis TA, de Waard H, Wu J, Yuan L, Citterio E, Houtsmuller AB, Neefjes J, Hoeijmakers JH, Vermeulen W, Dantuma NP. DNA damage triggers nucleotide excision repair-dependent monoubiquitylation of histone H2A. Genes Dev. 2006;20(10):1343–52.

58. Doil C, Mailand N, Bekker-Jensen S, Menard P, Larsen DH, Pepperkok R, Ellenberg J, Panier S, Durocher D, Bartek J, Lukas J, Lukas C. RNF168 binds and amplifies ubiquitin conjugates on damaged chromosomes to allow accumulation of repair proteins. Cell. 2009;136(3):435–46.

59. Mailand N, Bekker-Jensen S, Faustrup H, Melander F, Bartek J, Lukas C, Lukas J. RNF8 ubiquitylates histones at DNA double-strand breaks and promotes assembly of repair proteins. Cell. 2007;131(5):887–900.

60. Huen MS, Grant R, Manke I, Minn K, Yu X, Yaffe MB, Chen J. RNF8 transduces the DNA-damage signal via histone ubiquitylation and checkpoint protein assembly. Cell. 2007;131(5):901–14.

61. Sin HS, Barski A, Zhang F, Kartashov AV, Nussenzweig A, Chen J, Andreassen PR, Namekawa SH. RNF8 regulates active epigenetic modifications and escape gene activation from inactive sex chromosomes in post-meiotic spermatids. Genes Dev. 2012;26(24):2737–48.

62. Eskandari-Shahraki M, Tavalaee M, Deemeh MR, Jelodar GA, Nasr-Esfahani MH. Proper ubiquitination effect on the fertilisation outcome post-ICSI. Andrologia. 2013;45(3):204–10.

63. Sutovsky P, Moreno R, Ramalho-Santos J, Dominko T, Thompson WE, Schatten G. A putative, ubiquitin-dependent mechanism for the recognition and elimination of defective spermatozoa in the mammalian epididymis. J Cell Sci. 2001;114(Pt 9):1665–75.

64. Sutovsky P. Ubiquitin-dependent proteolysis in mammalian spermatogenesis, fertilization, and sperm quality control: killing three birds with one stone. Microsc Res Tech. 2003;61(1):88–102.

65. Hongmei W, Changcheng S, Chongwen D, Weixian S, Cunxi L, Dayuan C, Yongchao W. Effects of ubiquitin proteasome pathway on mouse sperm capacitation, acrosome reaction and in vitro fertilization. Chin Sci Bull. 2002;47:127–32.

66. Muratori M, Marchiani S, Forti G, Baldi E. Sperm ubiquitination positively correlates to normal morphology in human semen. Hum Reprod. 2005;20(4):1035–43.

67. Haraguchi CM, Mabuchi T, Hirata S, Shoda T, Tokumoto T, Hoshi K, Yokota S. Possible function of caudal nuclear pocket: degradation of nucleoproteins by ubiquitin-proteasome system in rat spermatids and human sperm. J Histochem Cytochem. 2007;55(6):585–95.

68. Meccariello R, Chianese R, Ciaramella V, Fasano S, Pierantoni R. Molecular chaperones, cochaperones, and ubiquitination/deubiquitination system: involvement in the production of high quality spermatozoa. Biomed Res Int. 2014;2014:561426.

69. Geiss-Friedlander R, Melchior F. Concepts in sumoylation: a decade on. Nat Rev Mol Cell Biol. 2007;8(12):947–56.

70. Hannoun Z, Greenhough S, Jaffray E, Hay RT, Hay DC. Post-translational modification by SUMO. Toxicology. 2010;278(3):288–93.

71. Wilkinson KA, Henley JM. Mechanisms, regulation and consequences of protein SUMOylation. Biochem J. 2010;428(2):133–45.

72. Vigodner M, Morris PL. Testicular expression of small ubiquitin-related modifier-1 (SUMO-1) supports multiple roles in spermatogenesis: silencing of sex chromosomes in spermatocytes, spermatid microtubule nucleation, and nuclear reshaping. Dev Biol. 2005;282(2):480–92.

73. Vigodner M, Ishikawa T, Schlegel PN, Morris PL. SUMO-1, human male germ cell development, and the androgen receptor in the testis of men with normal and abnormal spermatogenesis. Am J Physiol Endocrinol Metab. 2006;290(5):E1022–33.

74. Shrivastava V, Pekar M, Grosser E, Im J, Vigodner M. SUMO proteins are involved in the stress response during spermatogenesis and are localized to DNA double-strand breaks in germ cells. Reproduction. 2010;139(6):999–1010.

75. Marchiani S, Tamburrino L, Giuliano L, Nosi D, Sarli V, Gandini L, Piomboni P, Belmonte G, Forti G, Baldi E, Muratori M. Sumo1-ylation of human spermatozoa and its relationship with semen quality. Int J Androl. 2011;34(6 Pt 1):581–93.

76. Vigodner M, Shrivastava V, Gutstein LE, Schneider J, Nieves E, Goldstein M, Feliciano M, Callaway M. Localization and identification of sumoylated proteins in human sperm: excessive sumoylation is a marker of defective spermatozoa. Hum Reprod. 2013;28(1):210–23.

77. Puscheck EE, Jeyendran RS. The impact of male factor on recurrent pregnancy loss. Curr Opin Obstet Gynecol. 2007;19:222–8.

78. Tesarik J, Greco E, Mendoza C. Late, but not early, paternal effect on human embryo development is related to sperm DNA fragmentation. Hum Reprod. 2004;19(3):611–5.

79. Palermo GD, Neri QV, Cozzubbo T, Rosenwaks Z. Perspectives on the assessment of human sperm chromatin integrity. Fertil Steril. 2014;102(6):1508–17.

80. Ramasamy R, Scovell JM, Kovac JR, Cook PJ, Lamb DJ, Lipshultz LI. Fluorescence in situ hybridization detects increased sperm aneuploidy in men with recurrent pregnancy loss. Fertil Steril. 2015;103(4):906-909.e1.

81. Carrell DT, Wilcox AL, Lowy L, Peterson CM, Jones KP, Erickson L, Campbell B, Branch DW, Hatasaka HH. Elevated sperm chromosome aneuploidy and apoptosis in patients with unexplained

recurrent pregnancy loss. Obstet Gynecol. 2003;101(6):1229–35.

82. Robinson L, Gallos ID, Conner SJ, Rajkhowa M, Miller D, Lewis S, Kirkman-Brown J, Coomarasamy A. The effect of spermDNA fragmentation on miscarriage rates: a systematic review and meta-analysis. Hum Reprod. 2012;27(10):2908–17.

83. Ribas-Maynou J, García-Peiró A, Fernandez-Encinas A, Amengual MJ, Prada E, Cortés P, Navarro J, Benet J. Double stranded sperm DNA breaks, measured by Comet assay, are associated with unexplained recurrent miscarriage in couples without a female factor. PLoS One. 2012;7(9), e44679.

84. Biermann K, Steger K. Epigenetics in male germ cells. J Androl. 2007;28(4):466–80.

85. Vieweg M, Dvorakova-Hortova K, Dudkova B, Waliszewski P, Otte M, Oels B, Hajimohammad A, Turley H, Schorsch M, Schuppe HC, Weidner W, Steger K, Paradowska-Dogan A. Methylation analysis of histone H4K12ac-associated promoters in sperm of healthy donors and subfertile patients. Clin Epigenetics. 2015;7(1):31.

86. Bestor TH. The DNA, methyltransferases of mammals. Hum Mol Genet. 2000;9(16):2395–402.

87. Hata K, Kusumi M, Yokomine T, Li E, Sasaki H. Meiotic and epigenetic aberrations in Dnmt3L-deficient male germ cells. Mol Reprod Dev. 2006 ;73(1):116–22.

88. Monk D. Germline-derived DNA methylation and early embryo epigenetic reprogramming: The selected survival of imprints.Int J Biochem Cell Biol. 2015;pii: S1357 2725(15)00115-6.

89. Ankolkar M, Salvi V, Warke H, Vundinti BR, Balasinor NH. Methylation status of imprinted genes DLK1-GTL2, MEST (PEG1), ZAC (PLAGL1), and LINE-1 elements in spermatozoa of normozoospermic men, unlike H19 imprinting control regions, is not associated with idiopathic recurrent spontaneous miscarriages. Fertil Steril. 2013;99(6):1668–73.

90. Houshdaran S, Cortessis VK, Siegmund K, Yang A, Laird PW, Sokol RZ. Widespread epigenetic abnormalities suggest a broad DNA methylation erasure defect in abnormal human sperm. PLoS One. 2007;2, e1289.

91. Nanassy L, Carrell DT. Abnormal methylation of the promoter of CREM is broadly associated with male factor infertility and poor sperm quality but is improved in sperm selected by density gradient centrifugation. Fertil Steril. 2011;95(7):2310–4.

92. Nanassy L, Carrell DT. Analysis of the methylation pattern of six gene promoters in sperm of men with abnormal protamination. Asian J Androl. 2011 ;13(2):342–6.

93. Aston KI, Punj V, Liu L, Carrell DT. Genome-wide sperm deoxyribonucleic acid methylation is altered in some men with abnormal chromatin packaging or poor in vitro fertilization embryogenesis. Fertil Steril. 2012;97(2):285–92.

94. Navarro-Costa P, Nogueira P, Carvalho M, Leal F, Cordeiro I, Calhaz-Jorge C, Gonçalves J, Plancha CE. Incorrect DNA methylation of the DAZL promoter CpG island associates with defective human sperm. Hum Reprod. 2010;25(10):2647–54.

95. Ankolkar M, Patil A, Warke H, Salvi V, Kedia Mokashi N, Pathak S, Balasinor NH. Methylation analysis of idiopathic recurrent spontaneous miscarriage cases reveals aberrant imprinting at H19 ICR in normozoospermic individuals. Fertil Steril. 2012;98(5):1186–92.

96. Paterson L, DeSousa P, Ritchie W, King T, Wilmut I. Application of reproductive biotechnology in animals: implications and potentials. Applications of reproductive cloning. Anim Reprod Sci. 2003;79 :137–43.

97. Lewis SE. Is sperm evaluation useful in predicting human fertility? Reproduction. 2007;134(1):31–40.

98. Collodel G, Giannerini V, Antonio Pascarelli N, Federico MG, Comodo F, Moretti E. TEM and FISH studies in sperm from men of couples with recurrent pregnancy loss. Andrologia. 2009;41(6):352–60.

99. Shamsi MB, Kumar R, Dada R. Evaluation of nuclear DNA damage in human spermatozoa in men opting for assisted reproduction. Indian J Med Res. 2008;127(2):115–23.

100. Oliva A, Spira A, Multigner L. Contribution of environmental factors to the risk of male infertility. Hum Reprod. 2001;16(8):1768–76.

101. Zini A, Libman J. Sperm DNA damage: clinical significance in the era of assisted reproduction. CMAJ. 2006;175(5):495–500.

102. Tan M, Luo H, Lee S, Jin F, Yang JS, Montellier E, et al. Identification of 67histone marks and histone lysine crotonylation as a new type of histone modification. Cell. 2011;146:1016–28.

Naama Steiner and Asher Bashiri

Background

Recently, society has become more aware of and concerned about lifestyle and environmental toxins. This is also true for RPL couples who are concerned that toxins within the environment may have contributed to their reproductive difficulty.

This chapter discusses the association between lifestyle and RPL including obesity, air pollution, cigarette smoking and caffeine and alcohol consumption. Except for obesity, all studies discuss mainly the association between lifestyle and spontaneous miscarriage. Nevertheless, this information is relevant, and an extrapolation for RPL should be made until there will be further studies. Hence, as a consequence, we should recommend change in lifestyle for prevention of another miscarriage.

In order to understand the impact of these on RPL, it is mandatory to understand some definitions:

N. Steiner, MD (✉)
Recurrent Pregnancy Loss Clinic, Department of Obstetrics and Gynecology, Soroka Medical Center, Be're Sheva, Israel
e-mail: Steinern@bgu.ac.il

A. Bashiri, MD
Director Maternity C and Recurrent Pregnancy Loss Clinic, Department of Obstetrics and Gynecology, Soroka Medical Center, Faculty of Health Science, Ben-Gurion University of the Negev, 84101 Be'er Sheva, Israel

Developmental toxicology is a basic term defined as the study of adverse effects on the developing organism occurring anytime during the life span of the organism that may result from exposure to chemical or physical agents before conception (either parent), during prenatal development, or postnatal until the time of puberty.

Teratology is defined as the study of defects induced during development between conception and birth. Six principles of teratology were introduced by Jim Wilson in 1959 in his monograph *Environment and Birth Defects* and are still applied today. Wilson's general principles of teratology: [1, 2]

1. Susceptibility to teratogenesis depends on the genotype of the conceptus and the manner in which this interacts with adverse environmental factors.
2. Susceptibility to teratogenesis varies with the developmental stage at the time of exposure to an adverse influence.
3. Teratogenic agents act in specific ways (mechanisms) on developing cells and tissues to initiate sequences of abnormal developmental events (pathogenesis).
4. The access of adverse influences to developing tissues depends on the nature of the influence (agent).
5. The four manifestations of deviant development are death, malformation, growth retardation, and functional defect.

© Springer International Publishing Switzerland 2016
A. Bashiri et al. (eds.), *Recurrent Pregnancy Loss*, DOI 10.1007/978-3-319-27452-2_9

6. Manifestations of deviant development increase in frequency and degree as dosage increases, from no effect to lethal level.

The criteria or principles by which an environmental factor is considered to be a human teratogen are: [3–5]

1. An increase in the frequency of the phenotypic effect in the exposed group should be seen above its frequency in the general population.
2. An animal model should exist such that when the same route of exposure is applied, it duplicates the effect observed in humans (i.e. there should be a plausible biologic explanation for the mechanism of action of the teratogen).
3. A dose–response relationship should be observed.
4. A genetically more susceptible group of exposed individuals should exist (i.e. genetic variability will determine the differences in placental transport, absorption, metabolism, and distribution of an agent accounting for the variation in teratogenic effect observed between species and individuals).
5. A threshold effect should be observed, implying that there is a level of exposure or dose below which the incidence of a phenotypic effect is not statistically greater than that of controls.
6. The teratogenic insult is stage sensitive, meaning that the effect varies depending on the stage of embryonic development at which the exposure occurs.

The effect of each teratogen depends on the period of exposure:

(a) Fertilisation—Early implantation (days 0–15 post-fertilisation), the effect of an insult is often all-or-nothing. Implantation failure or spontaneous miscarriage when teratogenic exposure occurs during the first 15 days of development or, if just some few cells would be affected, the embryo would able to effectively repair itself.
(b) Organogenesis (day 18 through day 60), anatomical malformations may be induced.
(c) Fetal development during the second and third trimesters of pregnancy, exposures may

lead to growth restriction, stillbirth, or impaired cognitive development.

In addition, Karnofsky's law is also important and relevant, and says that any substance "administered at the proper dosage, at the proper stage of development to embryos of the proper species will be effective in causing disturbances in embryonic development" [6].

Finally, the United States Food and Drug Administration (FDA) lists five categories of labelling for drug use in pregnancy:

(a) Controlled studies in women fail to demonstrate a risk to the fetus in the first trimester, and the possibility of fetal harm appears remote;
(b) Animal studies do not indicate a risk to the fetus; there are no controlled human studies or animal studies that show an adverse effect on the fetus, but well-controlled studies in pregnant women have failed to demonstrate a risk to the fetus;
(c) Studies show the drug to have animal teratogenic or embryocidal effects, but no controlled studies are available in women, or no studies are available in either animals or women;
(d) Positive evidence of human fetal risk exists, but benefits in certain situations (e.g. life-threatening situations or serious diseases for which safer drugs cannot be used or are ineffective) may make use of the drug acceptable despite its risks;
(e) Studies in animals or humans have demonstrated fetal abnormalities, or evidence demonstrates fetal risk based on human experience, or both, and the risk clearly outweighs any possible benefit [7].

Obesity

Obesity has become a major health problem worldwide. The World Health Organization defined normal weight as BMI of 18.5–24.9 kg/m^2, overweight as BMI of 25–29.9 kg/m^2, and obesity as a BMI over 30 kg/m^2. Obesity was further divided into three classes: BMI 30.0–34.9 kg/

m^2 (class I), BMI 35.0–39.9 kg/m^2 (class 2), and BMI 40 kg/m^2 and over (class 3 or morbid obesity). Obesity in pregnancy is defined as a BMI of 30 kg/m^2 or more at the first antenatal consultation [8, 9].

Many studies were published in recent years discussing the association of obesity with adverse pregnancy outcomes. In 2015, a systematic review of reviews was conducted to compare pregnant women of healthy weight with women with obesity, and measure a health outcome for mother and/or baby. Narrative analysis of the 22 reviews shows gestational diabetes, pre-eclampsia, gestational hypertension, depression, instrumental and caesarean birth, and surgical site infection to be more likely to occur in pregnant women with obesity compared with women with a healthy weight. Maternal obesity is also linked to greater risk of preterm birth, large-for-gestational-age babies, fetal defects, congenital anomalies, and perinatal death [10].

Studies that were published during the last decade demonstrate clear association between obesity and RPL. A case–control study that included a total of 1644 obese (BMI >30 kg/m^2) women and 3288 age-matched normal weight controls (BMI 19–24.9 kg/m^2) found that the risks of early miscarriage and recurrent early miscarriages (three or more miscarriages between 6 and 12 weeks) were significantly higher among the obese patients (OR 1.2 and 3.5, 95 % CI 1.01–1.46 and 1.03–12.01, respectively; $p = 0.04$, for both) [11].

Metwally et al. conducted a prospective study of a total of 844 pregnancies from 491 patients with recurrent miscarriage to investigate the effect of overweight and obesity on the risk of miscarriage in the subsequent pregnancy in women with recurrent miscarriage. Obese patients had a significantly higher odds of miscarriage (OR 1.71; 95 % CI 1.05–2.8); however, no significant association was found between overweight women and RPL (OR 1.02; 95 % CI 0.72–1.45). They concluded that in women with recurrent miscarriage, a mild increase in the body mass index does not increase the risk of miscarriage, whereas obese patients have a small but significant increased risk of miscarriage in the subsequent pregnancy [12].

In 2012 a systematic review of published studies was performed. Data were compared for obese (BMI ≥28 or 30 kg/m^2), overweight (BMI 25–29 kg/m^2), and normal-weight (BMI <25 kg/m^2) women, with pooled odds ratios (ORs). Six studies met the criteria for a cohort of 28,538 women. Pooled analysis revealed a higher miscarriage rate of 13.6 % in 3800 obese versus 10.7 % in 17,146 normal-BMI women (OR 1.31; 95 % CI 1.18–1.46). Although the cohort was small, there was a higher prevalence of recurrent early miscarriage in obese versus normal-BMI women (0.4 % versus 0.1 %; OR 3.51; 95 % CI 1.03–12.01). In women with recurrent miscarriage, there was a higher miscarriage rate in the obese versus nonobese women (46 % versus 43 %; OR 1.71) [13].

Lo et al. determined the relationship between maternal BMI and future outcome of pregnancy in 696 couples with unexplained recurrent miscarriage. Logistic regression demonstrated that maternal obesity (BMI ≥ 30 kg/m^2) significantly increased the risk of miscarriage (OR 1.73; 95 % CI 1.06–2.83). No difference in the miscarriage rate was found among those who were overweight (OR 1.27, 95 % CI 0.89–1.83) [14]. Sugiura-Ogasawara summarised those four studies in recent review on RPL and obesity, published at 2015 (See Table 9.1) [15].

In an observational cohort study using prospectively collected data, Boots et al. determined whether the frequency of euploid miscarriage is increased in obese women with recurrent early pregnancy loss. Conventional cytogenetic analysis and, when indicated, microsatellite analysis and/or comparative genomic hybridisation, was performed in aborted conceptuses of a total of 372 women with recurrent early pregnancy loss (defined as ≥2 pregnancy losses <10 weeks), and at least one ultrasound-documented miscarriage with chromosome results. Of the 117 subsequent miscarriages with chromosome results, the frequency of a euploid miscarriage among obese (BMI ≥30 kg/m^2) women was 58 % compared with 37 % of nonobese (BMI <30 kg/m^2) women (relative risk = 1.63; 95 % CI 1.08–2.47) [16].

Several mechanisms were reported in the literature with regard to the effect of obesity on

Table 9.1 Studies concerning the association between obesity and recurrent pregnancy loss

	Study design	No. of patients	Definition of obese	Definition of RM	Or (95 % CI)
Lashen et al. [11]	Case–control study	1644 obese women: 3288 age-matched with normal BMI	Obese BMI >30 kg/ m^2 normal BMI 19–24.9 kg/m^2	Early (6–12 weeks) three or more	Early miscarriage: 1.2 (1.01–1.46) early RM: 3.5 (1.03–12.0)
Metwally et al. [12]	Prospective cohort	844 subsequent pregnancies in 491 patients with RM			Obese: 1.71 (1.05–2.8) Underweight: 3.98 (1.06–14.92)
Lo et al. [14]	Prospective cohort	First subsequent pregnancy in 696 patients with unexplained RM	Obese BMI ≥30 kg/ m^2 Overweight BMI 25.0–29.99 kg/m^2 Normal BMI 18.5–24.99 kg/m^2 Underweight BMI <18.5 kg/m^2	Three or more	Obese: 1.73 (1.06–2.83) Asian: 2.87 (1.52–5.39) Age: 1.99 (1.45–2.73) No. of previous miscarriages: 2.08 (1.42–3.06)
Boots et al. [15]	Prospective cohort	117 Aborted conceptuses of subsequent miscarriage	Obese BMI ≥30 kg/ m^2 nonobese BMI <30 kg/m^2	Two or more RPL <10 weeks	Relative risk of euploid rate 1.63 (1.08–2.47)

RM recurrent miscarriage [adapted from Sugiura-Ogasawara M. Recurrent pregnancy loss and obesity. Best Pract Res Clin Obstet Gynaecol. 2015;29(4):489–97. With permission from Elsevier]

miscarriages. One of them is an adverse impact on endometrial development or a detrimental effect on ovaries, affecting oocyte quality and hence embryo viability or combination of both. Another potential mechanism is an increased production of inflammatory and prothrombotic agents produced by adipose tissue or released from endothelium secondary to stimulation by adipocyte-derived factors. It has been suggested that plasminogen activator inhibitor type 1 (PAI-1) is associated with increased rates of miscarriage in association with maternal obesity [17].

Clark et al. reported that weight loss among women with elevated BMI is associated with decreased pregnancy loss rate in anovulatory obese women [18]. The potential effect of weight loss on the RPL should be assessed in future studies.

Air Pollution

Air pollution, one of the most prevalent environmental hazards, which affects up to 100 % of the population living in urban areas, has gained considerable interest because of the multiple adverse

effects reported on human health [19]. It is a known risk factor for cardiovascular [20–22] and respiratory disease [23–25], and the International Agency for Research on Cancer (IARC), the division of the World Health Organization (WHO) that coordinates cancer research, has classified outdoor air pollution as carcinogenic to humans [26].

The associations between air pollution and adverse reproductive outcomes have also been described, including a restricted fetal growth leading to low birth weight newborns small for gestational age, and preterm birth [27–31].

Air pollutants that have mainly been studied in relation to adverse birth outcomes are particulate matter with aerodynamic diameter of less than 2.5 μm (PM 2.5), NO_2, CO, SO_2, PAHs (polycyclic aromatic hydrocarbons), and ozone (O3).

The associations between air pollution and miscarriages also have been described by several authors. Faiz et al. examined the risk of fetal loss associated with ambient air pollution during pregnancy. Using live birth and fetal death data, the authors assigned daily concentrations of air pollution to each birth or fetal death. The relative odds of fetal loss in the first trimester were significantly increased with each 10-ppb increase in mean nitrogen dioxide concentration (OR = 1.16, 95 % CI 1.03–1.31) and each 3-ppb increase in mean sulphur dioxide concentration (OR = 1.13, 95 % CI 1.01–1.28) [32].

Mohorovic et al. conducted a retrospective epidemiological study to evaluate the role of environmental factors in miscarriages. Methaemoglobin in the bloodstream was used as the biomarker. The frequencies of miscarriages were significantly lower in the control than in the exposure period ($p < 0.05$) [33].

In a cohort study, living within 50 m of a road with maximum annual average daily traffic was significantly associated with spontaneous miscarriage among African Americans (OR = 3.11; 95 % CI 1.26–7.66) and non-smokers (OR = 1.47; 95 % CI 1.07–2.04) [34].

With regard to studies conducted in women undergoing IVF/ET, a significant increase in miscarriage rate among women in the quartile with higher exposure to PM10 (OR 5.05, 95 % CI 1.04–24.51) was observed by Perin et al. [35].

In a recent retrospective case–control study, 959 fetal losses and 959 normal intrauterine pregnancies (controls) were selected. The association between ambient air pollutants and fetal loss was examined. Logistic regression suggested that fetal loss within 14 weeks was associated with higher exposure to SO_2 (OR = 19.76, 95 % CI 2.34–166.71) in the first month of pregnancy [36].

Several mechanisms were reported in the literature with regard to the effect of air pollutants on pregnancy outcomes including miscarriages.

1. Reduction of oxygen-carrying capacity of maternal haemoglobin, which could adversely affect oxygen delivery to fetal circulation. This is represented, for example, by CO. CO crosses the placental barrier and disturbs oxygen delivery to the fetal tissues (because fetal haemoglobin has greater affinity for binding CO than does adult haemoglobin) [37–41].
2. Oxidative stress. Kannan et al. have, however, suggested that PM exposure may cause oxidative stress, induce pulmonary and placental

inflammation, alter blood coagulation factors, influence endothelial functions, and trigger haemodynamic responses that restrict fetal growth through impaired transplacental oxygen and nutrient exchange [42].
3. Impaired trophoblast proliferation. Dejmek et al. indicated that PAHs may directly affect early trophoblast proliferation. This is due to their reaction with placental growth factor receptors, thereby hampering feto-placental exchange of oxygen and nutrients, and consequently impairing fetal growth [43].
4. DNA damage. Others have also hypothesised that PAHs and/or their metabolites may bind to the aryl hydrocarbon receptor, resulting in anti-estrogenic effects thereby disrupting the endocrine system and interfering with uterine growth during pregnancy [44, 45]. Fetal toxicity from DNA damage and resulting activation of apoptotic pathways have also been proposed [46].

Caffeine

Animal data on the toxicity of caffeine have demonstrated teratogenicity from caffeine only at very high doses. The teratogenic effect of caffeine has been clearly demonstrated, for example in rodents. Consumption of caffeine by oral-gastric intubation or intraperitoneal injection with doses ranging from 6 to 250 mg/kg indicate that at a dose of 250 mg/kg, 50 % of the mothers die, and at 200 mg/kg survivors frequently develop seizures within minutes of dosing. Evidence of teratogenesis was seen when dosing rose above 75–80 mg/kg. This dose also resulted in a doubling of the number of fetal deaths. The incidence of congenital malformations was not significantly different from that in controls until a dose of 125 mg/kg was exceeded [47].

Caffeine can cross the placental and blood brain barriers and the human fetus may not have developed enzymes for detoxification of caffeine via demethylation [48]. It has been hypothesised that caffeine inhibits cyclic nucleotide phosphodiesterases with a consequent increase in cellular cyclic adenosine monophosphate (cAMP), [49] and the rise in cAMP may interfere with fetal cell growth and development [50].

Several studies have shown the association between caffeine exposure and miscarriage. In 1998, a meta-analysis of 12 studies, which compared a caffeine-exposed group (>150 mg/d) and controls (0–150 mg/d), concluded that the Mantel-Haenszel odds ratio (95 % CI) for spontaneous miscarriage in 42,988 pregnancies was 1.36 (1.29–1.45) [51].

In 2003, A case–control study of 474 women indicated that high caffeine consumption during pregnancy (>300 mg/day), in particular coffee consumption, is an independent risk factor for increased risk of miscarriage. Adjusted odds ratios were 1.94 [95 % CI 1.04–3.63] for 301–500 mg/day and 2.18 [95 % CI 1.08–4.40] for >500 mg/day [52].

In a prospective cohort study involving 3135 women, the relative risk for spontaneous miscarriage for women consuming over 150 mg of caffeine daily was 1.73 ($p = .03$) [53]. In a case–control study, Kline et al. [54] karyotyped 900 pregnancy losses prior to 28 weeks of gestation and employed 1423 controls. In women who consumed more than 225 mg of caffeine daily during pregnancy, the adjusted odds ratio for chromosomally normal losses versus controls was 1.9 (1.3–2.6), which was statistically significant.

A case–control study of 331 women with spontaneous miscarriage showed that caffeine intake before and during pregnancy was associated with an increased risk of fetal loss. After controlling for confounding factors, there was a strong association of caffeine intake during pregnancy and fetal loss, compatible with a linear trend on the logistic scale in which ORs increased by a factor of 1.22 (1.10–1.34) for each 100 mg of caffeine ingested daily during pregnancy. Consumption of less than 162 mg/day were not associated with an increased risk of fetal loss [55].

Another case–control study of 330 women with spontaneous miscarriages found that consumption of 375 mg or more caffeine per day during pregnancy may increase the risk of spontaneous miscarriage OR 2.21 (1.53–3.18) [56].

In a recent prospective cohort study that included 5132 women planning pregnancy, women reported their daily caffeine and caffeinated beverage consumption on questionnaires before conception and during early pregnancy; 732 women (14.3 %) had spontaneous miscarriages. In the preconception period, caffeine consumption was not materially associated with spontaneous miscarriage risk (Hazard Ratio comparing ≥300 with <100 mg/day: 1.09; 95 % CI 0.89–1.33). In early pregnancy, the Hazard Ratios for 100–199, 200–299, and ≥300 mg/day of caffeine consumption were 1.62 (95 % CI 1.19–2.22), 1.48 (95 % CI 1.03–2.13), and 1.23 (95 % CI 0.61–2.46), respectively, compared with <100 mg/day. They concluded that preconception caffeine consumption was not materially associated with an increased risk of spontaneous miscarriage, but consumption during early pregnancy was associated with a small increased risk, although the relation was not linear [57].

It is important to emphasise that in regard to caffeine consumption there may be several confounders that may be relevant: In a cohort study, an increased mean daily caffeine intake in women with spontaneous abortions was reported. But, heavier caffeine consumers were also significantly older and more likely to smoke cigarettes, which could have confounded the results of this study [58]. Successful pregnancies may also be more often associated with food aversion, nausea, and vomiting than pregnancies destined to result in miscarriage, and because coffee is one of the foods most commonly found unappealing under these circumstances, women with successful pregnancies may therefore decrease their coffee intake, whereas women destined to early pregnancy loss may not [59]. Therefore, even though several studies have reported an association between higher caffeine intake and spontaneous miscarriage, the relationship may not necessarily be causal.

Cigarette Smoking

Maternal cigarette smoking is a well-known cause associated with adverse reproductive outcomes including increases incidence of abruptio placentae, placenta previa, bleeding during pregnancy, premature rupture of membranes, and reduced fertility [60]. Exposed infants are more likely to be of low birth weight (<2500 g) and have twice the risk of infant mortality from all causes, specifically from sudden infant death syndrome [61].

Cigarette smoking contains plenty of toxic components. Nicotine, the main addictive compound, is a strong vasoconstrictor that reduces uterine and placental blood flow. Other toxic components include carbon monoxide, which binds to haemoglobin and decreases the availability of oxygen to the fetus and cyanide, which depletes vitamin B 12, a necessary cofactor for fetal growth and development [62]. Cigarette smoking is measured in the studies by self-reports or by urine analysis (urine cotinine concentrations).

Several studies have shown the association between cigarette smoking and miscarriage, but not all of them. In 1996, in a systematic review of the literature, including seven studies evaluating spontaneous miscarriage, suggested a small increased risk among female smokers (OR 0.83–1.8). The dose–response effect was consistent [63]. A retrospective study of 12,914 pregnancies found a significant increase in risk for spontaneous miscarriage with maternal cigarette smoking. The risk of spontaneous miscarriage for smokers was as much as 1.7 times that of the nonsmoker group [64].

Harlap et al. in a prospective study of 32,019 women, found after adjustment for alcohol use, that the only subgroup in which smoking had a significant adverse effect was in those women smoking more than two packs of cigarettes per day. In this group, the odds ratio for second-trimester pregnancy loss was 2.02 (95 % CI 1.01–4.01) [65].

In another prospective study of 970 women, the presence of cotinine in urine was independently associated with an increased risk of spontaneous miscarriage (OR 1.8; 95 % CI 1.3–2.6) [66].

Armstrong et al. analysed data of occupational factors and pregnancy outcome from 47,146 women, to examine the effects of cigarette smoking on pregnancy outcome. Clear and statistically significant associations were found between cigarettes and spontaneous miscarriage. If the associations were causal, 11 % of the spontaneous miscarriages could be attributed to smoking [67].

On the other hand, Wisborg et al. in a prospective study found no association between smoking and first- and second-trimester miscarriages. Adjustment for alcohol, coffee, maternal age, marital status, occupation, education, prepregnancy body mass index, and parity did not change the result substantially [68].

What about environmental tobacco smoke and passive smoking? The chemical exposure from passive smoking is qualitatively similar but quantitatively different from that of the smoker. The undiluted sidestream smoke contains many harmful chemicals in greater amounts than the inhaled cigarette smoke. For example, the amount of nicotine in the undiluted sidestream is seven times more [69]. But when it is diluted, the concentration in the air is low. In meta-analyses, the scientific evidence on the effects of preconception and prenatal exposure to environmental tobacco smoke on reproductive health has been described. The associations noted between passive exposure and spontaneous miscarriage are of similar magnitude as the associations found between spontaneous miscarriage and active smoking, although the effect of passive exposure might be expected to be much lower than that of active smoking [70].

In summary, the data evaluating smoking and miscarriage suggest an increased risk for early pregnancy loss that is dose dependent. The evidence on the effects of environmental tobacco smoke on spontaneous miscarriage is weak but a potential relationship between exposure and spontaneous miscarriage cannot be excluded.

Alcohol

Maternal alcohol consumption is known to be teratogenic and associated with fetal alcohol syndrome. Fetal alcohol syndrome includes growth restriction, a pattern of craniofacial anomalies, neurological effects, and behavioural effects [71]. In 1983, Kaufman described that ethanol consumption at the time of conception may be the cause of certain types of chromosomal defects commonly observed in human spontaneous miscarriages [72]. Animal data on the toxicity of ethanol have demonstrated the risk for pregnancy failure. Animals were given a 1.8 g/kg dose of ethanol once per week for the first 3, 6, or 24 weeks (full gestation) of pregnancy. Peak plasma ethanol levels ranged from 175 to 250 mg/dl. Weekly maternal exposure to this intoxicating dose of ethanol, starting early in pregnancy, did not influence risk of pregnancy failure during the first 30 days of gestation but appeared to be associated with an increased risk of miscarriage occurring between gestational days 30 and 160 [73]. Studies on the association between alcohol consumption and miscarriage have yielded inconsistent results:

Harlap et al. in a prospective study of 32,019 women, found that the adjusted relative risks of second-trimester losses (15–27 weeks) were 1.03 (not significant) for women taking less than 1 drinks daily, 1.98 ($p < 0.01$) for women taking 1–2 drinks daily, and 3.53 ($p < 0.01$) for women taking more than 3 drinks daily, compared with non-drinkers. The increased risk of second-trimester miscarriage in drinkers was not explained by age, parity, race, marital status, smoking, or the number of previous spontaneous miscarriages or induced abortions [65].

In a large case–control study of spontaneous miscarriages (626 cases, 1,300 controls), the odds ratio for alcohol consumption of seven or more drinks per week was 1.9 (95 % CI 1.1–3.4) when adjusted for maternal smoking, passive smoking, and maternal age [74].

Armstrong et al. analysed data of occupational factors and pregnancy outcome from 47,146 women to examine the effects of alcohol on pregnancy outcome. Clear and statistically significant associations were found between alcohol consumption and spontaneous miscarriage (odds ratios increased on average by a factor of 1.26 (1.19–1.33) for each drink per day). If the associations were causal, 5 % of the spontaneous miscarriages could be attributed to alcohol consumption [67].

Another case–control study of 330 women with spontaneous miscarriages found that consumption of 5 or more units of alcohol per week during pregnancy may increase the risk of spontaneous miscarriage (OR 4.84, 95 % CI 2.87–8.16) [56].

In a cohort study, women consuming ≥ 5 drinks/week are at increased risk of first trimester spontaneous miscarriage. No association was found between alcohol intake and spontaneous miscarriage during the second trimester [75].

Very few studies described no association between alcohol consumption and pregnancy loss. Halmesmaki et al. found that moderate maternal or paternal alcohol consumption does not increase the risk of miscarriage. There were no significant differences between the incidence of alcohol consumption in the miscarriage (13 %) and the control (11 %) groups [76]. In a case–control study, the relation between alcohol consumption and the risk of recurrent miscarriage was analysed. Cases were 94 women who had two or more "unexplained" miscarriages (after exclusion of genetic, endocrine, and Müllerian factors). Controls were 176 women admitted for normal delivery without previous miscarriages. Compared with non-drinkers the risk of recurrent miscarriage was 0.9 for regular drinkers [77].

Alcohol consumers may be older, more often smokers, and caffeine consumers, which could have confounded the results of some studies. Alcohol consumption is also known to be underreported in questionnaires.

References

1. Curtis D, Klaassen. Casarett and Doull's toxicology, the basic science of poisons. 6th ed. New York: McGraw-Hill; 2011.
2. Wilson JG. Environment and birth defects (environmental science series). London: Academic; 1973.

3. Wilson JG. Embryotoxicity of drugs in man. In: Wilson JG, Fraser FC, editors. Handbook of teratology, vol. 1. New York: Plenum; 1977. p. 309–55.

4. Brent RL. Editor's note. Teratology. 1978;17:183–4.

5. Beckman DA, Brent RL. Mechanisms of teratogenesis. Ann Rev Pharmacol Toxicol. 1984;24:483–500.

6. Karnofsky CA. Mechanisms of action of certain growth-inhibiting drugs. In: Wilson JG, Warkany J, editors. Teratology: principles and techniques. Chicago: University of Chicago Press; 1965. p. 185–213.

7. Teratology Society Public Affairs Committee. FDA classification of drugs for teratogenic risk. Teratology. 1994;49:446.

8. National Institute for Health and Clinical Excellence. Obesity. Guidance on the prevention, identification, assessment and management of overweight and obesity in adults and children. London: National Institute for Health and Clinical Excellence (NICE); 2006.

9. World Health Organization. Obesity: preventing and managing the global epidemic. Geneva: World Health Organization; 2000.

10. Marchi J, Berg M, Dencker A, Olander EK, Begley C. Risks associated with obesity in pregnancy, for the mother and baby: a systematic review of reviews. Obes Rev. 2015;16(8):621–38.

11. Lashen H, Fear K, Sturdee DW. Obesity is associated with increased risk of first trimester and recurrent miscarriage: matched case-control study. Hum Reprod. 2004;19:1644–6.

12. Metwally M, Saravelos SH, Ledger WL, Li TC. Body mass index and risk of miscarriage in women with recurrent miscarriage. Fertil Steril. 2010;94:290–5.

13. Boots C, Stephenson MD. Does obesity increase the risk of miscarriage in spontaneous conception: a systematic review. Semin Reprod Med. 2011;29:507–13.

14. Lo W, Rai R, Hameed A, Brailsford SR, Al-Ghamdi AA, Regan L. The effect of body mass index on the outcome of pregnancy in women with recurrent miscarriage. J Family Community Med. 2012;19:167–71.

15. Sugiura-Ogasawara M. Recurrent pregnancy loss and obesity. Best Pract Res Clin Obstet Gynaecol. 2015;29(4):489–97.

16. Boots CE, Bernardi LA, Stephenson MD. Frequency of euploid miscarriage is increased in obese women with recurrent early pregnancy loss. Fertil Steril. 2014;102:455–9.

17. Lim CC, Mahmood T. Obesity in pregnancy. Best Pract Res Clin Obstet Gynaecol. 2015;29(3):309–19.

18. Clark AM, Ledger W, Galletly C, Tomlinson L, Blaney F, Wang X, Norman RJ. Weight loss results in significantly improvement in pregnancy and ovulation rates in anovulatory obese women. Hum Reprod. 1995;10:2705–12.

19. Brunekreef B, Holgate ST. Air pollution and health. Lancet. 2002;360:1233–42.

20. Beelen R, Stafoggia M, Raaschou-Nielsen O, Andersen ZJ, Xun WW, Katsouyanni K, et al. Long-term exposure to air pollution and cardiovascular mortality: an analysis of 22 European cohorts. Epidemiology. 2014;25:368–78.

21. Shah AS, Langrish JP, Nair H, McAllister DA, Hunter AL, Donaldson K, et al. Global association of air pollution and heart failure: a systematic review and meta-analysis. Lancet. 2013;382:1039–48.

22. Uzoigwe JC, Prum T, Bresnahan E, Garelnabi M. The emerging role of outdoor and indoor air pollution in cardiovascular disease. N Am J Med Sci. 2013;5:445–53.

23. Sava F, Carlsten C. Respiratory health effects of ambient air pollution: an update. Clin Chest Med. 2012;33:759–69.

24. Laumbach RJ, Kipen HM. Respiratory health effects of air pollution: update on biomass smoke and traffic pollution. J Allergy Clin Immunol. 2012;129:3–11.

25. Pope III CA, Dockery DW, Spengler JD, Raizenne ME. Respiratory health and PM10 pollution. A daily time series analysis. Am Rev Respir Dis. 1991;144:668–74.

26. Loomis D, Grosse Y, Lauby-Secretan B, El Ghissassi F, Bouvard V, Benbrahim-Tallaa L, et al. The carcinogenicity of outdoor air pollution. Lancet Oncol. 2013;14:1262–3.

27. Dadvand P, Parker J, Bell ML, Bonzini M, Brauer M, Darrow LA, et al. Maternal exposure to particulate air pollution and term birth weight: a multi-country evaluation of effect and heterogeneity. Environ Health Perspect. 2013;121:267–373.

28. Pedersen M, Giorgis-Allemand L, Bernard C, Aguilera I, Andersen AM, Ballester F, et al. Ambient air pollution and low birthweight: a European cohort study (ESCAPE). Lancet Respir Med. 2013;1:695–704.

29. Laurent O, Wu J, Li L, Chung J, Bartell S. Investigating the association between birth weight and complementary air pollution metrics: a cohort study. Environ Health. 2013;12:18.

30. Estarlich M, Ballester F, Aguilera I, Fernández-Somoano A, Lertxundi A, Llop S, et al. Residential exposure to outdoor air pollution during pregnancy and anthropometric measures at birth in a multicenter cohort in Spain. Environ Health Perspect. 2011;119:1333–8.

31. Candela S, Ranzi A, Bonvicini L, Baldacchini F, Marzaroli P, Evangelista A. Air pollution from incinerators and reproductive outcomes: a multisite study. Epidemiology. 2013;24:863–70.

32. Faiz AS, Rhoads GG, Demissie K, Kruse L, Lin Y, Rich DQ. Ambient air pollution and the risk of stillbirth. Am J Epidemiol. 2012;176:308–16.

33. Mohorovic L, Petrovic O, Haller H, Micovic V. Pregnancy loss and maternal methemoglobin levels: an indirect explanation of the association of environmental toxics and their adverse effects on the mother and the fetus. Int J Environ Res Public Health. 2010;7:4203–12.

34. Green RS, Malig B, Windham GC, Fenster L, Ostro B, Swan S. Residential exposure to traffic and spontaneous abortion. Environ Health Perspect. 2009;117:1939–44.

35. Perin PM, Maluf M, Czeresnia CE, Januário DA, Saldiva PH. Impact of shortterm preconceptional exposure to particulate air pollution on treatment

outcome in couples undergoing in vitro fertilization and embryo transfer (IVF/ET). J Assist Reprod Genet. 2010;27:371–82.

36. Hou HY, Wang D, Zou XP, Yang ZH, Li TC, Chen YQ. Does ambient air pollutants increase the risk of fetal loss? A case-control study. Arch Gynecol Obstet. 2014;289:285–91.

37. Salam MT, Millstein J, Li YF, Lurmann FW, Margolis HG, Gilliland FD. Birth outcomes and prenatal exposure to ozone, carbon monoxide, and particulate matter: results from the Children's Health Study. Environ Health Perspect. 2005;113(11):1638–44.

38. Sangalli MR, Mclean AJ, Peek MJ, Rivory LP, Le Couteur DG. Carbon monoxide disposition and permeability-surface area product in the fetal circulation of the perfused term human placenta. Placenta. 2003;24(1):8–11.

39. Longo LD. The biological effects of carbon monoxide on the pregnant woman, fetus, and newborn infant. Am J Obstet Gynecol. 1977;129(1):69–103.

40. Di Cera E, Doyle ML, Morgan MS, De Cristofaro R, Landolfi R, Bizzi B, et al. Carbon monoxide and oxygen binding to human hemoglobin F0. Biochemistry. 1989;28(6):2631–8.

41. Bosley ARJ, Sibert JR, Newcombe RG. Effects of maternal smoking on fetal growth and nutrition. Arch Dis Child. 1981;56:727–9.

42. Kannan S, Misra DP, Dvonch JT, Krishnakumar A. Exposures to airborne particulate matter and adverse perinatal outcomes: a biologically plausible mechanistic framework for exploring potential effect modification by nutrition. Environ Health Perspect. 2006;114(11):1636–42.

43. Dejmek J, Solanský I, Benes I, Leníček J, Sra´m RJ. The impact of polycyclic aromatic hydrocarbons and fine particles on pregnancy outcome. Environ Health Perspect. 2000;108(12):1159–64.

44. Carpenter DO, Arcaro K, Spink DC. Understanding the human health effects of chemical mixtures. Environ Health Perspect. 2002;110 Suppl 1:25–42.

45. Bui QQ, Tran MB, West WL. A comparative study of the reproductive effects of methadone and benzo[a] pyrene in the pregnant and pseudopregnant rat. Toxicology. 1986;42(2–3):195–204.

46. Nicol CJ, Harrison ML, Laposa RR, Gimelshtein IL, Wells PG. A teratologic suppressor role for p53 in benzo[a]pyrene-treated transgenic p53-deficient mice. Nat Genet. 1995;10(2):181–7.

47. Bertrand M, Schwam E, Frandon A, Vagne A, Alary J. Surun effet teratogene systematique et specifique de la cafeinechez les rongeurs. C R Soc Biol (Paris). 1965;159:2199–202.

48. Eteng MU, Eyong EU, Akpanyung EO, Agiang MA, Aremu CY. Recent advances in caffeine and theobromine toxicities: a review. Plant Foods Hum Nutr. 1997;51:231–43.

49. Morris MB, Weinstein L. Caffeine and the fetus: is trouble brewing? Am J Obstet Gynecol. 1981;140: 607–10.

50. Weathersbee PS, Lodge R. Caffeine: its direct and indirect influence on reproduction. J Reprod Med. 1977;19:55–63.

51. Fernandes O, Sabharwal M, Smiley T, Pastuszak A, Koren G, Einarson T. Moderate to heavy caffeine consumption during pregnancy and relationship to spontaneous abortion and abnormal fetal growth: a meta-analysis. Reprod Toxicol. 1998;12:435–44.

52. Giannelli M, Doyle P, Roman E, Pelerin M, Hermon C. The effect of caffeine consumption and nausea on the risk of miscarriage. Paediatr Perinat Epidemiol. 2003;17(4):316–23.

53. Srisuphan W, Bracken MB. Caffeine consumption during pregnancy and association with late spontaneous abortion. Am J Obstet Gynecol. 1986;154:14–20.

54. Kline J, Levin B, Silverman J, Kinney A, Stein Z, Susser M, Warburton D. Caffeine and spontaneous abortion of known karyotype. Epidemiology. 1991;2:409–17.

55. Infante-Rivard C, Fernandez A, Gauthier F, David M, Rivard G. Fetal loss associated with caffeine intake before and during pregnancy. JAMA. 1993;270: 2940–3.

56. Rasch V. Cigarette, alcohol, and caffeine consumption: risk factors for spontaneous abortion. Acta Obstet Gynecol Scand. 2003;82(2):182–8.

57. Hahn KA, Wise LA, Rothman KJ, Mikkelsen EM, Brogly SB, Sørensen HT, et al. Caffeine and caffeinated beverage consumption and risk of spontaneous abortion. Hum Reprod. 2015;30(5):1246–55.

58. Mills JL, Holmes LB, Aarons JH, Simpson JL, Brown ZA, Jovanovic-Peterson LG, et al. Moderate caffeine use and the risk of spontaneous abortion and intrauterine growth retardation. JAMA. 1993;269:593–7.

59. Stein Z, Susser M. Miscarriage, caffeine, and the epiphenomena of pregnancy: the causal model. Epidemiology. 1991;2:163–7.

60. Fielding JE. Smoking and women: tragedy of the majority. N Engl J Med. 1987;317:1343–5.

61. McIntosh ID. Smoking and pregnancy: attributable risks and public health implications. Can J Public Health. 1984;75:141–8.

62. Walsh RA. Effects of maternal smoking on adverse pregnancy outcomes: examination of the criteria of causation. Hum Biol. 1994;66:1059–92.

63. Hughes EG, Brennen BG. Does cigarette smoking impair natural or assisted fecundity? Fertil Steril. 1996;66:679–89.

64. Himmelberger DU, Brown BW, Cohen EN. Cigarette smoking during pregnancy and the occurrence of spontaneous abortion and congenital abnormality. Am J Epidemiol. 1978;108:470.

65. Harlap S, Shiono PH. Alcohol, smoking, and incidence of spontaneous abortions in the first and second trimester. Lancet. 1980;2:173–8.

66. Ness RB, Grisso JA, Hirschinger N, Markovic N, Shaw LM, Day NL, Kline J. Cocaine and tobacco use and the risk of spontaneous abortion. N Engl J Med. 1999;340:333–9.

67. Armstrong BG, McDonald AD, Sloan BA. Cigarette, alcohol, and coffee consumption and spontaneous abortion. Am J Public Health. 1992;82:85–7.

68. Wisborg K, Kesmodel U, Henriksen TB, Hedegaard M, Secher NJ. A prospective study of maternal smoking and spontaneous abortion. Acta Obstet Gynecol Scand. 2003;82(10):936–41.

69. National Research Council. Environmental tobacco smoke: measuring exposures and assessing health effects. Washington, DC: National Academy Press; 1986.

70. Lindbohm ML, Sallmen M, Taskinen H. Effects of exposure to environmental tobacco smoke on reproductive health. Scand J Work Environ Health. 2002;28:84–6.

71. Streissguth AP, LaDue RA. Fetal alcohol: teratogenic causes of developmental disabilities. In: Schroeder S, editor. Toxic substances and mental retardation. Washington, DC: American Association on Mental Deficiency; 1987.

72. Kaufman MH. Ethanol-induced chromosomal abnormalities at conception. Nature. 1983;302:258–60.

73. Clarren SK, Astley SJ. Pregnancy outcomes after weekly oral administration of ethanol during gestation in the pig-tailed macaque: comparing early gestational exposure to full gestational exposure. Teratology. 1992;45:1–9.

74. Windham GC, Fenster L, Swan SH. Moderate maternal and paternal alcohol consumption and the risk of spontaneous abortion. Epidemiology. 1992;3(4): 364–70.

75. Kesmodel U, Wisborg K, Olsen SF, Henriksen TB, Secher NJ. Moderate alcohol intake in pregnancy and the risk of spontaneous abortion. Alcohol. 2002;37(1):87–92.

76. Halmesmaki E, Valimaki M, Roine R, Ylikahri R, Ylikorkala O. Maternal and paternal alcohol consumption and miscarriage. Br J Obstet Gynaecol. 1989;96:188–91.

77. Parazzini F, Bocciolone L, La Vecchia C, Negri E, Fedele L. Maternal and paternal moderate daily alcohol consumption and unexplained miscarriages. Br J Obstet Gynaecol. 1990;97:618–22.

The Common Characteristics Between Infertility and Recurrent Pregnancy Loss

10

Avi Harlev, Deepak Kumar, and Ashok Agarwal

Introduction

Recurrent pregnancy loss (RPL) and infertility are two entities sharing a patient's common unfulfilled desire to conceive and successfully deliver a baby. RPL is most commonly defined as two or more failed clinical pregnancies as documented by either ultrasonography or approved in a histopathologic examination [1]. Infertility is defined as "failure to achieve a successful pregnancy after 12 months or more of appropriate, timed unprotected intercourse or therapeutic donor insemination" [1].

Recently the definition of RPL has been significantly modified and reevaluated. Traditionally, RPL was defined by the European Society of human and the Royal College of Obstetricians and Gynecologists (RCOG) as three consecutive pregnancy losses at less than 20 weeks of gestation [2, 3]. Despite that strict definition for RPL, many caregivers initiated clinical investigation after the second pregnancy loss because an investigation after a third loss occurred, added little clinical insight little clinical insight [4]. Thus, in 2008, the American Society of Reproductive Medicine (ASRM) published the previously mentioned updated definition of RPL [5]. Despite the revised definition, the ASRM still recommends to carefully assess the necessity of any specific evaluation after two losses, but a thorough evaluation of RPL is recommended only after three pregnancy losses [1].

Adhering to the criteria and definitions mentioned above, RPL and infertility are treated as different entities, despite the fact that both are defined as diseases by the ASRM. However, there is an undefined border that brings those entities closer: the pre-clinically documented pregnancy, also known as biochemical pregnancy or a non-visualized pregnancy. This is a type of pregnancy in which a positive pregnancy test confirms the occurrence of fertilization but neither an intrauterine nor an ectopic pregnancy is visualized before a decline in HCG levels are documented indicating the termination of the pregnancy [6–9]. In these pregnancies, although fertilization occurs, complete implantation does not. Thus, these pregnancy losses are considered significant when the prognosis of future pregnancies is evaluated [7–9].

A. Harlev, MD (✉)
Recurrent Pregnancy Loss Clinic, Fertility and IVF Unit, Department of Obstetrics and Gynecology, Soroka University Medical Center, Ben Gurion University of the Negev, Be'er Sheva, Israel

D.N Negev 3, Sansana, 85334, Israel
e-mail: harlev@bgu.ac.il

D. Kumar
Cleveland Clinic, Center for Reproductive Medicine, Cleveland, OH, USA

A. Agarwal, PhD
American Center for Reproductive Medicine, Cleveland Clinic, 10681 Carnegie Avenue, Desk X11, Cleveland, OH 44195, USA

© Springer International Publishing Switzerland 2016
A. Bashiri et al. (eds.), *Recurrent Pregnancy Loss*, DOI 10.1007/978-3-319-27452-2_10

The apparent artificial disparity between RPL and infertility makes it difficult to appropriately interpret and manage cases involving both entities. For example, if fertilization occurs, patients do not meet the criteria of infertility, but at the same time, if no clinical pregnancy is documented, patients do not fit the RPL criteria. These cases of early terminated pregnancies bolstered a broader line of thought by challenging the commonly accepted division between populations with RPL and infertility. Therefore, this chapter aims to address this disparity by reviewing the common etiologies and recommended workup. Further inquiry into this topic will still be required in order to establish a practice which will enable evaluation and treatment of both RPL and infertility under the same multidisciplinary clinic.

The Etiologic Linkage Between RPL and Infertility

Uterine Factors

The uterus and the endometrium play a major role in implantation, which is highly important for successful pregnancy. Uterine anomaly may cause implantation failure either via a mechanical obstacle or through impaired endometrial receptivity (Table 10.1).

Congenital Uterine Anomalies

Congenital uterine anomalies, also known as Mullerian anomalies are the result of an incomplete fusion of the mesonephric ducts [10]. The prevalence of the Mullerian anomaly is debatable as a result of the imprecision of the commonly used diagnostic methods and the lack of widely accepted standard classification. Moreover, since many of the Mullerian anomaly cases are asymptomatic [11], the true prevalence of the anomaly in the general population is difficult to determine [12]. The commonly cited prevalence of uterine anomalies observed in the fertile population is 3.2 % [11]. Reviewing five different studies of

almost 3000 cases, Grimbizis et al. [13] reported an overall incidence of 4.3 % indicating it is relatively common.

The etiology of the congenital uterine anomalies remains unclear with the exception of maternal exposure to diethylstilbestrol (DES) [14].

The Mullerian anomalies are classified according to the severity of the anomaly, the clinical manifestation, treatment, and prognosis. Regrettably, there is no commonly acknowledged classification system for the Mullerian anomalies. The American Fertility Society classification was published on 1988 [15]. In this system the anomalies are classified from type I representing Müllerian agenesis or hypoplasia through type VI representing DES-related anomalies with all the range of anomalies in-between. Likewise, the European Society of Human Reproduction and Embryology (ESHRE) and the European Society for Gynaecological Endoscopy (ESGE) issued in 2013 their classification system [16] ranging from class U0 as the normal uterus to class U5 as the aplastic uterus.

The association between both the congenital and acquired uterine anomalies was reviewed thoroughly in Chap. 7. As concluded there, both congenital and acquired uterine structural anomalies of the uterus play a major role in the pathophysiology of RPL. The diagnostic modality will be a 2D followed by 3D trans-vaginal ultrasonography with a diagnosis rate of more than 95 % of the cases.

The association between congenital uterine anomalies and infertility is less established, creating a debate regarding the approach to uterine anomalies in infertile patients. Several studies suggested that uterine anomalies distort the uterine cavity and as a result increase infertility rates [13, 17, 18], cause RPL [14, 18] and impose perinatal risk of preterm labor amongst other obstetric complications [19, 20] while other studies claim that uterine anomalies cause trouble in maintaining the pregnancy but not in the actual conception [14, 21, 22]. However, accumulating evidence including recent data indicates that resection of a uterine septum may be beneficial in cases of infertile patients [23–25].

Table 10.1 Basic evaluation tests for RPL and infertility

	Test	Aim	Performed
Uterine assessment	2D Ultrasound	Myometrium, endometrium, ovaries, pelvis	RPL + infertility
	3D Ultrasound	Uterine cavity (congenital anomalies), myometrium, endometrium	RPL + infertility
	Hysteroscopy	Uterine cavity, myomas, endometrium (Ashreman syndrome)	RPL + infertility
	Hysterosalpingography	Uterine cavity	Infertility
	Laparoscopy	Endometriosis, tubal potency	Infertility
Fallopian tubes assessment	Hysterosalpingography	Fallopian tubes potency	Infertility
	3D ultrasound	Hydrosalpyx	RPL + infertility
Endocrine assessment	Thyroid function, prolactin	Ovulation dysfunction, implantation failure	RPL + infertility
	Diabetes mellitus screening	Glucose intolerance, hyperandrogenemia	RPL + infertility
Male evaluation	Basic semen analysis	Sperm count and basic function	Infertility
	Advanced semen analysis	DNA fragmentation, sperm immunoglobulin, reactive oxygen species and antioxidants capacity	RPL + infertility
Ovaries	FSH, antral follicular count or AMH	Ovarian reserve assessment	Infertility
Genetic	Karyotype of the couple	Translocations, deletions	RPL
	Karyotype and micro-deletions of the male	Assessment of azoospermia	Infertility
Autoantibodies and immune function	Anti-cardiolipin antibody and lupus anticoagulant	Autoimmune disorders	RPL

RPL recurrent pregnancy loss, *AMH* anti-Mullerian hormone

Leiomyoma

Uterine leiomyomas, also known as leiomyomatas or fibroids, are benign solid tumors of the uterus. They are usually slow-growing and asymptomatic. Myomas are common in woman of reproductive age with prevalence as high as 70–80 % in woman aged 50 years [26]. The myomas differ in their symptoms according to their anatomic location, specifically in the uterine subserosa, intra-myometria or sub-mucous layers. Myomas have been previously reported to be associated with break-through uterine bleeding and symptoms caused by the enlarged uterus imposing on neighboring organs, such as the urinary bladder or the bowel.

Beside the symptoms discussed above, uterine leiomyomas were also reported to be associated with RPL and infertility. Myomas, especially sub-mucous myomas, may distort the endometrial cavity, negatively impacting the implanta-

tion of the embryo. Although the mechanism by which the myomas impact implantation is not completely understood, it is estimated that atrophy of the endometrium overlaying the myoma is the cause for the implantation failure [27]. A systemic review reported a significantly higher rate of pregnancy losses in women with sub-mucous myomas [28]. While atrophic endometrium may cause implantation failure, the distorted shape of the uterus was suggested to alter the gametes and embryo transport through blockage of the tubal ostia, decreasing chance of fertilization and implantation [29, 30].

Myomas altering reproduction can be surgically removed. The surgical approach is determined by the location and size of the myoma. Sub-mucosal myomas can be hysteroscopically removed while intra-mural and sub-serosal myomas can be laparoscopically approached. The impact of the removal on reproduction, however, is still debatable. While the sub-serosal myomas probably do not impact reproduction considerably, their removal question-ably improves reproductive outcome [31]. However, in cases of sub-mucosal myomas and intra-mural myomas, which alter the uterine cavity, surgical resection of the myomas may improve reproduction scores both for infertility and RPL. The same applies to cases of unexplained infertility in the presence of myoma in which myomectomy appears to be beneficial [31–34].

Male Factor

The male factor is a well-established and an obvious cause of infertility. Male factor includes not only the sperm production and function but also other factors such as erectile dysfunction, anatomic alterations like hypospadias or micropenis, endocrine disorders, and others. It was commonly believed that if fertilization did occur, the inability of the fetus to undergo a successful implantation or to maintain the pregnancy was associated with only female factors.

The association between basic semen parameters and RPL is still widely debated [35]. As more advanced tests for male factor were developed, especially in male DNA structures and their impact on the embryonic development, this association changed.

Accumulating evidence supports the link between male factors and RPL. Several studies reported a positive association between paternal age and the risk of RPL [36, 37]. Chromosomal aberrations in the sperm are associated with embryonic developmental arrest or implantation failure and consequently, early pregnancy loss [38]. Male factors are now known to play a key role in fertilization, implantation, embryo development and placental development [39, 40].

The association between male DNA dysfunction and RPL supports the notion that regular work-up should not exclude male factor as an etiology of RPL. Hence, the discovered positive association between sperm dysfunction and RPL led some of the researchers to recommend routine advanced male factor assessment in cases of RPL even in the presence of a normal male infertility basic workup [38].

Endocrine Factors

Polycystic Ovary Syndrome (PCOS), diabetes mellitus, hyperprolactinemia, luteal phase defect, and thyroid antibodies and disease are commonly encountered endocrine factors in cases of both RPL and infertility. Although the exact pathophysiology underlying these disorders in relation to RPL and infertility still remains elusive, experts have determined commonly accepted mechanisms of action. Together, these five disorders serve to establish the endocrinological connection between women with RPL and infertility in terms of shared mechanisms, diagnosis, treatment, and prognosis.

Diabetes Mellitus

There are two types of diabetes mellitus: Type 1 diabetes (T1D) and Type 2 diabetes (T2D). T1D is a disorder in which the body cannot produce sufficient insulin. The more prevalent T2D occurs via the onset of insulin resistance and can be caused by high-fat diets and sedentary lifestyles [41]. Adequate insulin production or supplementation is necessary for the maintenance of a healthy female reproductive system [42]. Females with uncontrolled T1D usually experience delayed menarche [42]. They may also be exposed to acute or chronic hyperglycemia, which has damaging effects on the embryo, particularly via intracellular glucose starvation.

Insulin resistance in T2D patients leads to hyperinsulinemia and can result in ovulatory dysfunction, hyperandrogenism, and infertility [42]. One mechanism in which hyperinsulinemia affects the reproductive hormonal axis is by reducing sex hormone-binding globulin (SHBG). Decreased SHBG activity is coupled with an increase in circulating testosterone levels. This can lead to anovulation because high testosterone levels can suppress FSH [43]. T2D also elevates the glucose production in the liver and increases insulin resistance from other tissue. Because the embryo is sensitive to insulin, inadequate glucose consumption due to hyperinsulinemia and hyperglycemia can lead to apoptosis, increasing the risk of miscarriage [41].

Many women with T2D are also obese and studies have indicated that obese patients usually take longer to conceive and have poorer blastocyst quality [43]. Women with diabetes who also had low BMI displayed high HbA1c levels and had menstrual irregularities [43]. Studies have shown that high HbA1c levels in diabetic pregnant women indicate poor pregnancy outcomes and increased miscarriage rates.

Thus, uncontrolled diabetes mellitus is considered a risk factor for both RPL and infertility primarily because of its association with hyperinsulinemia, hyperglycemia, and obesity and high HbA1c levels.

Polycystic Ovary Syndrome

Polycystic Ovary Syndrome (PCOS) is considered the most common endocrine abnormality, affecting 5–10 % of women of reproductive age [44, 45]. The Rotterdam Criteria for diagnosing PCOS has to fulfill at least two out of the three following criteria: oligo/anovulation, hyperandrogenism, and presence of polycystic ovaries. Women with PCOS display elevated levels of LH and thereby have an increased androgen production in theca cells. Hyperandrogenism can then cause increases in estrone levels, which suppresses FSH production, leading to ovarian dysfunction, oligo/amenorrhea, anovulation, and subsequently, infertility. The prevalence of PCOS in women with RPL is as high as 56 %. Obesity and supraphysiological levels of LH can impair ovarian folliculogenesis and increase risk of miscarriage. Studies have further implicated an association between PCOS and hyperinsulinemia/insulin resistance, obesity, and hyperhomocysteinemia. Hyperinsulinemia and insulin resistance are shown to negatively affect pre-implantation, by decreasing the activity of proteins involved in feto-maternal adhesion. Hyperhomocysteinemia may also have adverse effects on embryo quality. These factors are considered the link between women with PCOS and RPL/infertility [46].

Thyroid Antibodies and Disease

The two main thyroid disorders are hypothyroidism and hyperthyroidism. Hyperthyroidism does not display significant connections to RPL or infertility. Hypothyroidism, primarily caused by Hashimoto's disease, however, affects 2–4 % of women of reproductive age and is associated with miscarriage, preeclampsia, and preterm birth [47]. Hypothyroidism can either be classified as overt (clinical) or subclinical, both of which can increase risk of first trimester loss and infertility. Subclinical hypothyroidism is more common and can directly lead to anovulation and increases in prolactin levels [48]. Women with hypothyroidism display high levels of thyroid-regulating hormone (TRH). TRH activates thyroid-stimulating hormone (TSH) and subsequently the main thyroid hormones, T3 and T4. TRH, additionally, causes idiopathic increases in prolactin levels, which in turn causes dysregulation of hypothalamic hormonal function and ovulatory dysfunction. Amenorrhea in hypothyroidism is linked to hyperprolactinemia, which causes a defect in estrogen to LH positive-feedback mechanism and also suppresses LH and FSH. Even in the absence of hyperprolactinemia, hypothyroidism can result in infertility because adequate thyroid activity is needed for greatest production of estradiol and progesterone [49]. Thyroid antibodies are usually higher in women with RPL and impact trophoblast survival and invasion. They can also cause dysregulation of inflammatory processes (i.e., pregnancy), which can lead to greater risk of miscarriage [50]. Overall thyroid antibodies and hypothyroidism are important common factors affecting women with RPL and infertile women.

Hyperprolactinemia

Hyperprolactinemia is a disorder, in which, there is an abnormally high level of prolactin in the bloodstream. Studies have shown that some of the women who have miscarried and/or considered RPL patients display high prolactin levels [51]. One study suggested that high concentrations of prolactin can inhibit progesterone secretion, leading to luteal insufficiency and resulting in infertility. Hyperprolactinemia can also cause hypothalamic dysfunction, defective ovulation and follicle activity, and reduced fecundability, indicative of miscarriage [51]. A possible mechanism for hyperprolactinemia is via dopamine suppression. As prolactin levels increase, dopamine suppresses prolactin production, but indirectly affects GnRH neurons, resulting in hypogonadotropic hypogonadism and possible anovulation. In another study with mice, an alternative mechanism was proposed. Hyperprolactinemia lowered levels of kisspeptin, a protein that stimulates GnRH secretion [52]. Both mechanisms show the same underlying result: hyperprolactinemia affects the hypothalamic-pituitary-ovarian axis, commonly affecting fertility and pregnancy outcomes.

Luteal Phase Defect

Luteal phase defect (LPD) or insufficiency is characterized by insufficient progesterone production and/or progesterone receptivity [53]. Normally, the corpus luteum produces adequate levels of progesterone to prepare the endometrium for blastocyst implantation, favor Th2 cytokines, which are supportive of pregnancy, with progesterone-induced blocking factor, and inhibit prostaglandins, which initiate uterine contractions, to create a stable environment for implantation. Studies have shown that women with luteal insufficiency can have poor luteal blood flow as well as lower FSH and LH signaling, which is vital for adequate folliculogenesis, oocyte maturation, ovulation, and implantation [54, 55]. LPD can engender anovulation, luteal atrophy, or implantation failure in the first trimester, becoming a potential cause of both infertility and recurrent pregnancy loss in premenopausal women.

Personal Habits

Personal habits such as smoking, alcohol consumption, intense exercise, and substance abuse can negatively impact the female reproductive health and function. Although the exact pathophysiology of these factors is unclear, there are many reports suggesting that these lifestyle choices are potential risk factors for infertility and RPL by causing oxidative stress (OS), hormonal disruption, or physical changes in the female reproductive system.

Smoking

Because of its prevalence, especially in women of reproductive age, cigarette smoking is one of the most clinically relevant risk factors [56]. Cigarette smoke (CS) contains over 4000 chemicals, many of which are known reproductive toxicants [57]. Smoking can lead to many hormonal changes. Research shows that CS causes increased FSH production, shortening the follicular phase and resulting in anovulation, poor luteal function, and menstrual irregularities [58]. Alkaloids present in CS can similarly decrease the production of progesterone, leading to luteal deficiency [59]. CS can also decrease estrogen levels by interfering with granulosa cells and aromatase enzyme, consequently disturbing the pituitary-gonadal axis. One study showed that women who smoked had a significantly increased risk of spontaneous abortion [60].

Harmful chemicals in smoking such as nicotine and polycyclic aromatic hydrocarbons can increase OS in the body by upregulating production of free radicals and/or decreasing antioxidant defenses [57, 61, 62]. Since OS is widely recognized to impair vital processes such as folliculogenesis, steroidogenesis, embryo transport, and uterine receptivity, CS can be highly detrimental to reproductive function. Thus, CS, via OS and hormonal alterations, can result in infertility and high risk pregnancies [63].

Alcohol

Alcohol consumption, like CS, can cause hormonal changes and OS, resulting in infertility and recurrent miscarriage. Alcohol intake is reported to decrease estrogen and progesterone concentrations, inhibit ovulation, and animal experiments have shown that it interferes with sperm passage through the fallopian tube. This can lead to infertility. Alcohol can also induce OS, which can affect oocyte DNA and cause luteal damage and apoptosis, resulting in implantation failure and subsequently, abortion [64].

Women who drink frequently display menstrual disorders such as amenorrhea and dysmenorrhea. Low to moderate alcohol intake is shown to reduce fecundability and in a dose-dependent fashion, can greatly increase risk of first-trimester miscarriage [65]. If even moderate alcohol consumption can lead to reproductive irregularities, alcohol consumption is an important risk factor in both infertile women and women with RPL.

Intense Exercise

Regular exercise is reported to have beneficial impacts on a woman's body and reproductive health and can exhibit protective effects, especially for obese patients [66]. Intense exercise, however, can have negative effects on female reproductive health [67].

Women who engage in strenuous exercise, especially in high-impact exercises, show increased risk of miscarriage [68]. Energy drain, in which energy expenditure overwhelms sufficient dietary reserves, is the primary cause of hormonal disruptions. This extra strain from high physical activity can decrease GnRH pulses, leading to lower levels of LH and FSH and causing anovulation, short luteal phase, mild hyperandrogenism, and amenorrhea. These changes can cause infertility and higher miscarriage rates [69].

Healthy exercise promotes good body health. Through hormonal alterations, however, strenuous exercise can have a detrimental impact on the female reproductive system, resulting in infertility and an increased risk of abortion.

Substance Abuse

Research on substance abuse has been limited due to ethical considerations [66]. Illicit drug use, however, does negatively affect reproductive health

and function. Women who smoked marijuana showed increased risk of developing infertility due to ovulatory irregularities [70]. Marijuana use is also linked with decreases in LH levels, which suggests a decline in uterine receptivity [71].

Cocaine use is reported to decrease responsiveness to gonadotropins and cause placental abruption [66, 72]. It can also cause physical abnormalities in the fallopian tubes increasing the risk of infertility [70]. Both cocaine and marijuana use have been associated with increased risk of miscarriage [73].

Although there is little information on this topic, there is still some evidence suggesting that the use of illicit drugs can lead to infertility and possible recurrent miscarriage either due to hormonal changes or physical alterations of the female reproductive system.

Conclusion and Future Considerations

This chapter aimed to challenge the traditional idea of viewing infertility and RPL as independent entities. The disparity results in completely separate evaluations and varied treatments of these populations by professionals of different disciplines. The challenge to this common concept arises in several aspects. Firstly, many common etiologies are shared by these presently separated populations (Fig. 10.1). Secondly, as a result of the common etiology, a common workup is shared in many cases by both RPL and infertile couples (Table 10.1). Thirdly, some of the cases, especially those involving chemical pregnancies, are difficult to manage appropriately because of the apparent distinction between RPL and infertility and inconsistent definitions and standards of approach for RPL.

One question remains, i.e., the significance of these observations. Obviously, chemical pregnancies should be better defined and the workup for RPL and infertile patients should be revised. From our experience and as a result of the described common characteristics we propose two immediate active measures to be taken. The first is to relate to chemical pregnancies in the same manner as we relate to clinical pregnancies

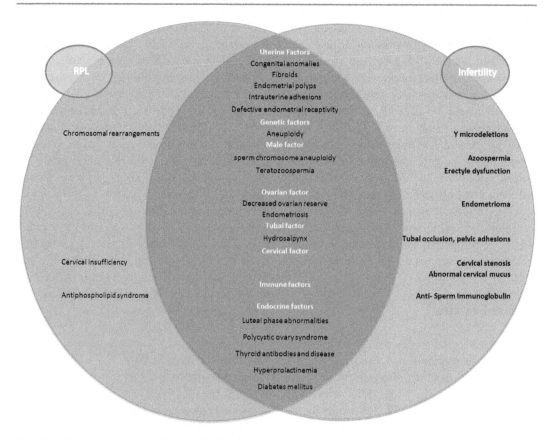

Fig. 10.1 Common causes of RPL and infertility

in terms of abortions. Hence, couples with two or three chemical pregnancies will be defined as RPL patients and undergo the RPL workup. The second is to evaluate and treat the RPL and consistent infertile patients in the same clinic in a multidisciplinary fashion involving both RPL and infertility experts.

References

1. Practice Committee of American Society for Reproductive Medicine. Definitions of infertility and recurrent pregnancy loss: a committee opinion. Fertil Steril. 2013;99(1):63.
2. Rai R, Regan L. Recurrent miscarriage. Lancet. 2006;368(9535):601–11.
3. Jauniaux E, et al. Evidence-based guidelines for the investigation and medical treatment of recurrent miscarriage. Hum Reprod. 2006;21(9):2216–22.
4. Jaslow CR, Carney JL, Kutteh WH. Diagnostic factors identified in 1020 women with two versus three or more recurrent pregnancy losses. Fertil Steril. 2010;93(4):1234–43.
5. Practice Committee of American Society for Reproductive Medicine. Definitions of infertility and recurrent pregnancy loss. Fertil Steril. 2008;90((Suppl 5)):S60.
6. Kirk E, Condous G, Bourne T. Pregnancies of unknown location. Best Pract Res Clin Obstet Gynaecol. 2009;23(4):493–9.
7. Kolte AM, et al. Non-visualized pregnancy losses are prognostically important for unexplained recurrent miscarriage. Hum Reprod. 2014;29(5):931–7.
8. Zeadna A, et al. A comparison of biochemical pregnancy rates between women who underwent IVF and fertile controls who conceived spontaneously. Hum Reprod. 2015;30(4):783–8.
9. Maesawa Y et al. History of biochemical pregnancy was associated with the subsequent reproductive failure among women with recurrent spontaneous abortion. Gynecol Endocrinol. 2015;31(4):306–8.
10. Rackow BW, Arici A. Reproductive performance of women with Mullerian anomalies. Curr Opin Obstet Gynecol. 2007;19(3):229–37.
11. Simon C, et al. Mullerian defects in women with normal reproductive outcome. Fertil Steril. 1991;56(6):1192–3.

12. Raga F, et al. Reproductive impact of congenital Mullerian anomalies. Hum Reprod. 1997;12(10): 2277–81.
13. Grimbizis GF, et al. Clinical implications of uterine malformations and hysteroscopic treatment results. Hum Reprod Update. 2001;7(2):161–74.
14. Propst AM, Hill 3rd JA. Anatomic factors associated with recurrent pregnancy loss. Semin Reprod Med. 2000;18(4):341–50.
15. The American Fertility Society classifications of adnexal adhesions, distal tubal occlusion, tubal occlusion secondary to tubal ligation, tubal pregnancies, Mullerian anomalies and intrauterine adhesions. Fertil Steril. 1988;49(6):944–55.
16. Grimbizis GF, et al. The ESHRE/ESGE consensus on the classification of female genital tract congenital anomalies. Hum Reprod. 2013;28(8):2032–44.
17. Grimbizis G, et al. Hysteroscopic septum resection in patients with recurrent abortions or infertility. Hum Reprod. 1998;13(5):1188–93.
18. Abrao MS, Muzii L, Marana R. Anatomical causes of female infertility and their management. Int J Gynaecol Obstet. 2013;123 Suppl 2:S18–24.
19. Fox NS, et al. Type of congenital uterine anomaly and adverse pregnancy outcomes. J Matern Fetal Neonatal Med. 2014;27(9):949–53.
20. Dhar H. Ruptured rudimentary horn at 22 weeks. Niger Med J. 2012;53(3):175–7.
21. Lin PC, et al. Female genital anomalies affecting reproduction. Fertil Steril. 2002;78(5):899–915.
22. Homer HA, Li TC, Cooke ID. The septate uterus: a review of management and reproductive outcome. Fertil Steril. 2000;73(1):1–14.
23. Mollo A, et al. Hysteroscopic resection of the septum improves the pregnancy rate of women with unexplained infertility: a prospective controlled trial. Fertil Steril. 2009;91(6):2628–31.
24. Tonguc EA, Var T, Batioglu S. Hysteroscopic metroplasty in patients with a uterine septum and otherwise unexplained infertility. Int J Gynaecol Obstet. 2011;113(2):128–30.
25. Freud A et al. Reproductive outcomes following uterine septum resection. J Matern Fetal Neonatal Med. 2015;28(18):2141–4.
26. AAGL practice report: practice guidelines for the diagnosis and management of submucous leiomyomas. J Minim Invasive Gynecol. 2012;19(2):152–71.
27. Deligdish L, Loewenthal M. Endometrial changes associated with myomata of the uterus. J Clin Pathol. 1970;23(8):676–80.
28. Pritts EA, Parker WH, Olive DL. Fibroids and infertility: an updated systematic review of the evidence. Fertil Steril. 2009;91(4):1215–23.
29. Farhi J, et al. Effect of uterine leiomyomata on the results of in-vitro fertilization treatment. Hum Reprod. 1995;10(10):2576–8.
30. Benecke C, et al. Effect of fibroids on fertility in patients undergoing assisted reproduction. A structured literature review. Gynecol Obstet Invest. 2005;59(4):225–30.
31. Carranza-Mamane B, et al. The management of uterine fibroids in women with otherwise unexplained infertility. J Obstet Gynaecol Can. 2015;37(3):277–88.
32. Begum N, et al. Pregnancy outcome following myomectomy. Mymensingh Med J. 2015;24(1):84–8.
33. Bosteels J, et al. Hysteroscopy for treating subfertility associated with suspected major uterine cavity abnormalities. Cochrane Database Syst Rev. 2015;2: CD009461.
34. Borja de Mozota D, Kadhel P, Janky E. Fertility, pregnancy outcomes and deliveries following myomectomy: experience of a French Caribbean University Hospital. Arch Gynecol Obstet. 2014;289(3):681–6.
35. Sbracia S, et al. Semen parameters and sperm morphology in men in unexplained recurrent spontaneous abortion, before and during a 3 year follow-up period. Hum Reprod. 1996;11(1):117–20.
36. Belloc S, et al. Effect of maternal and paternal age on pregnancy and miscarriage rates after intrauterine insemination. Reprod Biomed Online. 2008;17(3):392–7.
37. Kleinhaus K, et al. Paternal age and spontaneous abortion. Obstet Gynecol. 2006;108(2):369–77.
38. PK, Malini SS, Positive association of sperm dysfunction in the pathogenesis of recurrent pregnancy loss. J Clin Diagn Res. 2014;8(11):OC07-10.
39. Check JH, Katsoff D, Check ML. Some semen abnormalities may cause infertility by impairing implantation rather than fertilization. Med Hypotheses. 2001;56(5):653–7.
40. Moomjy M, et al. Sperm integrity is critical for normal mitotic division and early embryonic development. Mol Hum Reprod. 1999;5(9):836–44.
41. Jungheim ES, Moley KH. The impact of type 1 and type 2 diabetes mellitus on the oocyte and the preimplantation embryo. Semin Reprod Med. 2008;26(2):186–95.
42. Nandi A, Poretsky L. Diabetes and the female reproductive system. Endocrinol Metab Clin North Am. 2013;42(4):915–46.
43. Livshits A, Seidman DS. Fertility issues in women with diabetes. Womens Health (Lond Engl). 2009;5(6):701–7.
44. T.E.A.-S.P.C.W. Group. Consensus on infertility treatment related to polycystic ovary syndrome. Hum Reprod. 2008;23(3):462–77.
45. Teede H, Deeks A, Moran L. Polycystic ovary syndrome: a complex condition with psychological, reproductive and metabolic manifestations that impacts on health across the lifespan. BMC Med. 2010;8:41.
46. Chakraborty P, et al. Recurrent pregnancy loss in polycystic ovary syndrome: role of hyperhomocysteinemia and insulin resistance. PLoS One. 2013;8(5):e64446.
47. Vissenberg R, et al. Treatment of thyroid disorders before conception and in early pregnancy: a systematic review. Hum Reprod Update. 2012;18(4):360–73.
48. Sarkar D. Recurrent pregnancy loss in patients with thyroid dysfunction. Indian J Endocrinol Metab. 2012;16 Suppl 2:S350–1.
49. Binita G, et al. Correlation of prolactin and thyroid hormone concentration with menstrual patterns in infertile women. J Reprod Infertil. 2009;10(3):207–12.

50. Thangaratinam S, et al. Association between thyroid autoantibodies and miscarriage and preterm birth: meta-analysis of evidence. BMJ. 2011;342:d2616.
51. Pluchino N, et al. Hormonal causes of recurrent pregnancy loss (RPL). Hormones (Athens). 2014;13(3): 314–22.
52. Kaiser UB. Hyperprolactinemia and infertility: new insights. J Clin Invest. 2012;122(10):3467–8.
53. Ford HB, Schust DJ. Recurrent pregnancy loss: etiology, diagnosis, and therapy. Rev Obstet Gynecol. 2009;2(2):76–83.
54. Takasaki A, et al. Luteal blood flow in patients undergoing GnRH agonist long protocol. J Ovarian Res. 2011;4(1):2.
55. Shah D, Nagarajan N. Luteal insufficiency in first trimester. Indian J Endocrinol Metab. 2013;17(1):44–9.
56. Medicine PCoASfR. Smoking and infertility. Fertil Steril. 2008;90 Suppl 5:S254–9.
57. Mai Z, et al. The effects of cigarette smoke extract on ovulation, oocyte morphology and ovarian gene expression in mice. PLoS One. 2014;9(4):e95945.
58. Windham GC, et al. Cigarette smoking and effects on menstrual function. Obstet Gynecol. 1999;93(1):59–65.
59. Windham GC, et al. Cigarette smoking and effects on hormone function in premenopausal women. Environ Health Perspect. 2005;113(10):1285–90.
60. Chatenoud L, et al. Paternal and maternal smoking habits before conception and during the first trimester: relation to spontaneous abortion. Ann Epidemiol. 1998;8(8):520–6.
61. Gannon AM, Stämpfli MR, Foster WG. Cigarette smoke exposure elicits increased autophagy and dysregulation of mitochondrial dynamics in murine granulosa cells. Biol Reprod. 2013;88(3):63.
62. Gannon AM, Stämpfli MR, Foster WG. Cigarette smoke exposure leads to follicle loss via an alternative ovarian cell death pathway in a mouse model. Toxicol Sci. 2012;125(1):274–84.
63. Phipps WR, et al. The association between smoking and female infertility as influenced by cause of the infertility. Fertil Steril. 1987;48(3):377–82.
64. Chang G, et al. Problem drinking in women evaluated for infertility. Am J Addict. 2006;15(2):174–9.
65. Andersen AM, et al. Moderate alcohol intake during pregnancy and risk of fetal death. Int J Epidemiol. 2012;41(2):405–13.
66. Sharma R, et al. Lifestyle factors and reproductive health: taking control of your fertility. Reprod Biol Endocrinol. 2013;11:66.
67. Penney DS. The effect of vigorous exercise during pregnancy. J Midwifery Womens Health. 2008;53(2):155–9.
68. Madsen M, et al. Leisure time physical exercise during pregnancy and the risk of miscarriage: a study within the Danish National Birth Cohort. BJOG. 2007;114(11):1419–26.
69. Warren MP, Perlroth NE. The effects of intense exercise on the female reproductive system. J Endocrinol. 2001;170(1):3–11.
70. Mueller BA, et al. Recreational drug use and the risk of primary infertility. Epidemiology. 1990;1(3): 195–200.
71. Park B, McPartland JM, Glass M. Cannabis, cannabinoids and reproduction. Prostaglandins Leukot Essent Fatty Acids. 2004;70(2):189–97.
72. Thyer AC, et al. Cocaine impairs ovarian response to exogenous gonadotropins in nonhuman primates. J Soc Gynecol Investig. 2001;8(6):358–62.
73. Lamy S, Laqueille X, Thibaut F. Consequences of tobacco, cocaine and cannabis consumption during pregnancy on the pregnancy itself, on the newborn and on child development: a review. Encephale. 2015;41 Suppl 1:S13–20.

Part III

Management of Recurrent Pregnancy Loss

Contemporary Prevention and Treatment of Recurrent Pregnancy Loss

11

Mayumi Sugiura-Ogasawara, Yasuhiko Ozaki, Kinue Katano, and Tamao Kitaori

Etiology

Recurrent miscarriage (RM) is classically defined as three or more consecutive pregnancy losses occurring before 20 weeks postmenstruation. However, many researchers have now revised the definition to two or more pregnancy losses, because of the recent increase in the prevalence of childless couples. Thus, recurrent pregnancy loss (RPL) which is defined as two or more pregnancy losses at any gestational age is used in this article. The estimated frequencies of three or more and two or more consecutive pregnancy losses are 0.9 and 4.2 % in the Japanese general population [1].

Antiphospholipid syndrome (APS), uterine anomalies, and abnormal chromosomes in either partner are established causes of RPL [2–4]. Only about 30 % of cases have an identifiable cause (Fig. 11.1a) [3], and it is well known that the cause remains unexplained in over a half of the cases [5]. The abnormal embryonic karyotype was found in 41.1 % of patients in whom both conventional causes and karyotype of

M. Sugiura-Ogasawara, MD, PhD (✉)
Y. Ozaki, MD, PhD • K. Katano, MD, PhD
Tamao Kitaori, MD, PhD
Department of Obstetrics and Gynecology, Graduate School of Medical Sciences, Nagoya City University, Kawasumi 1, Mizuho-ku, Nagoya, Aichi 4678601, Japan
e-mail: og.mym@med.nagoya-cu.ac.jp

aborted conceptus could be examined in our previous study (Fig. 11.1b) [6]. Therefore, the prevalence of truly unexplained, of cases with normal embryonic karyotype, was only 24.5 %. An abnormal embryonic karyotype is usually included in unexplained because the embryonic karyotype is seldom analyzed clinically.

The distribution of each cause depends on the characteristics of patients such as women's age or the number of previous miscarriages. Patients over 40 years old increase year by year in Japan and identifiable causes cannot be found in such patients.

The clinical tests for antiphospholipid antibodies, uterine anomaly, and chromosome karyotype in both partner and the aborted concepti are recommended.

We examined blood test for hypothyroidism and diabetes mellitus and ultrasonography for polycystic ovarian syndrome. Endocrine disturbances have also been postulated to cause RPL, but few randomized controlled trials or cohort studies reporting endocrine disturbances as a cause have withstood scrutiny. It has not been established whether endocrine disturbances, thrombophilia, immune dysfunction, infection, and psychological stress may contribute to RPL [5].

Antiphospholipid Syndrome

The clinical criteria for the diagnosis of APS include the following[7]:

© Springer International Publishing Switzerland 2016
A. Bashiri et al. (eds.), *Recurrent Pregnancy Loss*, DOI 10.1007/978-3-319-27452-2_11

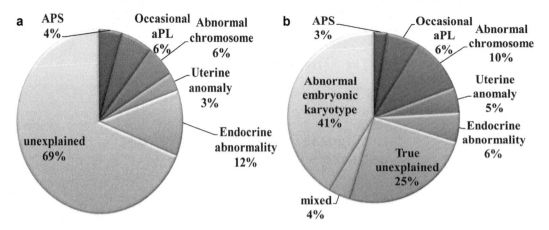

Fig. 11.1 Comparison of the distribution of causes. (**a**) 1676 patients in our previous study (based on data from Ref. [3]). (**b**) 482 patients with RPL, including those with an abnormal embryonic karyotype (based on data from Ref. [6])

1. Three or more consecutive unexplained miscarriages before the 10th week of gestation
2. One or more unexplained death of a morphologically normal fetus at 10 weeks of gestation or later
3. One or more premature births of a morphologically normal fetus at 34 weeks of gestation or earlier, associated with severe preeclampsia or placental insufficiency

Lupus anticoagulant (LA) by two kinds of reagent such as dilute activated partial thromboplastin time (aPTT) and dilute Russell viper venom time (RVVT) should be examined [8]. β2glycoprotein I (β2GPI) dependent anticardiolipin antibodies (aCL) IgG/IgM or anti-β2glycoprotein I (β2GPI) antibodies IgG/IgM are recommended [7].

Patients can be diagnosed as having APS when positivity for at least one antiphospholipid antibodies (aPLs) persistent for 12 weeks, according to the revised international criteria. The 99th percentile in healthy controls is recommended as the cutoff for the assays.

The reported incidence of APS is 5–15 % [5]. However, the references quoted in this review were published before the International Criteria for APS were published [7]. The incidence of APS was 4.5 % in our previous study though the study included RPL [3].

APS is the most important treatable cause of RPL. Low-dose aspirin plus heparin combined therapy is accepted as the standard treatment for patients with APS [9–17]. The previous studies are listed in Table 11.1. There were difference of assays and cutoff values to diagnose for APS among all facilities. Not only treatment but also difference of assays might influence on the pregnancy outcome.

LA is well known to be better correlated with pregnancy morbidity than aCL [18, 19]. The PROMISS study concluded that LA, but not classical aCL, was a predictor of adverse pregnancy outcomes [18]. Harris et al. also confirmed that classical CL IgG and IgM were rarely associated with adverse pregnancy outcomes [19]. Both aPTT and RVVT are suitable for assay of LA, and two tests with different assay principles are recommended [7, 8]. Therefore, a combination of aPTT-based LA and dRVVT-based LA could be used in daily clinical practice.

We conducted a prospective study to examine whether a positive test result for β2GPI-dependent aCL might predict adverse pregnancy by 10 weeks of gestation in 1,125 pregnant women without complications; results obtained using a cutoff value of 1.9 (99th percentile in healthy volunteers) were found to have a predictive value for intrauterine fetal death, intrauterine growth restriction, and preeclampsia [20]. However, in

Table 11.1 Assays for antiphospholipid antibodies and cutoff values and live birth rate according to treatment in patients with antiphospholipid antibodies

	aCL	LA	Case (n)	Control (n)	Live birth rate %	
Cowchock et al. (1992) [9]	IgG >30 IgM >11	dRVVT or aPTT	A+scUFH (26)	A+PSL (19)	73.1	68.4
Silver et al. (1993) [10]	IgG >8 IgM >5	dRVVT	A+PSL (12)	A (22)	100	100
Kutteh et al. (1996) [11]	IgG >=27 IgM >=27	No	A+scUFH (25)	A (25)	80.0[a]	44.0
Rai et al. (1996) [12]	IgG >5 IgM >3	RVVT aPTT (exclude SLE)	A+scUFH (45)	A (45)	71.1[a]	42.2
Pattison et al. (2000) [13]	IgG >=5 IgM >=5	aPTT, dRVVT, KCT	A (20)	A (20)	80	85
Farquharson et al. (2002) [14]	IgG >9 IgM >5	dRVVT	A+scLMWH (51)	A (47)	78.4	72.3
Franklin and Kutteh (2002) [15]	IgG >20 IgM >20	dRVVT	A+scUFH (25)		76.0	
Noble and Kutteh (2005) [16]	IgG >20 IgM >20	dRVVT, aPTT	A+scLMWH (25)	A+scUFH (25)	84	80
Laskin et al. [17]	IgG >15 IgM >25	dRVVT, aPTT, KCT, dPT (include ANA, thrombophilia)	A+scLMWH (45)	A (43)	77.8	79.1

A Low-dose aspirin, *scUFH* subcutaneous unfructionated heparin, *PSL* prednisolone, *LMWH* low-molecular-weight heparin
[a]Significant difference

the study, it could not be ascertained whether β2GPI-dependent aCL might have been of predictive value for early miscarriage, because the sampling was conducted only at about 10 weeks of gestation. On the other hand, we established a test for LA by 5×-diluted aPTT with the mixing test (LA-aPTT) and proved that treatment could improve the subsequent live birth in patients with a positive test result [21]. The ascertainment of each assay to improve live birth rate is important in obstetric APS. The true antigens of aPL are not phospholipids, but phospholipid-binding plasma proteins such as β2GPI, prothrombin, kininogen, protein C, and protein S [22, 23]. In fact, there are over 10 commercially available methods in Japan. Standardization is needed for detecting obstetric APS to improve the live birth rate.

Laskin et al. concluded that there was no difference in the live birth rates between treatment with low-molecular-weight heparin plus aspirin (77.8 %) and aspirin alone (79.1 %) based on the detection of aPLs, inherited thrombophilia, and antinuclear antibodies (Table 11.1) [17]. The live birth rate in patients treated with aspirin alone was high as compared with the rates reported

from Rai's or Kutteh's study [11, 12]. In our study, the frequency of antinuclear antibody (ANA) in 225 RPL patients was significantly higher than that in 740 normal pregnant controls; however, there was no significant difference in the subsequent miscarriage rate between the ANA-positive and ANA-negative cases [24].

We usually carry out LA-aPTT, LA-RVVT, and β2GPI-dependent aCL in clinical practice. The prevalence of at least one positive test is 10.7 %, and in 4.5 %, the positive finding is sustained for 12 weeks until APS is diagnosed. Precise calculation of the gestational weeks can be made from the basal body temperature chart. Combined treatment with low-dose aspirin and heparin calcium at 10,000 IU/day (twice a day) should be started from 4 weeks of gestation. We discontinue aspirin by 35 weeks of gestation and continue heparin until the onset of labor. A live birth can be expected in 70–80 % of the patients treated thus [11, 12].

We found that the live birth rate in 52 patients with occasional aPL, but not APS, treated with aspirin alone was significantly higher than that in 672 patients with unexplained RPL who received no medication [25]. The live birth rate was 84.6 % (44/52) and that was 95.7 % (44/46) when miscarriage cases caused by an abnormal embryonic karyotype were excluded. However, it is not yet established how to treat patients with occasional aPL.

Congenital Uterine Anomaly

Women with a history of RPL have been estimated to have a 3.2–10.4 % likelihood of having a major uterine anomaly except arcuate uterus, the variation largely depending on the methods and the criteria selected for the diagnoses [26–29]. The associations between arcuate uterus and RPL and between anomalies and infertility remain controversial.

Affected patients have been offered surgery in an attempt to restore the uterine anatomy. The live birth rates after surgery in studies including a relatively large number of patients are summarized in Table 11.2 [26, 30–37]. 35.1–65.9 % of patients with bicornuate or septate uteri give live births after correctional surgery. While this may provide hope that the operations would increase the rate of successful pregnancies, to the best of our knowledge, there have been no prospective studies comparing the pregnancy outcomes between cases of RPL with uterine anomalies treated and not treated by surgery.

We conducted a case-control study of 1676 patients with a history of 2–12 consecutive miscarriages whose subsequent pregnancies were ascertained at least one time in our medical records [3]. Uterine anomalies were diagnosed by HSG and laparoscopy/laparotomy.

Of the total, 3.2 % (54) had major uterine anomalies, including 38 with a partial bicornis unicolli, 10 with a septum, 5 with a unicornis, and 1 with a didelphys. Of the 42 patients with a septate or bicornuate uterus not treated by any kind of surgery, 59.5 % (25) had a successful outcome, while this was the case in 71.7 % (1096/1528) women with normal uteri at the subsequent first pregnancy ($p=0.084$). The normal chromosomal karyotype rates in the aborted concepti in cases with anomalies were significantly higher than that in those without anomalies (84.6 % vs. 42.5 %, $p=0.006$).

In 78.0 % of patients (32/41) with anomalies, one patient was treated by surgery after further miscarriage, and 85.5 % of patients (1307/1528) with normal uteri could cumulatively have live babies within the follow-up period (not significant). Live birth rates in patients with congenital uterine anomalies tended to be lower both at the first pregnancy after diagnosis and from the cumulative standpoint.

The defect/cavity ratio was also significantly higher in the subsequent miscarriage group than that in the live birth group. Because of a value of 0.8 for the area under curve of the ROC, major uterine anomalies clearly have a negative impact on the reproductive outcome in women with RPL, being associated with a higher risk of further miscarriage with a normal embryonic karyotype.

We conducted the first multi-center prospective study to examine whether surgery for a bicornuate or septate uterus might improve the live birth rate in 170 patients with RPL [38]. In 124 patients with a septate uterus, the live birth rate at the first pregnancy after ascertainment of anomalies with surgery tended to be higher than that in those without surgery (81.3 % vs. 61.5 %). The infertility rates were similar in both groups, while the cumulative live birth rate tended to be higher than without surgery (76.1 % vs. 60.0 %). Surgery showed no benefit in 46 patients with a bicornuate uterus for having a baby, but tended to decrease the preterm birth rate and the low birth weight. The possibility that surgery has benefits for having a baby in patients with a septate uterus suffering recurrent miscarriage could not be excluded.

A randomized control trial (RCT) is necessary to compare the live birth rates between patients with and without surgery, also taking into consideration the infertility rate.

Table 11.2 Live birth rate with and without surgery in patients with congenital uterine anomalies

	surgery							No surgery	
	Makino et al. 1992 (n=71) [30]	Candiani et al. 1990 (144) [31]	Ayhan et al. 1992 (89) [32]	DeCherney et al. 1986 (103) [33]	Daly et al. 1989 (55) [34]	Hickok et al. 2000 (40) [35]	Kormányos et al. 2006 (94) [36]	Sugiura-Ogasawara et al. 2010 (42) [3]	Ghi et al. 2012 (24) [37]
Type of anomaly	Arcuate, septate	Septate Bicornuate	Septate Bicornuate	Septate	Septate	Septate	Septate	Septate Bicornuate	Septate Subseptate
Indication	Recurrent SAB	Recurrent SAB Infertility	Recurrent SAB Preterm delivery	Recurrent SAB	Recurrent SAB Preterm delivery	Pregnancy loss Complication of pregnancy Infertility	2 or more SAB	2 or more SAB	First pregnancy
Method of surgery	Abdominal	Tompkins Jones Te Linde Strassman	Tompkins Jones Strassman	Resectoscope	Scissors	Resectoscope	Resectoscope	–	–
Live birth rate per pregnancy	84.8% (39/46)	68% (45/66) septate 76% (50/66) bicornuate	65% (30/46) septate 83% (45/54) Bicornuate	80% (63/72) successful resection	80% (60/75)	77.3% (17/22)	68.8% (33/48) Cumulative 71.8% (51/71)		
Live birth rate per patient	54.9 %	65.9 %		61.2 %		64.3 %	35.1 % Cumulative 54.3 %	59.5% Cumulative 78.0%	33.3%

Abnormal Chromosomes in Either Partner

De Braekeler et al. concluded that the rate of chromosomal structural rearrangements in couples with a history of two or more spontaneous abortions was 4.7 %, based on a review of the data of 22,199 couples [39].

We conducted the first prospective study of 1284 couples to examine whether translocations constituted a risk factor for RPL [4]. Our findings indicated a successful pregnancy rate of 31.9 % (15/47) in the first pregnancy after ascertainment of the carrier status, which is much less than that reported in cases with normal chromosomes (71.7 %, 849/1184), and a cumulative successful pregnancy rate of 68.1 % (32/47). We concluded that the prognosis of RPL patients with reciprocal translocations is poor, given that the study was conducted over a 17-year period, and included severe cases with a history of 10–13 miscarriages.

Franssen et al. reported cumulative successful pregnancy rates in RPL patients with reciprocal translocations, Robertsonian translocations, and a normal karyotype of 83.0, 82.0, and 84.1 %, respectively, based on a prospective case-control study [40]. They concluded that the chance of having a healthy child was as high as that in non-carrier couples, despite the higher risk of miscarriage.

The live birth rate with preimplantation genetic diagnosis (PGD) was reported to be 14–58 % [41–46]. The live birth rate with natural conception was reported to be 32–65 % on the first trial and 68–83 % cumulatively [4, 40]. The live birth rates with PGD in reciprocal translocation carriers are comparable to or sometimes lower than those with a subsequent first natural conception. The live birth rate with the use of new technology, microarray comparative genomic hybridization (array CGH) or single nucleotide polymorphism microarray, is also comparable to those with a subsequent first natural conception [3, 45]. It is difficult, however, to simply compare IVF plus PGD and natural conception in translocation carriers. To date, there has been no cohort study.

Thus, we compared the live birth rate of 37 patients with RPL associated with a translocation undergoing PGD *matched for age and number of previous miscarriages* with that of 52 patients who chose natural conception [47]. The live birth rates on the first PGD trial and the first natural pregnancy after ascertainment of the carrier status were 37.8 and 53.8 %, respectively. Cumulative live birth rates were 67.6 and 65.4 %, respectively, in the groups undergoing and not undergoing PGD. The time required to become pregnancy was similar in both groups. PGD was found to reduce the miscarriage rate significantly. The prevalence of twin pregnancies was significantly higher in the PGD group. The cost of PGD was US$7956 per patient.

While PGD significantly prevented further miscarriages, there was no difference in the live birth rate. Couples should be fully informed of the similarity in the live birth rate, the similarity in time to become pregnant, the advantages of PGD, such as the reduction in the miscarriage rate, as well as its disadvantages, such as the higher cost, and the advantages of a natural pregnancy, such as the avoidance of IVF failure. The findings should be incorporated into the genetic counseling of patients with RPL and carrying a translocation.

Abnormal Embryonic (Fetal) Karyotypes

Embryonic aneuploidy is the most common cause of sporadic spontaneous abortion before 10 weeks of gestation. A recent array CGH approach indicated about 80 % of abnormality in the aborted embryo.

Regarding RPL, both the live birth rate and the normal embryonic karyotype decreased according to the number of previous miscarriages in our previous study [48]. The study also indicated that the live birth rate of patients with a previous abnormal embryonic karyotype was significantly higher than that in patients with a previous normal embryonic karyotype. The embryonic karyotype can be a good predictor of subsequent success. Our another study showed that 41 % of patients had an abnormal embryonic karyotype [6]. However, this cannot be conclusive, because the aborted concepti are seldom karyotyped clinically.

The live birth rate with preimplantation genetic screening for aneuploidy (PGS) was reported to be 4–47 % [49–51]. PGS could never improve the live birth rate in patients with unexplained RPL though it could reduce the miscarriage rate, because the live birth rate in patients with a history of five miscarriages was 51 % [48]. The previous studies with the use of PGS lack appropriate controls. The RCT is necessary since the live birth rate depends on women's age and the number of previous miscarriages.

The True Unexplained Recurrent Pregnancy Loss

The subsequent live birth rates in unexplained patients, including patients caused by an abnormal embryonic karyotype, with previous 2, 3, 4, and 5 miscarriages are 80, 70, 60, and 50 % with no medication, respectively [52]. However, patients with unexplained RPL also desire to receive medication. Paternal immunization, or low-dose aspirin and heparin combined therapy had no effect on improving the live birth rate in patients with unexplained RM [53, 54]. It is important to make the patients aware that no medications have been established to improve the live birth rate shown above.

Recently, an association between about 100 kinds of polymorphisms and RPL has been reported. Factor V Leiden mutation is well known to be associated with RPL [55]. The study design of almost all manuscripts concerning this issue was cross-sectional. The clinical significance of examination of the mutations is not yet well established in patients with RPL [5].

Annexin A5 is a placental anticoagulant protein and is reported to be one of the true antigens of aPLs. Four cross-sectional studies have shown positive associations between *ANXA5* SNPs and RPL. Our previous cross-sectional study confirmed *ANXA5* SNP5 as a risk factor for RPL [56]. However, the subsequent live birth rate was 84.0 and 84.3 % in patients with and without the risk allele of SNP5 [56].

Coagulation factor XII activity is also well known to be associated with RPL. Our recent study proved that but LA-aPTT not β2GPI-dependent aCL reduced about 20 % of XII activity [57]. Our cross-sectional study suggested CT genotype of XII gene as a risk factor for RPL [57]. The subsequent live birth rates were similar in patients with and without the risk alleles [57].

This may mean that risk factors with small ORs identified in the cross-sectional study may be of little clinical relevance. It is speculated that patients with a number of risk alleles with small relative risks might be more likely to suffer from unexplained RPL.

Several couples in our experience divorced or gave up trying to conceive after RPL, because they had the misconception that it would be impossible for them to have a living baby [1]. Psychological support with tender loving care might be the most important to encourage such couples to continue to conceive until a live birth results.

References

1. Sugiura-Ogasawara M, Suzuki S, Ozaki Y, Katano K, Suzumori N, Kitaori T. Frequency of recurrent spontaneous abortion and its influence on further marital relationship and illness: The Okazaki Cohort Study in Japan. J Obstet Gynaecol Res. 2012;39(1):126–31.
2. Farquharson RG, Pearson JF, John L. Lupus anticoagulant and pregnancy management. Lancet. 1984;28: 228–9.
3. Sugiura-Ogasawara M, Ozaki Y, Kitaori T, Kumagai K, Suzuki S. Midline uterine defect size correlated with miscarriage of euploid embryos in recurrent cases. Fertil Steril. 2010;93:1983–8.
4. Sugiura-Ogasawara M, Ozaki Y, Sato T, Suzumori N, Suzumori K. Poor prognosis of recurrent aborters with either maternal or paternal reciprocal translocation. Fertil Steril. 2004;81:367–73.
5. Branch DW, Gibson M, Silver RM. Clinical practice: recurrent miscarriage. N Engl J Med. 2010;363:1740–7.
6. Sugiura-Ogasawara M, Ozaki Y, Katano K, Suzumori N, Kitaori T, Mizutani E. Abnormal embryonic karyotype is the most frequent cause of recurrent miscarriage. Hum Reprod. 2012;27:2297–303.
7. Miyakis S, Lockshin MD, Atsumi T, et al. International consensus statement of an update of the classification criteria for definite antiphospholipid syndrome (APS). J Thromb Haemost. 2006;4:295–306.
8. Pengo V, Tripod A, Reber G, Rand JH, Ortel TL, Galli M, De Groot PG. Update of the guidelines for lupus

anticoagulant detection. J Thromb Haemost. 2009; 7:1737–40.

9. Cowchock FS, Reece EA, Balaban D, Branch DW, Plouffe L. Repeated fetal losses associated with antiphospholipid antibodies: a collaborative randomized trial comparing prednisone with low-dose heparin treatment. Am J Obstet Gynecol. 1992;166(5): 1318–23.

10. Silver RK, MacGregor SN, Sholl JS, Hobart JM, Neerhof MG, Ragin A. Comparative trial of prednisone plus aspirin versus aspirin alone in the treatment of anticardiolipin antibody-positive obstetric patients. Am J Obstet Gynecol. 1993;169(6):1411–7.

11. Kutteh WH. Antiphospholipid antibody-associated recurrent pregnancy loss: treatment with heparin and low-dose aspirin is superior to low-dose aspirin alone. Am J Obstet Gynecol. 1996;174:1584–9.

12. Rai R, Cohen H, Dave M, Regan L. Randomised controlled trial of aspirin and aspirin plus heparin in pregnant women with recurrent miscarriage associated with phospholipid antibodies (or antiphospholipid antibodies). BMJ. 1997;314:253–7.

13. Pattison NS, Chamley LW, Birdsall M, Zanderigo AM, Liddell HS, McDougall J. Does aspirin have a role in improving pregnancy outcome for women with the antiphospholipid syndrome? A randomized controlled trial. Am J Obstet Gynecol. 2000;183(4): 1008–12.

14. Farquharson RG, Quenby S, Greaves M. Antiphospholipid syndrome in pregnancy: a randomized, controlled trial of treatment. Obstet Gynecol. 2002;100(3):408–13.

15. Franklin RD, Kutteh WH. Antiphospholipid antibodies (APA) and recurrent pregnancy loss: treating a unique APA positive population. Hum Reprod. 2002 Nov;17(11):2981–5.

16. Noble LS, Kutteh WH, Lashey N, Franklin RD, Herrada J. Antiphospholipid antibodies associated with recurrent pregnancy loss: prospective, multicenter, controlled pilot study comparing treatment with low-molecular-weight heparin versus unfractionated heparin. Fertil Steril. 2005;83(3):684–90.

17. Laskin CA, Spitzer KA, Clark CA, Crowther MR, Ginsberg JS, Hawker GA, Kingdom JC, Barrett J, Gent M. Low molecular weight heparin and aspirin for recurrent pregnancy loss: results from the randomized, controlled HepASA trial. J Rheumatol. 2009;36(2):279–87.

18. Lockshin MD, Kim M, Laskin CA, Guerra M, Branch DW, Merrill J, Petri M, Porter TF, Sammaritano L, Stephenson MD, Buyon J, Salmon JE. Prediction of adverse pregnancy outcome by the presence of lupus anticoagulant, but not anticardiolipin antibody, in patients with antiphospholipid antibodies. Arthritis Rheum. 2012;64(7):2311–8.

19. Harris EN, Spinnato JA. Should anticardiolipin tests be performed in otherwise healthy pregnant women? Am J Obstet Gynecol. 1991;165(5 Pt 1):1272–7.

20. Katano K, Aoki K, Sasa H, et al. beta 2-Glycoprotein I-dependent anticardiolipin antibodies as a predictor of adverse pregnancy outcomes in healthy pregnant women. Hum Reprod. 1996;11:509–12.

21. Ogasawara MS, Aoki K, Katano K, et al. Factor XII but not protein C, protein S, antithrombin III or factor XIII as a predictor of recurrent miscarriage. Fertil Steril. 2001;75:916–9.

22. Matsuura E, Igarashi Y, Fujimoto M, Ichikawa I, Koike T. Anticardiolipin cofactor(s) and differential diagnosis of autoimmune disease. Lancet. 1990;21:177–8.

23. Roubey RAS. Autoantibodies to phospholipid-binding plasma proteins: a new view of lupus anticoagulant and other "antiphospholipid" autoantibodies. Blood. 1994;84:2854–67.

24. Ogasawara M, Aoki K, Kajiura S, et al. Are antinuclear antibodies predictive of recurrent miscarriage? Lancet. 1996;347:1183–4.

25. Sugiura-Ogasawara M, Ozaki Y, Nakanishi T, Sato T, Suzumori N, Nozawa K. Occasional antiphospholipid antibody positive patients with recurrent pregnancy loss also merit aspirin therapy: a retrospective cohort-control study. Am J Reprod Immunol. 2008; 59:235–41.

26. Sugiura-Ogasawara M, Ozaki Y, Suzumori N. Müllerian anomalies and recurrent miscarriage. Curr Opin Obstet Gynecol. 2013;25:293–8.

27. Sugiura-Ogasawara M, Ozaki Y, Katano K, Suzumori N, Mizutani E. Uterine anomaly and recurrent pregnancy loss. Semin Reprod Med. 2011;29:514–21.

28. Chan YY, Jayaprakasan K, Zamora J, Thornton JG, Raine-Fenning N, Coomarasamy A. The prevalence of congenital uterine anomalies in selected and high-risk populations: a systematic review. Hum Reprod Update. 2011;17:761–71.

29. Saravelos SH, Cocksedge KA, Li TC. Prevalence and diagnosis of congenital uterine anomalies in women with reproductive failure: a critical appraisal. Hum Reprod Update. 2008;14:415–29.

30. Makino T, Umeuchi M, Nakada K, Nozawa S, Iizuka R. Incidence of congenital uterine anomalies in repeated reproductive wastage and prognosis for pregnancy after metroplasty. Int J Fertil. 1992 May-Jun;37(3):167–70.

31. Candiani GB, Fedele L, Parazzini F, Zamberletti D. Reproductive prognosis after abdominal metroplasty in bicornuate or septate uterus: a life table analysis. Br J Obstet Gynaecol. 1990 Jul;97(7):613–7.

32. Ayhan A, Yücel I, Tuncer ZS, Kişnişçi HA. Reproductive performance after conventional metroplasty: an evaluation of 102 cases. Fertil Steril. 1992 Jun;57(6):1194–6.

33. DeCherney AH, Russell JB, Graebe RA, Polan ML. Resectoscopic management of müllerian fusion defects. Fertil Steril. 1986 May;45(5):726–8.

34. Daly DC, Maier D, Soto-Albors C. Hysteroscopic metroplasty: six years' experience. Obstet Gynecol. 1989 Feb;73(2):201–5.

35. Hickok LR. Hysteroscopic treatment of the uterine septum: a clinician's experience. Am J Obstet Gynecol. 2000 Jun;182(6):1414–20.

36. Kormányos Z, Molnár BG, Pál A. Removal of a residual portion of a uterine septum in women of advanced reproductive age: obstetric outcome. Hum Reprod. 2006 Apr;21(4):1047–51.

37. Ghi T, De Musso F, Maroni E, Youssef A, Savelli L, Farina A, Casadio P, Filicori M, Pilu G, Rizzo N. The pregnancy outcome in women with incidental diagnosis of septate uterus at first trimester scan. Hum Reprod. 2012 Sep;27(9):2671-5. doi.

38. Sugiura-Ogasawara M, Lin BL, Aoki K, Maruyama T, Nakatsuka M, Ozawa N, Sugi T, Takeshita T, Nishida M. Does surgery improve live birth rates in patients with recurrent miscarriage caused by uterine anomalies? J Obstet Gynaecol. 2015;35(2):155–8.

39. De Braekeler M, Dao TN. Cytogenetic studies in couples experiencing repeated pregnancy losses. Human Reprod. 1990;5:519–28.

40. Franssern MTM, Korevaar JC, van der Veen F, et al. Reproductive outcome after chromosome analysis in couples with two or more miscarriages: case-control study. BMJ. 2006;332:759–62.

41. Lim CK, Jun JH, Min DM, Lee HS, Kim JY, Koong MK, Kang IS. Efficacy and clinical outcome of preimplantation genetic diagnosis using FISH for couples of reciprocal and Robertsonian translocations: the Korean experience. Prenat Diagn. 2004;24:556–61.

42. Otani T, Roche M, Mizuike M, Colls P, Escudero T, Munne S. Preimplantation genetic diagnosis significantly improves the pregnancy outcome of translocation carriers with a history of recurrent miscarriage and unsuccessful pregnancies. Reprod Biomed Online. 2006;13:869–74.

43. Feyereisen E, Steffann J, Romana S, Lelorc'h M, Äôh M, Ray P, Kerbrat V, Tachdjian G, Frydman R, Frydman N. Five years-experience of preimplantation genetic diagnosis in the Parisian Center: outcome of the first 441 started cycles. Fertil Steril. 2007;87:60–7.

44. Fischer J, Colls P, Escudero T, Munné S. Preimplantation genetic diagnosis (PGD) improves pregnancy outcome for translocation carriers with a history of recurrent losses. Fertil Steril. 2010;94:283–9.

45. Fiorentino F, Bono S, Biricik A, Nuccitelli A, Cotroneo E, Cottone G, Kokocinski F, Michel CE, Minasi MG, Greco E. Application of next-generation sequencing technology for comprehensive aneuploidy screening of blastocysts in clinical preimplantation genetic screening cycles. Hum Reprod. 2014; 29(12):2802–13.

46. Idowu D, Merrion K, Wemmer N, Mash JG, Pettersen B, Kijacic D, Lathi RB. Pregnancy outcomes following 24-chromosome preimplantation genetic diagnosis in couples with balanced reciprocal or Robertsonian translocations. Fertil Steril. 2015;103(4):1037–42.

47. Ikuma S, Sato T, Sugiura-Ogasawara M, Nagayoshi M, Tanaka A, Takeda S. Preimplantation genetic diagnosis and natural conception: a comparison of live birth rates in patients with recurrent pregnancy loss associated with translocation. PlosOne. 2015 Jun 17;10(6):e0129958.

48. Ogasawara M, Aoki K, Okada S, Suzumori K. Embryonic karyotype of abortuses in relation to the number of previous miscarriages. Fertil Steril. 2000;73:300–4.

49. Platteau P, Staessen C, Michiels A, Van Steirteghem A, Liebaers I, Devroey P. Preimplantation genetic diagnosis for aneuploidy screening in patients with unexplained recurrent miscarriages. Fertil Steril. 2005;83:393–7.

50. Wilding M, Forman R, Hogewind G, Di Matteo L, Zullo F, Cappiello F, Dale B. Preimplantation genetic diagnosis for the treatment of failed in vitro fertilization-embryo transfer and habitual abortion. Fertil Steril. 2004;81(5):1302–7.

51. Munné S, Chen S, Fischer J, Colls P, Zheng X, Stevens J, Escudero T, Oter M, Schoolcraft B, Simpson JL, Cohen J. Preimplantation genetic diagnosis reduces pregnancy loss in women aged 35 years and older with a history of recurrent miscarriages. Fertil Steril. 2005;84(2):331–5.

52. Katano K, Suzuki S, Ozaki Y, Suzumori N, Kitaori T, Sugiura-Ogasawara M. Peripheral natural killer cell activity as a predictor of recurrent pregnancy loss: a large cohort study. Fertil Steril. 2013; 100(6):1629–34.

53. Ober C, Karrison T, Odem RR, Barnes RB, Branch DW, Stephenson MD, Baron B, Walker MA, Scott JR, Schreiber JR. Mononuclear-cell immunisation in prevention of recurrent miscarriages: a randomised trial. Lancet. 1999;354(9176):365–9.

54. Kaandorp SP, Goddijn M, van der Post JAM, Hutten BA, Verhoeve HR, Hamulyak K, Mol BW, Folkeringa N, Nahuis M, Papatsonis DNM, et al. Aspirin plus heparin or aspirin alone in women with recurrent miscarriage. N Engl J Med. 2010;362:1586–96.

55. Kupferminc MJ, Eldor A, Steinman N, Many A, Bar-Am A, Jaffa A, et al. Increased frequency of genetic thrombophilia in women with complications of pregnancy. N Engl J Med. 1999;340:50–2.

56. Hayashi Y, Sasaki H, Suzuki S, Nishiyama T, Kitaori T, Mizutani E, Suzumori N, Sugiura-Ogasawara M. Genotyping analyses for polymorphisms of ANXA5 gene in patients with recurrent pregnancy loss. Fertil Steril. 2013;100(4):1018–24.

57. Asano E, Ebara T, Yamada-Namikawa C, Kitaori T, Suzumori N, Katano K, Ozaki Y, Nakanishi M, Sugiura-Ogasawara M. Genotyping analysis for the 46 C/T polymorphism of coagulation factor XII and the involvement of factor XII activity in patients with recurrent pregnancy loss. PLoS One. 2014;9(12): e114452.

Part IV

Psychological and Supporting Aspects of Recurrent Pregnancy Loss

The Health Caregiver's Perspective: The Importance of Emotional Support for Women with Recurrent RPL

Hanna Ziedenberg, Iris Raz, and Asher Bashiri

Introduction

Background

> And God blessed man and God said Be fruitful and multiply and replenish the earth [1] (Genesis 1:28).

To give birth and reproduce is the first commandment in Genesis. To fulfill this commandment is both a privilege and an obligation. Fertility, reproduction, parenthood, and family are central values in Jewish and Israeli society. A woman who has recurring miscarriages is afraid of infertility which is seen as a situation in which a person is robbed of significance and experiences which are central to life and without which life is: worthless. The right to parenthood is protected under the Basic Law Human Dignity and Liberty in Israel. "The yearning for a child is so well-known it needs no evidence." A couple that has trouble in having children makes every effort in order to have offspring [2, 3].

The process of socialization prepares a person for parenting. When a woman has recurrent miscarriages, she experiences anxiety and feels helpless in her ability to accomplish her goal of motherhood as well as fulfill the expectations of society from which she derives the craving for motherhood. This awareness stems from the fact that the society has created a framework which sees the construction of family and fertility the continued existence and its basic duty of an adult. The right to be a biological parent awkward is impaired in about 10–15 % of the population in the USA and Israel [2, 4].

The State of Israel has implemented since its inception a policy which encourages fertility both on a personal level and on an institutional level [2, 3, 5, 6]. This concept is a characteristic of the Jewish Israeli experience and is driven by two main forces which define motherhood as a supreme value—the Jewish religious tradition and the Israeli-Zionist heritage. It is expressed in the first chapter of the Bible in the commandment "Be fruitful and multiply and replenish the earth" [1] and in many other places in the biblical text. Rachel requests from Jacob "Give me children or I'll die" [7] which expresses the view that the need for children is more intense than the desire to live, that there is no point to life without children [6]. This outlook has been observed in many studies which discuss the intensity of the feelings and the stress of couples in a situation of recurring miscarriages. According to such studies, the

H. Ziedenberg, PhD (✉)
Nursing Department, Faculty of Health Sciences,
Recanati School for Community Health Professions,
Ben-Gurion University of the Negev,
Biet Kama 1, Kibutz Beet Kama 85325, Israel
e-mail: hannaz@bgu.ac.il

I. Raz, CNM, MHA • A. Bashiri, MD
Department of Obstetrics and Gynecology, Faculty of
Health Sciences, Soroka University Medical Center,
Ben-Gurion University of the Negev,
Be'er Sheva, Israel

© Springer International Publishing Switzerland 2016
A. Bashiri et al. (eds.), *Recurrent Pregnancy Loss*, DOI 10.1007/978-3-319-27452-2_12

degree of distress in these situations is very high and is characterized by depression and anxiety which influence all areas of life including the couple's relationships, their sex life, the quality of life, and, in men, the quality of the sperm [3, 6, 8].

Women who experience multiple natural miscarriages are in a complicated medical and emotional state due to the need for a complete medical evaluation as well as worry regarding the next pregnancy. The fear of the next pregnancy heightens anxiety and even contributes to depression [9, 10]. The emotional state of these women demands professional attention. They need emotional support to improve their quality of life during this difficult period [11].

Recurrent Miscarriages/Recurrent Pregnancy Losses

The notion of recurring miscarriages is defined by the ASRM (American Society for Reproductive Medicine) as a situation in which a woman has two or more repeated miscarriages before the pregnancy reaches 20 weeks [11]. Bashiri and his colleagues [9, 10] offer a definition of the concept of RPL (recurrent pregnancy loss) going beyond its purely medical aspects to include the feelings of loss and the emotional aspects associated with this problem. The rate of recurring miscarriages is about 3–5 % of pregnancies. The risk of recurrent miscarriages after three miscarriages rises to 30 % or more. Nevertheless about 75 % of women who experience recurrent miscarriages do finally become pregnant and have a live birth even without treatment. The majority of medical centers customarily begin a medical evaluation after two consecutive miscarriages [9, 10].

Causes for Miscarriages

The reasons for recurrent miscarriages are determined in only 50 % of the cases, 50 % are defined as "unexplained" and that it seems is related to the phenomenon of the multiple factors related to miscarriages [9–11]. There are a number of factors for RPL such as: congenital anatomical reasons, developed defects, endocrine disorders including hyperprolactinemia, polycystic ovary syndrome, insulin resistance, poorly treated diabetes, luteal phase defect in thyroid function, thyroid antibodies, obesity, genetic factors, clotting syndromes, etc. In this chapter we put the emphasis on miscarriages from unknown causes and the problems relating to clotting and the neuro-immune-endocrine axis [9].

Unexplained Recurrent Miscarriages

As mentioned 50 % of recurrent pregnancy losses are due to unknown causes. The treatment of RPL is a great challenge both for the woman and for her physician. The treatment is shrouded in darkness, and involves much trial and error. The high uncertainty increases the stress and anxiety for the women [5, 12]. Women after unexplained RPL continue to search for the cause of the problem and find it difficult to believe in the success of the current pregnancy. The probability of another miscarriage after RPL is high compared to women who have had only one miscarriage. The fact of not having a clear reason leaves the woman feeling helpless, frustrated, and anxious. The rate of live births among women who experience unexplained RPL is still about 50–54 % [5, 12].

The neuro-immune-endocrine axis emphasizes the impact of the relationship between systems, neurological system, endocrine and immune system, and recurrent miscarriages. Many studies have described the emotional responses displayed by the women experiencing recurrent miscarriages. It has been found that socio-psychological factors influence the woman and affect her immune system. It is assumed that there exists an immune factor in the relationship of the mother and the fetus. There is a connection between the mother's immune system and the fetal antigens. Recently, importance has been placed on the existence of natural killer lymphocyte cells in the uterine mucosa and they it seems can infiltrate the fetal trophoblast cells. Research shows that in women who experience RPL a high level of these cells are found in the uterine mucosa and therefore they are at high risk of losing the fetus in the absence of treatment. In addition, women with RPL tend to generate an immune reaction characterized by TH1 cell dominance during the period of implantation as opposed to the situation characteristic of a normal pregnancy where the TH2 cells are dominant. It has also been found that in women who experience a single miscarriage there is a rise in the endometrium of factors of the immune system of the type CD8 and TNF alpha and tryptase positive mast cells. In addition it has been found that a rise in stress related hormones (catecholamine and cortisol) can reduce the supply of blood to the fetus and can even influence the development of embryonic blood cells thereby increasing the chance of a miscarriage [12, 13]. These findings support the view which argues that immune tolerance disorders can contribute to recurrent miscarriages [12, 13].

Emotional Aspects Associated with Recurrent Miscarriages

Every miscarriage is accompanied by a feeling of loss, loss of the fetus, loss of confidence in the integrity of the body and its ability to give birth [14]. Studies show that there is a psychological morbidity in the first few weeks after a miscarriage. It has been found that about 40 % of women after a miscarriage will suffer from symptoms of bereavement immediately after a miscarriage [15]. It has also been found that about 43–70 % suffer from repeated bouts of mild to severe depression during the 6 months after a pregnancy loss [12].

RPL evokes a variety of responses such as anxiety, depression, denial, anger and a feeling of bereavement and loss. For the woman who miscarries in the early stages, the pregnancy loss is similar to the loss of a body part. Women feel that part of their body has been lost which brings on a feeling of deep emptiness and she feels damaged and incomplete. The process of separation between the mother and fetus begins to occur only after the women feel fetal movement [16]. Studies show that about 30 % of women treated in fertility clinics or pregnancy loss clinics suffer from clinical depression according to indices of the DSM, the Diagnostic and Statistical Manual of Mental Disorders. It has been found that every fifth woman in recurrent pregnancy loss clinics is diagnosed as suffering from anxiety [9, 10]. Women

after an unexplained RPL develop more psychological symptoms compared to women whose problem has been diagnosed. These women experience more anxiety since they are unable to believe in their ability to conceive and complete a pregnancy. When the reason for the miscarriage is not known women feel helpless and do not know the cause of the problem or what they must do to prevent a miscarriage in the future [16]. In a study of 39 women who had experienced two or more miscarriages conducted at the Recurrent Pregnancy Loss Clinic at Soroka Medical Center, Israel, the connection between the RPL and anxiety, the quality of sleep and quality of life was scrutinized. It was found that all the women who had had two miscarriages or more suffered from a moderate to high level of general and situational anxiety as well as from sleep disturbances and a lower quality of life [17] (Fig. 12.1).

There are two factors influencing the emotional responses of the women with recurring miscarriages. The first is connected with mourning for the loss and not knowing the cause; these women develop greater anxiety disorders. The second factor is connected to medical anamnesis. The conventional wisdom is that women who have given birth in the past are more resilient to anxiety stemming from RPL. However there is no research supporting this view. Also, the literature describes serious traumatic reactions to the degree of PTSD (Posttraumatic stress disorders) [12].

There is a long term study examining the prevalence of PTSD in response to RPL. About 1370 women were enrolled in the study during the early stages of their pregnancies and 113 experienced RPL. The interviews to evaluate the extent of the trauma and depression were conducted after 1 month and again after 4 months and the frequency of PTSD was 25 %, and the severity of the symptoms was similar to other trauma populations. Women with PTSD were at a high risk for depression: 34 % of the PTSD cases and 5 % of cases that did not report depression. At 4 months, 7 % met the criteria for PTSD, and half were chronic. In contrast the rate of depression did not decrease. The results show that pregnancy loss has the traumatic potential to contribute to the development of PTSD [17].

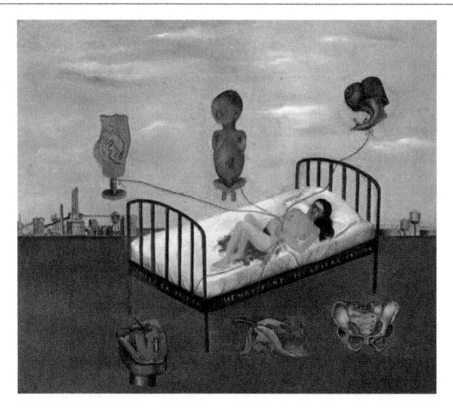

Fig. 12.1 Frida Kalo, 1929. This is how she drew the experience of her miscarriage. [Reprinted with permission from Frida Kahlo Museums Trust. Av. 5 de Mayo No. 2, Col. Centro, Del. Cuauhtémoc 06059, México, D. F &Banco de México Diego Rivera © 2015]

A study that examined the difference in the level of anxiety among women after one miscarriage compared to those who experienced two miscarriages shows that the second miscarriage had a stronger effect on the women's emotional state. In the same study it was found that while the first miscarriage was accompanied by less anxiety there was more anxiety during the next pregnancy. A connection was found between the degree of depression and anxiety in women after a miscarriage and a higher risk to miscarry in the next pregnancy [12, 18].

In a study of 205 women who experienced unexplained RPL 116 got emotional support and the rest didn't. It was found that among the women who received psychological support the rate of subsequent successful pregnancies resulting in a live birth was 85 % while among those who got no support only 36 % succeeded in becoming pregnant. This study was terminated due to ethical issues but illustrates the significance of psychological support [17, 18].

Understanding the connection between the emotional state of the women and miscarriages brought the European Society of Human Reproduction and Embryology (ESHRE) and the Royal College of Obstetricians and Gynecologists (RCOG) to recommend supportive care during the next pregnancy for women with unexplained miscarriages [11]. There is also a recommendation to offer emotional support during the first 4 weeks after a miscarriage in order to reduce anxiety and the chances for further mental morbidity [16].

As yet there are no set protocols for supportive treatment after recurring miscarriages. In their work Muster et al. [11] examined the preference of women for support during pregnancy after recurring miscarriages. Women were offered about 20 types of support. All indicated that emotional support immediately after a miscarriage at a time when anxiety and the feeling of loss of control was high was very important. Also, they stressed the importance of continuous communication with the attending physician which would allow them to report the next pregnancy immediately in order to plan monitoring and to consult with him during the pregnancy. The women reported that the ultrasound test which showed the fetus and the fetal pulse gave them support and faith in their bodies. In addition to emotional support they wanted the physician to be serious, available, attentive and understanding of their difficulties. They also noted the importance of the support from the social worker, their family and friends and especially from their husband [11]. They derived great support from the relaxation exercises and from the emotional support which alleviated their feeling of bereavement and anxiety [5, 11].

There is a connection between pregnancy loss and feelings of anxiety and depression after RPL. The literature shows a strong connection between the neuro-immune system, the emotional state of the women and RPL [9, 10, 13]. One of the factors which cause stress and anxiety in Israel is the social pressure from a society which expects a couple to have a baby [3, 4].

Social Aspects of Recurring Miscarriages

Social pressure is a significant factor in the couple's emotional response after a recurring miscarriage [6]. A couple which experiences difficulty in conceiving is inclined to relate to the fertility problem as a kind of disease due to their experience of malaise, connected on the one hand to the couple's self image as being infertile, a feeling of lack of control of the body, and on the other hand to the social pressure connected to society's expectation that they have children [3, 4, 6, 8]. The difficulty in having a baby is interpreted as not meeting the expectations of society, a culture that values heterosexual parenting [19]. Reproduction is perceived as self-evident and the primary and essential factor for a woman's self-realization, with motherhood perceived as her central function. Many women in Israel put their commitment to their family above their commitment to a career or to developing other fields of interest [3, 4, 7].

A voluntary choice not to have children is almost inconceivable. Society sees such a choice as socially deviant [3, 4, 7]. Studies show that women who have experienced recurring miscarriages experience a personal and social crisis due to the stigma. A woman who despite efforts to have children sees herself as one who is not whole, is damaged and sometimes even inferior. This feeling spreads and infiltrates aspects of her personal and sexual identity and all aspects of life. The stigma of infertility causes couples to try to hide their condition [3, 4, 8].

The health care system needs to respond to the emotional stress, depression and anxiety of these RPL women and recommend emotional counseling without the harmfulness of a diagnosis of mental illness [11, 12].

Emotional Support After RPL

Support Tools
Women occasionally are reluctant to seek emotional support due to a feeling of being labeled mentally ill [11]. As the literature shows, emotional support for women after RPL is related to many areas in a woman's life. There are many ways to tender support. In this paper we will describe a number of useful tools.

1. NLP (Neuro Linguistic Programming) and Guided Imagery.
2. CBT (Cognitive Behavior Therapy).
3. Mindfulness Based Stress Reduction MBSR.

It is possible to use one method or to use them in combination according to the patient.

The literature stresses that women with RPL can experience trauma, anxiety, depression, and even PTSD [13]. Studies show that there is an improvement in the emotional state and a decrease in the stress level in therapy for anxiety disorders and PTSD using NLP and CBT [20]. There are no articles describing the use of these methods specifically for treating women with RPL.

NLP (Neuro Linguistic Programming) and Guided Imagery

NLP is a scientific method whose aim is to help a person achieve a change in his perceptions and experience. It is a collection of processes observed in areas of the brain (neurology) and in the use of language (linguistics) and their programming (the manner in which such information is organized in the brain). This method was developed in the 1970s by Professor John Grinder, a linguistics professor and Dr. Richard Bandler a computer specialist and a psychotherapist [21–23]. They determined the concept of NLP.

The term *NLP* is comprised of:

N-Neuro reflects the nervous system (the brain) through which our experiences are processed by the senses: vision, hearing, touch, smell, and taste. They are processed and translated into experiences. For example, when we watch a movie and cry the information is comprehended through the senses of sight and hearing and it is translated into an experience which stimulates our neurological system [22, 23].

L-Linguistic—comprises verbal communications, how we express our thoughts and feelings; how language structures reflect internal and external communications which include thought processes and oral communication as formulated by the person. It is possible to express the same idea in a number of ways where each way creates a different experience. For example, you can say to a woman with unexplained RPL that it is a great challenge to succeed in achieving a live birth. Or you can say to her that although her miscarriage is a result of unexplained reasons experience shows that in similar situations over 75 % succeed in having a successful pregnancy with a live birth. The same statement but the experience is different. When the experience is different the neurological system responds differently [22, 23].

P-Programming—The encounter between what is understood by the neurological system through the five senses, and from language. The programming organizes the results of the analysis of neurological and linguistic events [22, 23].

NLP serves as a diagnostic tool and treatment method for problems requiring a change in behavior and habits, phobias, anxieties, PTSD, allergies,

transferring excellence, etc. This therapeutic approach works within a short time and the therapy is very brief [23]. In the case of Bigley [22] it was found that the treatment by NLP effectively dealt with patients who suffered from anxiety attacks and claustrophobia during MRI testing [23]. In one pilot study it was tested whether NLP could lessen symptoms of PTSD among soldiers and those in emergency services. Twenty-nine subjects participated in the study. Their level of anxiety and depression was tested before and after the intervention which included a variety of NLP techniques. It was found that the anxiety level decreased significantly after the NLP consultation [20, 21].

NLP uses the healing power of the imagination. The human brain does not make distinctions between the real and the imaginary. In many different studies similar neural responses have been observed (using MRI) whether the action was purely imaginary using all the senses or it was something that happened in reality. In both cases, the brain chemistry changes and organizes cells and the connections between the cells to create appropriate motor or verbal skills, in order to perform the same action [24, 25]. A woman with RPL begins to write herself a "script" imagining a variety of future catastrophes. Understanding that the brain does not distinguish between the imaginary and the real allows us to help women imagine for themselves better scripts which improve the neurological system and improve their chances for success [24–27]. Through NLP and guided imagery people suffering from depression and anxiety can be treated and supported using tools which identify their internal resources and strengthen them. The use of imagination to raise consciousness and achieve personal well-being has been in use for a long time in the therapeutic professions treating both body and soul [25–27].

Cognitive Behavior Therapy (*CBT*) is a treatment aimed at lessening psychological distress. The treatment is goal oriented. The cognitive behavior approach diagnoses the psychological problem according to measurable criteria based on research and defines the success of the treatment according to these criteria. The treatment is brief. The patient is an active participant in the treatment process [28].

CBT is a technique which emphasizes the connection between an event, its meaning and its emotional and behavioral consequences. The basic assumption is that thought is the interpretation of the event. The thought creates emotion and the emotion generates behavior. From the beginning of the treatment the therapist shares the logic of the therapeutic process with the patient aiming to make him an active partner in the process and to be aware of its results.

CBT therapy is found to be effective in a wide variety of problems such as different anxiety disorders, depression, eating disorders, and PTSD [28]. The aim of the treatment is to teach the patient to pay attention to negative feelings and thoughts, to deal with them and regulate them while simultaneously paying attention to positive feelings and to grant them significance [28]. The thoughts which accompany a woman with RPL are generally negative. Mostly the woman feels "certain and believes" that she is not able to stay pregnant and will not be able to and therefore she miscarries. This kind of thinking is accompanied by negative feelings of fear and anxiety concerning another failure, frustration, anger, loss, despair, depression, lack of self-esteem [11, 17, 29].

The main goal of cognitive therapy is to assist in understanding the thoughts behind the emotions. This understanding allows for the construction of new alternate ways of thinking which cast doubt on the negative thoughts. This leads to better feelings and a reduction in feelings of unworthiness, fear, anxiety, depression, and more [28].

Mindfulness

One of the first to develop the idea of mindfulness in the west is Prof. Jon Kabat-Zinn. Kabat-Zinn developed a therapy method, MBSR-Mindfulness Based Stress Reduction, to deal with emotional pain and anxiety. The method involves group work for 9 weeks training in meditation and exercises derived from cognitive behavior psychology. Studies show that Mindfulness improves the state of health by reducing depression and anxiety. People who practice Mindfulness meditation daily are more self-aware; they are calmer and exhibit fewer symptoms of stress and burnout at work [30].

Mindfulness exercises are exercises which allows one to enter a state of consciousness of "paying attention aiming at the present moment without judgment and without reaction," a state in which one listens to what catches ones attention at the moment—"outside" (such as a sound, wind) or "inside" (such as physical feeling, emotions, or thoughts) and adopting an approach which does not judge or classify [30, 31].

Supportive Processes for Women with RPL

Women in therapy at the RPL Clinic at the Soroka Medical Center in Israel undergo a comprehensive evaluation as to the reasons for the RPL. These women receive treatment according to the results of the evaluation such as Tender loving care (TLC) which includes personal attention, empathy, listening and availability of treatment, participation in decisions regarding the treatment program, support from the clinic's entire staff and the participation of the husband [12]. In addition at the beginning of the therapy it is suggested that she seek emotional support from psychotherapists and practitioners in CBT, NLP and Guided Imagery. The treatment aims to reduce anxiety, to treat depression, and to improve her sense of well being and that of her husband.

During the treatment and support for women with RPL each of the methods can be used individually or in combination. The decision as to which method to use depends on each specific woman, her difficulties, her emotional state, and her coping resources.

From the accumulated experience of working with the women who come to us we have discerned a number of key problems. These women come with high anxiety; they are desperate and angry. They have lost confidence in their bodies as well as in their physicians. They no longer believe they have a chance to conceive and carry a child to term. Most of them have been running from one medical center to another, from one doctor to another. They are very critical of themselves and of their surroundings. They describe feelings of loneliness and of being misunderstood. These women will tell you they have an understanding supportive husband, but in fact he does not exactly understand what they are really going through and they do not exactly tell him everything. They want to become pregnant and are afraid to.

Here are some of the stories we have heard during our meetings with these women.

Patient "A" came for emotional support in the 11th week of her present pregnancy. She has three living children and has had three miscarriages. She reports that since the last miscarriage a year earlier, she is afraid, anxious, and doesn't sleep at night. She says "I see pictures of the miscarriage, the blood, the fetus suspended on the cord emerging from the vagina over the water in the toilet. I feel helpless, out of control and disappointed…I feel a compulsive need to check the pulse of my fetus every day."

Patient "B" came in for support 3 months after her third miscarriage. She seems confused, anxious, with heart palpitations and stomach aches and does not believe in her ability to become a mother. She says, "I am very angry with myself, I did not look after myself as I should have, I worked too hard, I am irresponsible." When asked what she wants from the treatment she says, "I want to stop having these negative thoughts about pregnancy and myself. I want to believe that 'I will be a mother'…I feel damaged, that I am not good enough, I don't deserve what is happening to me…I feel disappointed, I hate myself and the others who succeed in getting pregnant."

Patient "C" was a religious woman who came for emotional support one and a half months after her third miscarriage which occurred in the 10th week of her pregnancy. "I feel that everyone is expecting me to be pregnant already. When they meet me that is their first question…Everyone looks at my stomach." She says "I went to the E.R. in the 10th week because of a bloody discharge. During the ultrasound the doctor said to me that there was no fetal pulse. I felt that I wanted to die. I said to the doctor that I wanted to die and started to cry. I felt hopeless; it was hard for me to look at pregnant women or babies. I am terribly anxious that it will happen again."

Patient "D" came for emotional support 7 months after an induced abortion in the 23rd week due to a genetic defect. The patient is a carrier of a defective gene. She was in great distress and said "I have a defect, I am defective, things are

not as simple as I would like, I am afraid of my next pregnancy. I am no longer naïve and do not think that pregnancy is a happy time full of love and happiness and thoughts of motherhood. I feel helpless. I am afraid of the next pregnancy."

The working assumption is that these women need emotional support personally customized so that they can function from day to day and so that they are able emotionally and physically to deal with their next pregnancy. The therapeutic contract promises emotional support but does not commit to a successful pregnancy despite the fact that the majority of women do conceive and give birth.

We defined a number of therapeutic targets:

1. To alleviate anxiety and anger aiming to allow the person to function normally day by day.
2. To explain the relation between thoughts, emotions, and behavior.
3. To provide a simple explanation of the interactions in psycho-neuro-immunology, the importance of peace of mind for the success of the process.
4. To help the patient restore her faith and love in herself and her body.
5. To help the patient believes in her doctor and the treatments offered.
6. To treat PTSD if diagnosed (Table 12.1).

Table 12.1 Emotional support for women with recurrent miscarriage

Treatment goals	Therapeutic actions offered
To alleviate anxiety and anger aiming to allow the person to function normally day by day	MBSR-, Guided Imagery, NLP, CBT
To explain the relation between thoughts, emotions, and behavior	Psycho-educational explanation of the process, its significance and importance
To provide a simple explanation of the interactions in psychoneuroimmunology, the importance of peace of mind for the success of the process	Psycho-educational explanation
To help the patient restore her faith and love in herself and her body	NLP, guided imagery, CBT

Treatment goals and therapeutic actions offered

Rachel's Story

Rachel was referred to us for emotional support in the 8th month of her fourth pregnancy. In the background was her first pregnancy which resulted in a normal birth to a healthy baby.

Two years later she had a miscarriage in the 10th week. Three months after that she again became pregnant. Her amniotic membrane is torn and there was a decline in amniotic fluid in week 18 and 2 days later she miscarried. About a year after this miscarriage Rachel turned to us to get emotional support. Rachel appeared uneasy, expressed high anxiety, her voice trembled and she choked back tears. She said the obstetrician referred her for emotional support to help her survive the pregnancy. She remarked that she could not believe there was a chance for this pregnancy to succeed and she so much wanted another child. Rachel's anxiety invaded all areas of her life. She did not sleep well, she did not eat and she found it hard to take care of her house. She found it difficult to communicate with her husband and was afraid to go to work. She reported that she was always checking for signs of a miscarriage, checking to see if her water broke, if the pad was wet or dry. In fact the experience of her last miscarriage was taking over her life.

As mentioned Rachel was under professional monitoring by her gynecologist who took responsibility for the medical side and was always available but also understood her need for emotional support in dealing with her difficult mental state.

At the start of the treatment goals were set: lessen anxiety, return her faith in mind and body and to do everything possible for her to give birth at full term.

The treatment began with two sessions per week with telephone support anytime it was needed. During the session we used methods of NLP and MBSR, relaxation and Guided Imagery. The aim was mainly to calm her down, to give Rachel an interlude of quiet repose.

As a resource we reminded her of the birth of her first daughter as proof that she can carry to term. At first Rachel answered that she has no imagination and this kind of treatment was not suited to her. This is a recognized reaction at this stage and demands repeated explanations of the aim and process of the therapy focusing chiefly on relaxation.

After two and a half weeks of therapy it was suggested to try the Swish NLP technique to change the scenario of failure. After mild relaxation exercises Rachel was asked to describe anew her anxiety regarding her water breaking, the moment when she realized that the pad was wet with amniotic fluid. She described feelings of suffocation and irritability. Again we practiced easy breathing and relaxation and then she was asked to imagine a blurred picture in faded colors and then create from this in her imagination another still blurred image. After imagining the picture she was asked to describe the scene that she would like to see… What would she like to happen at the end? What is the destination she wants to arrive at? At first Rachel hesitated and refused saying she was afraid to think about it. Then Rachel described very carefully that she wants to see herself walking in her yard with a baby carriage accompanied by her daughter Ronit. She was encouraged and asked to give details, such as a description of the yard where this was happening, the smells, the colors, shapes, time of day, weather, and color of the baby carriage. Rachel succeeded in imagining herself as if after the birth walking with her daughter and the new baby in the carriage. At this point she was asked to formulate from this scenario a still picture. After we had two pictures, one blurry associated with a bad experience (which led to anxiety) and another picture of the future where she is with a baby in a carriage. Using the Swish NLP technique the dreadful picture is blurred and the picture of a successful future is brought into focus. We did this a number of times until the terrible picture became blurred and disappeared.

The session ended and another appointment was made 3 days hence. Rachel did not communicate with us during those 3 days. She came to the session smiling and relaxed, reporting that she had begun eating and sleeping normally, and had stopped checking the pads.

Rachel gave birth in week 39 to a healthy wonderful infant. Three weeks later she came to thank us and brought us a picture of herself, with the baby in a carriage and her daughter at her side in the yard of their house.

Conclusions

The experience of RPL represents about 5 % of all pregnancies [9, 10, 12]. There are many factors contributing to RPL but today there is much more awareness of the woman's psychological state and its effect on her mental health and on those coming in contact with her. Today there is also more appreciation of the connection between a woman's mental state and the risks of her having another miscarriage [12].

Recurrent miscarriages can cause psychological trauma and other emotional phenomena such as anxiety, depression, denial, anger, marriage problems, and PTSD. RPL women see themselves as inferior and defective. Pregnancy loss is always accompanied by a sense of bereavement and loss of confidence in the body's ability to carry a baby to term [5–7]. The human socialization process prepares a person for parenting. Failure to bring a child into the world is connected to one's ability to fulfill one's personal right to be a parent. When a woman experiences recurrent miscarriages she feels anxiety and helplessness regarding her ability to realize her rights as a mother. She also feels frustration in face of society's expectation for her to become a mother. In this situation she can experience emotional pain, a feeling of losing control, and helplessness [2, 6, 7]. These women experience a great conflict between their desire to be pregnant and the difficulties in coping with a pregnancy. Each new pregnancy finds them anxious and uncertain about their chances of success. Being pregnant in such a condition increases the risk of miscarriage and a miscarriage is seen as a disaster. A deep understanding of the needs of these women demands the formation of a support system.

Emotional support methods for these women, such as NLP, CBT, MBSR, relaxation, and Guided Imagery assist them in lessening anxiety and relieving depression by strengthening their ability to develop their inner resources which will help them get through another pregnancy with a feeling of confidence and faith in the process. If the treatment for recurrent miscarriage fails after the woman has received emotional support to reinforce her inner resources there is a good chance that she will cope with the loss more effectively and it will be less traumatic due to her being more resilient and better at coping rather than dealing with the situation from a position of weakness. This topic is currently being studied.

Psychological support after RPL increases in importance with the understanding of the psychoneuroimmunology axis which shows a strong association between the woman's anxiety and her immune system and which increases the chance of miscarriage. It has been found that a spike in the hormones connected to stress can reduce the blood supply to the fetus and can even influence fetal blood cell development thereby increasing the probability of miscarriage [12]. In addition, support is crucial to the woman's general well-being and her daily functioning.

Today's medical services are becoming more aware of and are taking into account the psychological aspects of RPL. At the Soroka Medical Center in the RPL Clinic a process has begun to locate those women who are suffering from psychological distress and referring them for psychological support outside of the hospital. Experience shows that women who get such emotional support experience less anxiety and are more able to cope with their next pregnancy.

Mental aspects research on recurrent pregnancy losses has not yet been performed adequately. This important issue deserves to be explored in terms of emotional and mental state of women, as well as in terms of methods and approaches to support women with recurrent pregnancy loss. Those studies raise awareness of health workers including doctors, nurses and social workers to the special needs of these women. It is very important that health care workers include in their treatment program, not only medical treatment to achieve live-birth but also emotional care support.

References

1. Genesis Chapter 1, Verse28.
2. Reed SA, Wan Horn AS. Medical and psychological aspects of infertility and assisted reproductive technology for primary care provider. Mil Med. 2001;166(11):1018–26.
3. Remennick L. Childless in the land of imperative motherhood: stigma and coping among infertility Israeli women. Sex Roles. 2000;43(11):821–41.

4. Remennick L. Between reproductive citizenship and consumerism: attitudes towards assisted reproductive technologies among Jewish and Arab Israeli women. Assist Reprod Testing Gene Global Encounters New Biotechnol. 2009;18:318.

5. Mevorach-Zussman N, Boiotin A, Shelev H, Bilenko N, Mazoor M, Bashiri A. Anxiety and deterioration of quality of life factors association with recurrent miscarriage in an observational study. J Perinat Med. 2012;40(5):495–501.

6. Haelyon H. Longing for a child, perception of Motherhood among Israeli-Jewish women undergoing in vitro fertilization (IVF) treatments. Nashim J Women's Studies Gender Issues. 2006;12:177–203.

7. Ziedenberg H. Gender differences in attitudes towards willingness to donate gametes in Israel, Thesis submitted in partial fulfillment of the requirements for the degree of Doctor of philosophy Submission to the Senate of Ben-Gurion University of the Negev. 2008; 22–90.

8. Dill SK. Surviving infertility. Creating families. The Infertility Awareness Association of Canada. 2005;1:6–8.

9. Shapira E, Ratzon R, Shoham-Vard I, Serjienko R, Mazor M, Bashiri A. Primary vs. secondary recurrent pregnancy loss – epidemiological characteristics, etiology, and next pregnancy outcome. J Perinat Med. 2012;40(4):389–96.

10. Bashiri A, Ratzon R, Amar S, Serjienko R, Mazor M, Shoham-Vardi I. Two vs. three or more primary recurrent pregnancy losses – are there any differences in epidemiologic characteristics and index pregnancy outcome? J Perinat Med. 2012;40(4):65–371.

11. Musters AM, Taminiau-Bloem EF, van den Boogaard E, van deb Veen Goddijn F. Supportive care for women with unexplained recurrent miscarriage: patient's perspective. Hum Reprod. 2011;26(4):873–7.

12. Lachmi-Epstin A, Mazor M, Bashiri A. Psychological and mental aspects and "tender loving care among women with recurrent pregnancy losses". Harefuah. 2012;151(11):633–7.

13. Hosaka T, Matsubayashi H, Sugiyama Y, Izumi S, Makino T. Effect of psychiatric group intervention on natural-killer cell activity and pregnancy rate. Gen Hosp Psychiatry. 2002;24:353–6.

14. Friedman T, Bagchi D. Psychological aspect of spontaneous and recurrent abortion. Curr Obstet Gynecol. 1999;9:9–22.

15. Ingrid HL, Neugebauer R. Psychological morbidity folioing miscarriage. Best Pract Res Clin Obstet Gynecol. 2007;21(2):229–47.

16. Broquet K. Psychological aspect of reaction to pregnancy loss. Psychiatry Adapts. 1999;6(1):12–5.

17. Engelhard MS, van den Hout MA, Arnoud A. Posttraumatic stress disorder after pregnancy loss. Gen Hosp Psychiatry. 2001;23(2):62–6.

18. Stirrat GM. Recurrent miscarriage II: clinical associations, causes, and management. Lancet. 1990;336(18717):728–33. Review Article.

19. Kernberg P. Complex adoption and assisted reproduction technology. Arch Gen Psychiatry. 2002;59(5): 27–47.

20. Wake L, Leighton M. Pilot study using neurolinguistic programming (NLP) in post-combat PTSD. Ment Health Rev J. 2014;19(4):251–64.

21. Bailey R. NLP Counselling. Vol 1. Hebrew ed. Bicester, Oxon, UK: Winslow Press Ltd., Telford Road, Ach Publishing House Ltd.; 1997. p. 10–41.

22. Truter I. Neuro-linguistic programming (NLP) – an attitude of mind leaving behind it a trail of techniques SA Pharm J. 2007;46–40.

23. Bigley J, Griffiths D, Prydderch A, Romanowski J. MilesL, Lidiard H, Hoggard N, Neurolinguistic programming used to reduce the need for an aesthesia in claustrophobic patients undergoing MRI. Br J Radiol. 2010;83(1):13–117.

24. Lahad M, Doron M. SEE FAR CBT: beyond cognitive behavior therapy, protocol for treatment of post-traumatic stress disorder, vol. 1. Amsterdam: Amsterdam IOS Press; 2010. p. 15–32.

25. Lahad M. Fantastic reality creative supervision in therapy. Http://www.nordbooks.co.il. Nordbooks, Printed in Israel; 2006. p. 15–52.

26. Elitzor B. Self-relaxation. www.ORAM.co.il. Oram: Imprint in Israel; 2010. p. 7–120.

27. Tsur A. Being a butterfly: imagination-the healing power, vol. 1. Israel: Modan Publishing House Ltd.; 2003. p. 15–26.

28. Marom S, Gilboa-Schechtman E, Mor N, Meijers J. Cognitive behavioral therapy for adults, therapeutic principles, vol. 1. Israel: Probook Publishing House Ltd.; 2011. p. 1–15.

29. Kersting A, Kroker K, Schlicht S, Baust B, Wagner B. Efficacy of cognitive behavioral internet-based therapy in parents after the loss of a child during pregnancy: pilot data from a randomized controlled trial. Arch Womens Men Health. 2011;14:465–77.

30. Kabat-Zinn J. Full catastrophic of living-using the wisdom of your body and mound to face stress, pain and illness, vol. 3. New York: Bantam Books Trade Paperbacks; 2013. p. 277–355.

31. Greenberg J, Nachshon M. Mindfulness meditation associated with "feeling Less?", vol. 5. New York: Springer Science + Business Media; 2013. p. 471–6. Original Paper.

A Patient's Perspective

Hildee Weiss

As a three-time survivor of pregnancy loss, I know all too well the pain and heartbreak that come with losing a much-wanted pregnancy. I say "survivor," because pregnancy loss is indeed a loss that is not only experienced in the present state but is a loss that has to be overcome and a loss that has a past, a present, and a future. It is a loss that is all too real and a loss that knows no bounds when it comes to race, religion, and social group. It is a loss that I have personally experienced and known three times within the course of a 5-year period. For better or for worse, I call myself a survivor.

Nothing prepared me for the blow that hit me each and every time I was told that my pregnancy was lost. Nothing prepared me for the aftermath of my loss, when I was expected to move onward and upward. And nothing prepared me for the silence that was so deafening, when I so desperately needed to be heard and at the same time hear from others.

I was 25 when I became pregnant for the first time. I had been married for four and a half years and my husband and I were eager and excited about becoming parents. While I didn't "feel" pregnant and I had been spared the horrors of morning sickness, I embraced this special time in my life. I had always loved children—babies, especially—and I couldn't wait to have a child of my own. I bought maternity clothes in my 10th week, keeping the price tags on and I looked forward to wearing them once we officially announced my pregnancy. Both my parents and my husband's parents knew of my pregnancy and they shared in our excitement. We kept the news quiet from our siblings and friends for the first trimester but we knew that they would be delighted with our news. My husband and I talked about names but didn't pick anything out of superstition. I just needed to get through the 12-week visit with my doctor, knowing everything was fine with our baby, and then we could go public and start our planning. It was just a matter of days until we could reveal our news and we couldn't have been more overjoyed.

I had known a few close friends who had suffered a first-trimester miscarriage, so going into my 12-week visit with my ob/gyn, I shared my nervousness about seeing my baby's heartbeat for the first time. I was sure everything was fine and I would see the fluttering and beating heart but until I saw it for myself I was anxious. My doctor examined me and checked the heartbeat but there seemed to be some kind of problem that I didn't understand with the equipment. I was told to go to the radiologist next door, all the while unaware that anything was wrong. (In my mind, I was going to the radiologist for an ultrasound with a "better view.") As it turned out, the office was closing and I was told to return first thing in the morning with my husband. I never suspected anything was amiss. In my mind, it

H. Weiss (✉)
2401 Blossom Lane, Beachwood, OH 44122, USA
e-mail: gweiss@roadrunner.com

© Springer International Publishing Switzerland 2016
A. Bashiri et al. (eds.), *Recurrent Pregnancy Loss*, DOI 10.1007/978-3-319-27452-2_13

was simply a matter of waiting a few hours until we would know that everything was fine and we could finally share our excitement with our extended family and friends.

We went back the next morning, as eager and excited as the previous day, if not more so. The radiologist performed the ultrasound and delivered the blow that broke my heart in half. "Your fetus isn't viable." Huh? I thought. The radiologist added, "There is no heartbeat. Your baby is dead."

Not viable. No heartbeat. Dead. Everything was a blur after hearing those cold and cruel words; yet I remember that day from more than 20 years ago as the day that I was forever changed. I had a D & C that afternoon and was un-pregnant once again.

I can look back at that time and say that my husband and I got through our loss but it came with so much heartache. Losing my first pregnancy didn't just mean losing the baby I was carrying. It meant losing someone I would never meet; someone who was a part of something my husband and I created together and someone I would never know. It meant losing my innocence as that day etched as March 1, 1994, meant I was hardened by my pain yet broken by my grief.

The hospital stay was somewhat of an out-of-body experience, in that I was there experiencing everything physically and emotionally and yet I was raw and not yet feeling the grief that would soon overwhelm me in the coming days, weeks, and months. It was as if I was standing in the corner of my hospital room and in the operating room, observing it all but not feeling it sink in. I was a bystander and a witness to all that was happening around me and yet there was absolutely nothing I could do to stop or go back in time.

The sinking-in part is what I can recall most of all and to this day what I recall with the most pain. There was so much I needed and there was so little I received. Life went on even though I felt I couldn't. I left the hospital empty-handed. I was no longer pregnant and I had nowhere to turn, other than going back to my home and resuming my life once again. There was a follow-up appointment scheduled with my doctor to make sure that everything was back to "normal" physically. There was no follow-up appointment with

anyone at all to make sure that everything was back to "normal" emotionally.

I had questions for my doctor; yet I was told that the miscarriage was "one of those things and probably wouldn't happen again." (It did happen again and a few years after, a third time. And because I had healthy, living children that came in between the losses, nothing was ever questioned or addressed regarding the cause or reason for my losses.)

I needed answers from my doctor and I didn't get them. I needed to know why I lost my baby and I needed to know what to do so that it didn't happen again. I needed words of support from her on that terrible day when she eventually confirmed the radiologist's diagnosis and told me that I would have to have a D & C. I understand that she sees this happen on a regular basis as the statistics in 1994 claimed that 1 out of 4 pregnancies ends in a loss. I recognize that it is a part of her job and yet this happened to ME and it affected ME. I needed her to offer me a hug or some words of comfort during my hospital stay and I needed her reassurance in the aftermath. I understand that she is a doctor and I am a patient but for just a few moments I needed her to reach out to me, woman to woman. I needed to know that yes, this hurts and it will continue to hurt but it is a hurt that is to be expected and it is a hurt that will eventually lessen with time.

I needed some direction to deal with my grief; unfortunately, I was given very little. While I was given home-going instructions to deal with the physical recovery of my miscarriage, I was given nothing to prepare me emotionally for the aftermath of my loss. I was told nothing about support groups at the local hospital where I had my surgery nor did I hear about anything offered at the two other nearby hospitals. I wasn't told about any pregnancy loss websites that existed and to be honest I didn't think to look for resources online that could offer me names of books to read for answers. I think what I wanted most was to hear from others who had been through a miscarriage and tell me that what I was experiencing—the guilt, the anger, the sadness, the questioning of my faith, the isolation—was normal and to be expected.

I didn't have many people to talk to and identify with my grief. My friends and family members were hearing about my miscarriage at the same time they were learning I had been pregnant. They all said, "I'm sorry" and that offered me consolation. What I was also hearing (and this was something that would be said over and over again) was "I'm so glad to hear you were pregnant." The first time someone said that to me, I didn't think much of it but then after hearing it a second time, a third time and so many times after that, I got angrier and angrier. I felt the same way when people told me that it was better to miscarry now than to lose the baby later. I know everyone meant well but the words were more harmful than helpful. Why was the news of my miscarriage a good thing? And what difference does it make if I lost my baby at 12 weeks instead of 24 weeks?

The friends who had suffered miscarriages in the past had gone on to have healthy babies and I didn't feel right approaching them with questions. My siblings had, thankfully, never experienced a pregnancy loss and so I couldn't expect them to understand what I was going through. My husband's brother and his wife did go through a miscarriage but I didn't feel comfortable talking to them and bringing up what I knew to be a painful time in their lives. I was hesitant to talk to my mother and mother-in-law as they had been so excited about my pregnancy and then so devastated when I miscarried. I had an aunt, with whom I had always been close, who confided in me about her own miscarriage. It was only with her and with my husband that I felt I didn't have to grieve in silence. They listened to me, they wiped my tears, and they truly understood my pain.

I went on to have two additional pregnancy losses and I have been blessed with five beautiful, healthy children. The second time I miscarried, I had been eight and a half weeks along and I had two very young children. When I suffered my third loss, I had been almost 6 weeks along and I was a mother to three children. While each loss occurred earlier on in the pregnancy than my first miscarriage and I did have living children to offer me a ray of comfort, I was nonetheless devastated. I heard the words, "at least you have other children" and "this was probably too much for

you, what with two small kids to run after." A part of me just took it and didn't respond, as I know that as with my first miscarriage, people meant well and they were merely trying to offer me comforting words. The other part of me wanted to scream that "yes, I do have a toddler and an infant AND I was looking forward to having this next baby." The loss is no easier with living children. There is no "easy" about pregnancy loss.

On the anniversary of what would have been my due dates, I spend a lot of time thinking about that baby I never birthed and the child I never had the chance to nurture and know. September is particularly a difficult month for me as I remember two of my "angels" within less than 2 weeks. I cry a bit, I ponder over the what-ifs, and I remember all too well those fateful days in 1994, 1997, and 1999, when I was told that those pregnancies had come to an end.

I have moved forward with my life and I am now in a place where I can look at my losses as life experiences that have shaped me and changed me in so many ways. I will never "get over" what I've lost. I am able to write about my losses, I can speak about my losses, and I can be a voice of experience to other grieving parents facing pregnancy loss. I don't pretend to be an expert but I do have the personal experience and I want others to know that they do not have to suffer in silence. I can listen, I can share my experience, and I can validate the loss. That is really all we grieving parents want.

I use the term "we" as I will forever include myself in the ties that bind me with bereaved parents worldwide. It is a "club" I never imagined I would join; yet it is a club that has enriched my life through the friendships I have made with other men and women facing pregnancy loss. There is no turning back the clock on what I experienced and I can only hope that I can offer that voice of experience and be their advocate. There are so many things we need and want when we learn that our pregnancies have been lost and I humbly make the following recommendations and suggestions.

First, I would encourage all doctors, midwives, and obstetrical nurses to have some training in dealing with pregnancy loss, whether it is an early trimester loss, miscarriage, or stillbirth. There should be courses in nursing/medical schools and in the medical residencies for diagnosing and treating pregnancy loss. Bereaved parents need doctors, midwives, and nurses who can offer empathy, support, and comfort in those moments of diagnosing, treating, and recovering from a pregnancy loss of any kind. When a medical assistant comes to the room to check the patient's vitals, he/she should offer a simple "I'm sorry for your loss." When the doctor or midwife confirms the diagnosis of a pregnancy loss, he/she should offer words of consolation, avoid any blame, assuage any guilt, and, to put it simply, be there. We know that the practitioner's time is limited and there are other patients waiting in the next examination room but we need your consideration, your attention, and your understanding that WE matter. The blow of a pregnancy loss is heartbreaking as it is; recognize this and show us that you understand and you will be there for us over the coming days and weeks. Call your patient the day after surgery and ask her how she is coping and LISTEN. Ask her how her husband or partner is coping. Let her know that you are there for her if she has questions or concerns.

We need to hear that we are not alone and we don't need to grieve in silence and isolation. We need to know that there are support groups in our community and there are books and counselors to offer us for resources. Every obstetrician and midwifery office should have lists readily available. I would even go so far as to suggest that there be something of a support system setup in which patients who have previously experienced pregnancy loss offer to be something of a support system to a new grieving parent. I hesitate to offer the word "sponsor" but in essence that is exactly what I needed at my times of loss.

I would strongly recommend that when a woman is admitted to the hospital with a miscarriage or stillbirth, she is situated as far away from the neonatal ward as possible. She is coming to say goodbye to a pregnancy and the one thing she does not need to hear is the sound of a newborn baby's cry. I experienced this personally when I was admitted for a D & C and the sounds of a crying baby still ring in my ears more than 20 years later.

A pregnancy loss packet would be most helpful for a grieving mother to take home. This could include information about local pregnancy loss support groups, a book, and a business card for a social worker or counselor who specializes in pregnancy loss. There are so many wonderful resources that are available and they need to be offered from the onset.

From our family members, friends, clergy, and co-workers, we need you to validate our losses. We do not want you to turn the other way when you see us coming. We do not want you to feel awkward and feel that you cannot acknowledge our loss. We do not need to have our losses trivialized or minimized. Whether we were five days pregnant, 5 weeks pregnant, or 5 months pregnant, we were looking forward to becoming parents. Whether this was a first pregnancy or a tenth pregnancy, we were excited about giving birth and holding our babies. Please do not say "it's for the best" or "God had another plan" or "You will have another one." Losing a much-wanted pregnancy is not for the best and there is no guarantee that there will be another pregnancy. Please do not say "I can't imagine what you're going through" because we hear it as "this could never happen to me." The one and only thing you should say is "I'm so sorry for your loss and I am here for you." Leave it at that. And when we come to you and we want to talk and share our grief, be there for us. Listen to us and let us cry and vent and say whatever we need to say and be there for us. You don't have to offer words … just listen and be there for us. Do not tell it's time to move on and urge us to "get over it." Pregnancy loss is not something that one gets over. We will move on but it will be on our time watch and not on anyone else's watch.

Part V

The Future

Asher Bashiri, Avishai Shemesh, Angel Porgador, Gershon Holcberg, and Maor Kabessa

Multifactorial Etiology of Recurrent Miscarriage

Despite the great advance in recurrent miscarriage (RM) research in the recent years, about 50 % of the cases are still without known etiology, demonstrating how much more information is needed.

Christiansen et al. [1] suggested changing the methods and goals of our research in RPL. Sporadic miscarriages happen in 10–20 % of the

A. Bashiri, MD (✉)
Director Maternity C and Recurrent Pregnancy Loss Clinic, Department of Obstetrics and Gynecology, Faculty of Health Sciences, Soroka University Medical Center, Ben-Gurion University of the Negev, P.O. Box 151, Be'er Sheva 84101, Israel
e-mail: abashiri@bgu.ac.il

A. Shemesh
The Shraga Segal Department of Microbiology, Immunology and Genetics, Ben Gurion University of the Negev, Be'er Sehva, Israel

A. Porgador, PhD
National Institute for Biotechnology in the Negev, Ben Gurion University of the Negev, Be'er Sheva, Israel

G. Holcberg, MD, PhD
Placental Research Laboratory, Maternity-C Department and High Risk Pregnancy, Faculty of Health Sciences, Soroka University Medical Center, Ben Gurion University of the Negev, Be'er Sheva, Israel

M. Kabessa
Faculty of Health Sciences, Ben Gurion University of Negrev, Be'er Sheva, Israel

population and if recurrent miscarriage was solely due to three sporadic miscarriages we would expect a prevalence <0.5 %. However, the observed prevalence is 1.4–1.8 % (defined as three or more consecutive miscarriages). From the 50 % with known etiology, the following reasons were identified: uterine abnormalities, parental chromosome aberrations, various endocrine disturbances, and antiphospholipid antibodies. This multifactorial etiology is accepted at the population level, but at the individual level RM is considered to be monofactorial. Some of the pathologies indeed are found in RM couples in increased prevalence, but they are also found in couples with completely normal fecundity [2, 3]. This and the fact that none of the quoted etiologies exhibit a high sensitivity or specificity, led a group of researchers to propose that RM can be considered multifactorial in each couple.

Miscarriages Can Be Divided into Fetally Caused and Maternally Caused

Fetally caused miscarriages include all the chromosomal aberrations, and account for 43 % of the miscarriages in the normal population [4]. Abnormal trophoblast invasion and development are included in maternally caused miscarriages. This impairment of the trophoblast growth can be related to polycystic ovary syndrome (PCOS) [5, 6], excessive prothrombic events in the maternal vessels and the fetal–maternal interface [7, 8], and local or systemic immunological reaction to the fetus or trophoblast. Although anatomical abnormalities are considered to be maternally caused RMs they are not included in this model.

Biomarkers

Recognizing that autoimmune diseases, thromboembolic diseases, and PCOS are associated with RM led to the investigation of nongenetic and genetic biomarkers. Polymorphisms in approximately 100 genes have already been investigated. It is believed that those three diseases are caused by many genes and environmental factors—each of them contributes a little, and they add up to the overall risk of developing a disease. Once this total disease risk has exceeded the disease threshold, the disease will become a reality. An interesting finding is that many diseases are associated with several relatively common genetic polymorphisms associated with modest risk of disease and several rare polymorphisms associated with higher risk of disease [9], and that carrying two genetic biomarkers for RM results in a higher overall total risk for RM than the additive risk of each factor [10–12]. Despite some observations that recognized the connection between some polymorphisms and RM, no genetic polymorphism has so far proven unequivocally to be associated with RM. Apparently, RM inheritance happens through a multifactorial mode and is not simply Mendelian [1].

Rull et al. [13] explain that the difficulties in finding genetic biomarkers are due to differences in study designs, definitions of RPL and control group, focus on RM women instead of couples or placenta, low statistical power due to small sample size, ethnic difference in risk variants, population-specific low-impact gene variants increasing RM risk *in consort,* contribution of lifestyle and environmental factors on the pregnancy course, and secondary pathways affecting protein translation/metabolism lead-

ing to discrepancies between genotype and respective protein levels, e.g., Factor XII, Protein Z [14, 15].

Implications for Research

Apparently, discovering new genes and other risk factors that are strongly associated with RM will be impossible, and small studies that will succeed in doing so won't be successfully replicated by subsequent studies. In order to successfully detect genetic polymorphism with a weak but statically significant association with RM, large sample size groups of patients and controls must be included. In order to screen for only one polymorphism, 1213 patients and 1213 controls are needed [8]. Researchers must also keep in mind the great genetic polymorphism diversity among different ethnic groups when doing meta-analyses, and include only patients from related ethnic backgrounds. The importance of combinations of genetic biomarkers for RM—immunological, thrombophilic, and endocrine—must be further investigated.

Implications for Clinical Practice

When a single risk factor for a patient with RM is detected, the explanation given to the patient is much easier, relieving for the patient and answering the patient's wish. However, as we saw, still, a great percentage of patients are with unknown etiology.

According to Christiansen's model, the optimal future scenario is the condition where for every couple, combining information about validated genetic biomarkers, their individual strengths of association with RM, and their degree of epistatic interaction, together with information about relevant clinical factors into a computer-based algorithm, will derive the etiological fractions that are immunological, thrombophilic, endocrine, and fetal.

This knowledge will provide the clinician with the optimal means of providing the treatment that has been proven to be most efficient in placebo-controlled trials in adequately selected patients as discussed.

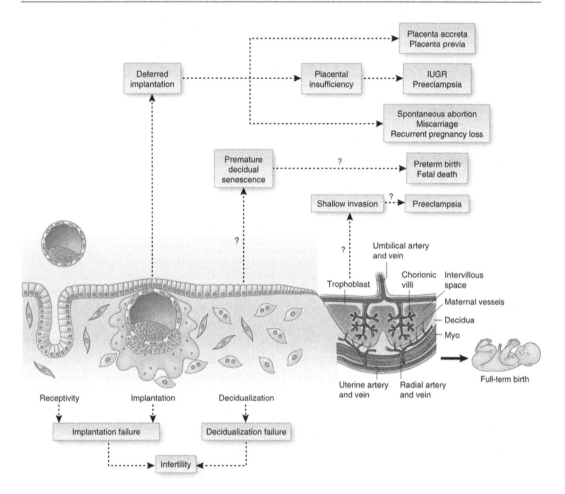

Fig. 14.1 Defective receptivity, implantation, and/or decidualization can lead to infertility. Deferred implantation past the window of receptivity can lead to misguided embryo placement and implantation, resulting in placenta previa, ectopic placentation (placenta accreta) or placental insufficiency resulting in intrauterine growth restriction (IUGR) and/or preeclampsia. Implantation beyond the normal window can also give rise to spontaneous abor-

tion, miscarriage and recurrent pregnancy loss, leading to infertility. Premature decidual senescence can lead to preterm birth and fetal death, whereas shallow trophoblast invasion into maternal decidua and/or blood vessels can lead to preeclampsia. [Reprinted Cha, J., X. Sun, and S.K. Dey, Mechanisms of implantation: strategies for successful pregnancy. Nature medicine, 2012. 18(12): p. 1754–1767. With permission Nature Publishing Group]

Window of Implantation

Human reproduction is very inefficient compared to other mammalian species, with many pregnancies being complicated or lost due to different disorders. A new research field might shed light on the implantation molecular events and try to understand some of those pathologies and their connection to RPL.

Recent publications have shown that implantation is a complex process, with many perils waiting to happen, such as preterm birth, IUGR, pre-

eclampsia, placenta accerta, placenta previa, and miscarriage, in a case implantation doesn't occur in its usual precise way (Fig. 14.1) [16]. Implantation is composed of two key components: the embryo and the receptive endometrium. This complex process depends on cross-talk between the embryo and the endometrium, and the very well synchronized progesterone-dependent changes in the endometrium to render it responsive to the embryonic signals. The concept of the "passive" deciduas and the "active" or "invasive" embryo is being challenged by recent research. Due to ethics issues and inaccessibility of implantation sites in humans, most of our knowledge of early pregnancy events is based on animal models and in vitro models. The window of implantation is a short time span starting ~6 days after ovulation and can last up to 5 days, in which the blastocyst is competent and the endometrium is at its receptive stage [17, 18]. In humans, compared to other mammals, the trophoblast invasion is deep, thus ensuring the endometrium has decidualized and is now ready for the embryo, can prevent failure in implantation, and be "selective" for the embryo quality [19].

Decidualization is a postovulatory process, driven mainly by the progesterone secretion from the corpus luteum, in which the endometrium is prepared for embryo implantation and pregnancy. Human endometrial stroma cells differentiate from fibroblast-like into secretory and receptive decidual endometrial stromal cells. It happens every cycle, during the mid-secretory phase, irrespective of pregnancy [20]. A novel hypothesis named "menstrual preconditioning" might have the answer for why the decidualization process happens each cycle, ending in most cases in menstrual bleeding and shedding of the decidua [21].

In "menstrual preconditioning" the repetitive, short exposures to harmful stimuli to a degree below the threshold for tissue injury will provide some degree of protection from subsequent injury—as will happen when the trophoblast deeply invades into the endometrium during pregnancy. It appears that decidualization grants valuable characteristics to the endometrium, including embryo defense against environmental and oxidative stress, regulation of trophoblast invasion, and protection of the uterus from aggressive invasion by the embryo.

Only after the decidualization process do the endometrium stroma cells have the ability to act as biosensors of the embryo quality and react to low quality embryos by shutting down production of key implantation mediators and immunomodulators such as IL-1b, -6, -10, -17, -18, eotaxin, and heparin-binding EGF-like growth factor, thus preventing it from implanting [22]. This process is considered to be "embryo selection" in humans.

What Happens When There Is Impaired Embryo Selection?

Understanding decidualization's important role led to the idea that aberrations during the decidualization and implantation might give rise to pregnancy with embryos who would otherwise be rejected by the decidua, resulting in early embryo loss. For example, a study of 221 women attempting to conceive demonstrated dramatic risk, increasing on a daily basis, of early miscarriage if pregnancy was established beyond the normal "implantation window" [23]. Correspondingly, recent observations succeeded in identifying several differences between women who suffer from RPL and no-RPL women: Women suffering from RPL express lower levels of mucin 1, an anti-adhesion molecule that contributes to the barrier function of luminal epithelium [24–26]. Another research showed different levels of two maker genes: higher levels of *prok1*, which encodes prok1, a cytokine that promotes endometrium receptivity, and lower levels of prolactin, a prototypic marker of decidualizing endometrial cells [27].

It was also shown that decidualized endometrial stromal cells from women who suffer from RPL fail to discriminate between low and high quality embryos when it comes to migrating towards the embryo at the site of implantation, unlike non-RPL women (as seen in Fig. 14.2) [28].

The lack of embryo natural selection might provide an explanation for chromosomal and nonchromosomal pregnancy failures.

Superfertility and RPL

One could describe clinical pregnancies as "the tip of the iceberg"—representing only 40 % of all conceptions, when 30 % of all conceptions are lost before implantation and an additional 30 % are lost before 6 weeks gestation [21].

The odds for a fertile couple to achieve pregnancy is ~20 % during one menstrual cycle, defined as the Monthly Fecundity Rate (MFR), odds that are considered to be very low compared to other mammalian species [29].

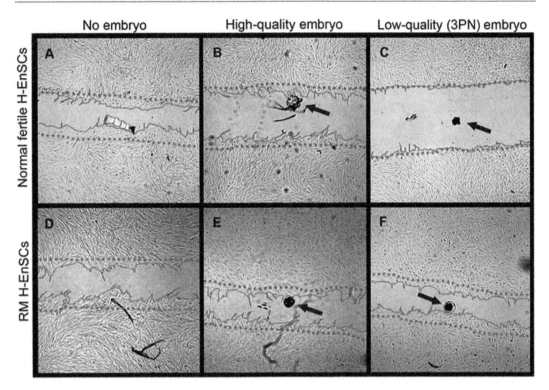

Fig. 14.2 The migration zone after adding a high-quality, low-quality or no embryo. The migratory response of decidualized H-EnSCs from normally fertile (**a–c**) and RM women (**d–f**) was analyzed in absence of a human embryo (**a, d**), in presence of a high-quality embryo (**b, e**) or a low-quality embryo (**c, f**). Phase contrast pictures were taken 18 h after creating the migration zone. The *dotted line* represents the front of the migration zone

directly after its creation. As a reference for the position of the embryo, the bottom of the plate was marked. The arrows indicate the position of the embryo. All pictures were taken with 25× magnification. [Reprinted from Weimar, C.H., et al., Endometrial stromal cells of women with recurrent miscarriage fail to discriminate between high-and low-quality human embryos. PLoS One, 2012. 7(7): p. e41424. With permission from PLoS One]

Using the MFR, a mathematical model predicts that 74, 93, and 100 % of normally fertile couples will achieve pregnancy in 6, 12, and 24 months.

Subfertility and superfertility have been defined by MFRs of 5 % or less, and 60 % or more, respectively [29]. According to the Tietze Model, it has been estimated that 79 % of the population is fertile, 18 % subfertile or infertile, and 3 % superfertile [30].

This relative inefficiency is sometimes considered to represent a strategy dealing with embryo chromosomal abnormalities, which is accepted as the most common cause for miscarriage, including recurrent miscarriage [31].

Recent observations have shown that as much as 40 % of the women with RPL can be defined as superfertile, with time-to-pregnancy (TTP) shorter than 3 months [27]. Rapid conceptions are associated with risk of early pregnancy loss even in low-risk populations, which can partly be explained by the lack of natural embryo selection.

In summary, we might learn from the low efficacy of human reproduction the role of cyclic decidualization of the endometrium and its importance.

Teklenburg et al. [22] coined the term "window of natural embryo selection," as it reflects the functional role of decidualizing stromal cells in assessing the implanting embryo's quality, and moreover the decidualizing stromal cells end the window of endometrial receptivity and enable the mother to dispose of embryos who are not "high quality."

The most significant conclusion might be preventing early pregnancy complications and failures by targeting the endometrial decidual response prior to pregnancy or immediately after implantation.

Heparin Use in Recurrent Pregnancy Loss

Heparin is a very widely used injectable anticoagulant and, according to the World Health Organization's List of Essential Medicines, it is one of the most important medications needed in a basic health system [32].

It was originally isolated from canine liver cells, hence its name (hepar is Greek for "liver") in 1916, but it wasn't until the mid-30s that heparin was manufactured in a safe, nontoxic form, easily available, thus making it a popular anticoagulant. In the human body, heparin is stored exclusively in the granules of subsets of mast cells [33]. Although it is used principally in medicine for anticoagulation, its true physiological role in the body is still uncertain, since blood anticoagulation is achieved mostly by heparan sulfate proteoglycans derived from endothelial cells [34].

Almost 100 years after heparin's discovery, nowadays best known for its first described anticoagulant ability, it is being researched for its other abilities as well. Heparin is useful in RPL in very specific indications but there is an option that some other less-known characteristics of the drug have impact on RPL outcome that come from other medical fields. Heparin is believed to possess many biological activities that include the ability to modulate embryonic development, neurite outgrowth, tissue homeostasis, wound healing, metastasis, cell differentiation, cell proliferation, and inflammation [33].

In this chapter we'll see which of those attributes is pertinent in the RPL clinic through heparin's effect on different molecules in in vitro studies and in vivo experiments.

Heparin's Effect on Different Molecules

Although our knowledge about heparin's anticoagulant properties has developed in the last century, discoveries about heparin's anti-inflammatory features are comparatively new (see Chap. 2 for elaborated information). Heparin affects several molecules, including cytokines, growth factors, adhesion molecules, cytotoxic peptides, and tissue-destructive enzymes, many of which are crucially involved in the inflammatory process. Each of these proteins might be essential in better understanding the inflammatory component in RPL, and might help to decrease this phenomenon.

During the process of implantation heparin, and heparin-derived molecules, affect through expression of adhesion molecules, matrix-degrading enzymes, and trophoblast phenotype and apoptosis [35].

LMWH was shown to increase matrix metalloproteinase (MMPs) concentrations and activity and reduce their tissue inhibitor (TIMP) in a dose-dependent manner. Two of those MMPs, a group of matrix-degrading enzymes, were found to be necessary for the embryo's ability to degrade the basement membrane of the uterine epithelium and to invade the uterine stroma [36]. Additionally, It was shown that LMWH induces an increased decidual expression and secretion of heparin-binding EGF-like growth factor (HB-EGF) and reduced TNF-alpha-induced apoptosis [37]. LMWH induces activation of a DNA-binding transcription factor that, once activated, enhances HB-EGF expression [38]; heparin has the ability to activate the EGF receptor in primary villous trophoblasts [39].

During the first trimester, fetal and placental development takes place in a low O_2 tension environment, which is important to prevent complications related to exposure with normal concentrations of oxygen, such as preeclampsia, IUGR, and miscarriage [40]. HB-EGF has an important role in preventing hypoxic-induced apoptosis in the early stages of placentation. Heparin was also found to prevent apoptosis in human trophoblasts triggered by pathological and other stimuli ((IFN)-γ, (TNF)-α, thrombin, staurosporine) and activated survival signal transduction pathways [39].

More information on the effects of heparin on different molecules is elaborated in Table 14.1.

In Vitro Models Succeeded in Showing Some of Heparin's Beneficial Effects

1. Dextran sulfate sodium (DSS)-induced colitis symptoms in a mouse model were found to be relieved by LMWH. It was found to inhibit the expression of IL-1b and IL-10 in the intestinal mucosa of DSS-induced colitis thus down-

Table 14.1 Proteins involved in the inflammatory response that are bound by heparin and related molecules

Examples of heparin-binding inflammatory mediators	(Patho)physiological significance	Examples	Comments
Adhesion molecules	Cell transport	CD11b/CD18 [132] (MAC1)	–
–	–	P-selectin [133, 134] L-selectin [133]	Specific residues that are found in P- and L- (but not E-) selectin are required for heparin/heparin-sulfate binding [135]. Inhibition of selectin-dependent leukocyte rolling by heparin and related molecules is directly related to sulphation [136]
Chemokines [137]	Inflammatory cell recruitment and activation; viral infection	RANTES, IL-8, MIP1, MCP1, eotaxin	–
–	–	PF4	A minimum length of GAG chain is required for binding of PF4, a property that is exploited in improving the side-effect profile of heparin as an anticoagulant [138]
Growth factors [137]	Tissue repair and repairing; angiogenesis	PDGF, VEGF, TGF-β	–
–	–	FGF2	Binding affinity is related to both length and composition (L-iduronic acid content) of the GAG chain [139]. FGF2 signal transduction requires binding of heparin-sulfate (or heparin) to both FGF2 and its receptor. 2-O-sulphation is essential for the former and 6-O-sulphation for the latter. Therefore, selectively 6-O-desulphated heparin competitively inhibits FGF2-induced angiogenesis [140]

(continued)

Table 14.1 (continued)

Examples of heparin-binding inflammatory mediators	(Patho)physiological significance	Examples	Comments
Enzymes [137]	Digestion of tissue/ECM structural components	Heparanase69 MMPs	–
–	–	Elastase cathepsin	As well as directly binding elastase and cathepsin G, heparin is thought to modulate the activity of these enzymes through potentiation of their natural inhibitor, SLPI. Heparin binds SLPI with greater affinity than less-sulphated GAGs, although within heparin, undersulphated chains bind with the highest affinity [141]
Cytotoxic mediators [137]	Destruction of parasites; tissue damage	ECP MBP	–

ECM extracellular matrix, *ECP* eosinophil cationic protein, *FGF2* fibroblast growth factor 2, *GAG* glycosaminoglycan, *IL-8* interleukin-8, *MAC1* macrophage 1, *MBP* major basic protein, *MCP1* monocyte chemotactic protein 1, *MIP1* macrophage inflammatory protein 1, *MMPs* matrix metalloproteases, *PDGF* platelet-derived growth factor, *PF4* platelet factor 4, *RANTES* regulated on activation, normal T-cell expressed and secreted, *SLPI* secretory leukocyte protease inhibitor, *TGF-β* transforming growth factor-β, *VEGF* vascular endothelial growth factor
Reprinted from Lever R, Page CP. Nonanticoagulant Effects of Heparin: An Overview. Handb Exp Pharmacol. 2012;(207):281–305. With permission from Springer Science

regulating the expression of inflammatory cytokine production [41].

2. When given after ischemia, heparin and *N*-acetylheparin were found to reduce the extent of myocardial injury associated with regional ischemia and reperfusion in the canine heart, in a mechanism of cytoprotection that is unrelated to alterations in the coagulation cascade and may involve inhibition of complement activation in response to tissue injury [42].

3. The effects of single administrations of aerosolized heparin, LMWH, were examined on antigen-induced airway hyperresponsiveness and leukocyte accumulation in neonatal immunized rabbits, and were found to significantly inhibit the development of airway hyperresponsiveness if given prior to antigen challenge [43].

In Vivo Experiments

Several small clinical trials have shown heparin can be helpful in several inflammatory diseases thanks to its anti-inflammatory qualities.

1. More than 20 years ago, it was discovered that inhaled heparin prevents exercise-induced asthma when given to the patients 45 min before their exercise. The researchers' hypothesis was that this non-anticoagulant ability was more likely related to heparin's modulation on mediator release rather than to an effect on smooth muscle [44].

2. In a reported study, patients with ulcerative colitis unresponsive to high dose corticosteroid therapy were treated with heparin. Twelve out of 16 patients showed marked improvement in the disease activity [45], although meta-analyses of this and similar trials have concluded that there is currently insufficient evidence to support the use of heparin for the treatment of active ulcerative colitis [46].

3. In a different study enoxaparin was shown to be of benefit when given to COPD patients and a significant increase in forced expiratory volume in 1 s (FEV1) over baseline was observed. A possible mechanism is heparin's ability to inhibit the activity of neutrophil-derived proteases such as elas-

tase and cathepsin G, or other neutrophil activities including degranulation, the respiratory burst, and processes involved in neutrophil trafficking into tissues. Given that COPD is an airways inflammatory disease with a predominance of neutrophils, the researchers hypothesized that heparin may have some therapeutic benefit in patients with COPD [47]. More diseases affected by non-anticoagulant attributes of heparin are elaborated in Table 14.2.

Table 14.2 Conditions (other than thrombosis) in which heparin has been reported to confer benefit

Condition level of evidence	Level of evidence
Acute respiratory distress syndrome/acute lung injury	Animal models [142, 143] Anecdotal report (human) [144]
Allergic encephalomyelitis	Animal models
Allergic rhinitis	Controlled trial (human)
Arthritis	Anecdotal report (human) [145]
Asthma	Animal models, controlled trials (human)
Cancer	Animal models, some trials (human) Some meta-analyses
Chronic obstructive pulmonary disease	Controlled trial (human)
Delayed-type hypersensitivity reactions	Animal models
Inflammatory bowel disease	Some controlled trials (human)
Interstitial cystitis	Human experimental model of condition [146] Related molecule (pentosan polysulphate) used clinically [147]
Transplant rejection	Animal models
Wound healing	Various reports in animals and humans

Reprinted from Lever R, Page CP. Novel drug development opportunities for heparin. Nature Reviews Drug Discovery 2002;1(2):140–148. With permission from Nature Publishing Group

Heparin and Recurrent Implantation Failure (RIF)

The term RIF has been used to describe IVF treatment failure due to embryos' failure to implant. The ESHRE PGD consortium document mentioned that RIF can be considered after more than three high-quality embryo transfers or implantation failure with transfer of ≥10 embryos in multiple transfers with exact numbers to be determined by each center [48]. A meta-analysis with systemic review of the literature compared the use of LMWH with placebo or no adjuvant treatment in women with RIF undergoing IIVF/ICSI. The results have shown that in women with at least three RIFs, the use of LMWH during IVF treatment improved the live birth rate in 79 %. These results show that heparin might have a useful and important role during IVF treatment and more research should be done.

Heparin and Recurrent Pregnancy Loss

The role of heparin and LMWH has long been investigated and published, mainly in the context of antiphospholipid syndrome and thrombophilia. As was shown in the LIVE-ENOX study, prophylactic administration of enoxaparin to women with RPL and thrombophilia was found to be effective and safe [49]. Several studies that investigated heparin's role when it comes to women who suffer with RPL with an unknown etiology didn't show heparin to be beneficial, despite heparin attributes described hitherto.

One research done in Israel in 2006 compared live birth rates in women who suffered from RPL. One group was administered enoxaparin (LMWH) while the other received aspirin. No statistical difference was found between the two groups when comparing live birth rates, but a difference was shown between the live birth rates as expected from the literature (60 % after three pregnancy failures, 40 % after four pregnancy failures) and their results in both groups with more than 80 % live birth rate.

In a study where enoxaparin was compared to placebo when treating women with RPL with unknown cause no significant difference in live birth rate was found between the two groups (66.6 and 72.9 %, respectively) [50].

A study that compared different treatment methods for women with unexplained RPL found no difference in live birth rate (written in brackets after each group) when comparing treatment regimens with aspirin (50.8 %), aspirin + (LMWH) nadroparin (54.5 %), and placebo (57.0 %) [51].

In conclusion, heparin has a place of honor in RPL treatment thanks to its anticoagulant ability; heparin's additional characteristics are the reason for the conclusion that it might be useful in RPL women who don't have thrombophilia. Hitherto, no conclusive evidence has yet supported this idea. Further research and investigation are needed to be sure that we do not inject heparin for no reason.

Involvement of Immunity in Recurrent Pregnancy Loss

Pregnancy: A Balancing Act of the Maternal Immune System

Pregnancy success requires suppression of the mother's immune system, enabling an immune-tolerant state [52]. The maternal immune system of endometrial and decidual tissues is primarily composed of immune cell populations that are myelomonocytic, T cells and decidual Natural Killer (dNK) cells. dNK cells are thought to play an important role, serving as the predominant cell type in this process [53]. These immune cell populations play an important role in placental tissue development, fetal growth, and establishment of immune-tolerance by secretion of various type-1 cytokines (IFN-γ, TNF-α, TNF-β, and IL-2) that contribute to cellular immunity, and type-2 cytokines (IL-4, IL-5, IL-6, IL-10, and IL-13) that encourage humoral immunity.

The balance between type-1 and type-2 cytokines is essential to the success of pregnancy [54–56]. IFN-γ supports remodeling of spiral arteries, promotes immune tolerance by inhibition of pro-inflammatory T_H17 cells, and encourages indole-

amine 2,3-dioxygenase (IDO) upregulation in myelomonocytic cells, which in turn induces Treg FOXP3$^+$ and suppress CD8$^+$ T cells [53, 57, 58]. IFN-γ also increases TRAIL-R expression on syncytiotrophoblasts, and human trophoblasts express FasL; both molecules can serve as a mechanism for protection against dNK and T cells. TNF-α mediates apoptosis of cytotrophoblasts and promotes the formation of syncytiotrophoblasts [59]. IL-10 inhibits the secretion of IFN-γ and TNF-α, modulating trophoblast invasion and suppressing T_H17 cells [60]. IL-10 also regulates the number of myelomonocytic cells that are the main antigen presenting cells in the decidua tissue (20–30 % throughout pregnancy) and have a role in defending against microbes. Type 3 cytokines, such as TGF-β, can regulate the balance between type-1 and type-2 cytokines. Secretion of TGF-β by decidual myelomonocytic cells leads to inhibition of dNK and prevents the killing of the cytotrophoblast by dNK [61]. Other cytokines and chemokines additionally have a role in placenta development and immune tolerance. For example, MIP-1α (CCL3) and MIP-1β (CCL4) are important to attract and activate maternal immune cells, while IL-8 promotes trophoblast migration. GM-CSF regulates decidual leukocyte populations and enhances placental growth and differentiation [62, 63] thereby, both type-1 and type-2 cytokines have a major role in regulating the development of placental tissue and establishment of an immune-tolerance towards the fetus.

Recurrent Pregnancy Loss and NK Cells: Breaking the Balance

Recurrent pregnancy loss (RPL) was recently suggested to be associated with superfertility. In a retrospective analysis of 560 RPL patients, Salker et al. showed that 40 % of the women were considered "superfertile," relative to the prevalence in the total population that is about 3 % [21, 64]. Superfertility refers to a longer "Implantation window" [65]. This interval in the menstrual cycle is a transient endometrial state with a high receptivity for the adherence of a blastocyst that is dependent on paracrine signals from stromal cells to the immune cell popu-

Fig. 14.3 Human natural killer cells interacting with CFSE-labeled cervical cancer (HeLa) cells (*green*) and nuclei dye (DAPI *blue*). Filamentus actin is labeled with Phalloidin (*yellow* to *red*) to show points of interaction. Acquires using FV1000 (Olympus) equipped with 100× oil objective. [Confocal Microscopy, Courtesy of Mr. Uzi Hadad, Ben-Gurion University of the Negev]

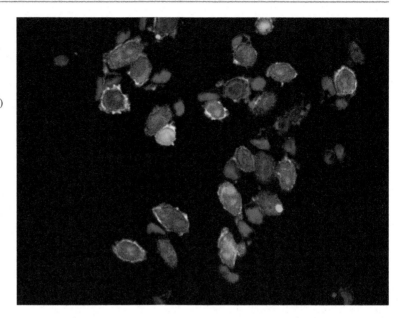

lations and is part of the decidualization process[66]. This prolonged blastocyst receptivity correlates with early pregnancy loss and superfertility [21].

During the first trimester of pregnancy, dNK cells are the dominant cell population and are about 50–70 % of leukocytes (Fig. 14.3) [67–69]. dNK cells secrete IFN-γ, TNF-α, GM-CSF, IP-10, MIP-1α (CCL3), MIP-1β (CCL4), IL-8, VEGF, PLGF, Ang-1, Ang-2, IL-10, and IL-1RA [70, 71]. Decidual stromal cells can regulate myelomonocytic cells and dNK cells by the IL-33/ST2L/sST2 axis. Upon decidualization, a mechanism that was disordered in stromal cells of women with RPL [72], the IL-33/ST2 axis, also promotes the temporal expression of receptivity genes in stromal cells; failure to restrain this axis leads to a longer implantation window [72]. IL-33 promotes proliferation of stromal cells, macrophages, and trophoblasts [73]. ST2, a receptor for IL-33, is expressed on dNK but not on peripheral blood NK cells (see Chap. 6 for elaborated information). Culture medium from decidual stromal cells inhibits the cytolytic activity of dNKs. Furthermore, it shifts the cytokines' balance of dNK from type-1 to type-2 by downregulating the secretion of IFN-γ and TNF-α, and upregulating IL-10 [74]. In mice, administration of IFN-γ and TNF-α promote abortions and both cytokines inhibit growth of human trophoblasts

in vitro [55]. IL-33 also up regulates the expression of PCNA in stromal cells, a nuclear protein that was shown to inhibit NK cell function by interaction with NKp44 [75–77].

Moreover, it was shown that decidual stromal cells and trophoblasts express ligands to DNAM-1, NKp30, and NKp44, which are activation receptors expressed on NK cells [71, 78]. Recently, it was suggested that women with RPL have impaired regulation of pregnancy-related cytokines [79, 80]. Analysis of peripheral blood NK cells and their NKp30, NKp44, and NKp46 receptors (NCRs) expression compared to intracellular cytokine expression (TNF-a, IFN-γ, IL-4, IL-10) after activation revealed a negative correlation between NCRs' protein expression and intracellular cytokine. Furthermore, the correlation between the mRNA expression of NKp30, NKp46, and pregnancy-related cytokines seems to be lost in placental tissue from RPL patients compared to elective abortions. Moreover, mRNA of IFN-γ, TNF-α, and IL-10 was higher in placenta tissue obtained from spontaneous miscarriage patients [81, 82].

Depletion of NK cells in a murine model did not have an effect on the outcome of pregnancy [83]. However, in an IL-10 KO murine model, NK cell activity was enhanced after LPS administration and led to pregnancy loss. Depletion of dNK or administration of anti-TNF-α or -IL-10 rescued pregnancies [84]. These observations point to the necessity of a balance between type-1 and type-2 cytokines, which in turn influence dNK cells activity and can lead to pregnancy loss [85].

Influencing the Balance: Target for Therapy

Immunologic etiologies can be attributed to 40 % of all RPL cases. There is a strong association between pregnancy loss and type-1 cytokines while a successful pregnancy is associated with type-2 cytokines [54–56]. In a murine model of antiphospholipid syndrome (APS), antiphospholipid (aPL) Abs increased in decidual and systemic TNF-α levels, which promote trophoblast apoptosis, identifying TNF blockade as a potential therapy for the pregnancy complications [86]. TNF-α activity can be blocked with monoclonal antibodies against the TNF-α molecule (adalimumab) or against soluble TNF-α receptors (etanercept) [87, 88]. TNF-α blockers administered with or without anticoagulants, or anticoagulants + IVIG treatments (control groups), were given to women with RPL history during pregnancy. The live birth rate of patients who received TNF-α blockers was 71 %, whereas the control groups showed rates of 19 and 54 %, respectively [89]. The same trend was observed in women undergoing IVF; TNF-α blockers improve the implantation rate [90].

G-CSF was also found to have a positive effect on RPL patients. G-CSF reduces the cytotoxicity and IFN-γ secretion of dNK cells, increases the number of Treg cells, and reduces the synthesis of various cytokines, among them TNF-α [91]. A randomized controlled trial of women with RM treated with G-CSF or a placebo showed that G-CSF administrations increased the live birth rate from 48.5 % (placebo group) to 82.8 % (G-CSF group) [92]. In a second study, treatment of RPL patients undergoing assisted reproductive treatment (IVIG, LMWH, cortisone) with G-CSF increased the live birth rate from 13 to 32 % [93].

The results of these few clinical studies reveal the necessity of maintaining a balance between

type 1 and type 2 cytokines in early pregnancy. TNF-α inhibition seems to have much potential in future clinical therapies.

RPL and Several Molecular Findings

Alijotas-Reig et al. list in their review three new risk factors: microparticles, glycoproteins, and leptin [94].

Microparticles—Microparticles (MPs) are a heterogeneous group of submicronic phospholipid vesicles, 0.1–1 μm in size, derived from different cell types including platelets, endothelial cells, leukocytes, and red blood cells besides several other cell types and are found also in normal healthy conditions. They are released from the cytoplasmic membranes during activation or apoptosis [94, 95]. They represent subcellular elements for cell signaling and intracellular communication in inflammation and thrombosis [96] and were found in increased numbers in several prothrombotic conditions such as deep vein thrombosis, pulmonary embolism, and stroke [97]. This proinflammatory attribute is believed to be due to MPs' expression of different anionic phospholipids such as phosphatidylserine [94]. MPs can also be found in increased numbers in normal pregnancy [98, 99] and in complicated pregnancy disorders, mainly severe preeclampsia [100, 101], which was recently discovered to be correlated to RPL in studies on trophoblastic circulating MPs [102, 103].

It is still unclear if this increase in MPs is a cause or consequence of RPL [94].

Glycoproteins—Glycoproteins expressed at the fetal–maternal interface have been shown to have immunomodulating effects. Human chorionic gonadotropin (hCG) and glycodelin (Gd) are glycoproteins secreted in large amounts by the trophoblast or the decidualized endometrium, mainly during the first trimester of pregnancy [104], but in RPL patients both proteins were found to be downregulated [105, 106].

It was found that glycodelin and hCG both inhibit the E-selectin-mediated cell adhesion, so this could indicate a possible role of these proteins in preventing leukocyte adhesion to the fetal trophoblast [107].

hCG—Our understanding of hCG has improved a lot during the last 15 years. Nowadays, we know that hCG consists of two different forms with different actions [108]. We will focus on the new immunological revelations: Lymphocytes from pregnant women express the hCG receptor gene [109]. High hCG levels at very early pregnancy stages ensure regulatory T-cell migration to the fetal–maternal interface, the contact site between paternal antigens and maternal immune cells, where it orchestrates the immunologic tolerance of the fetus [110]. Thus, reduced expression of hCG in patients with recurrent miscarriage affects the process of fetal tolerance.

Leptin—The hormone leptin, a 16 kDa polypeptide, is mainly synthesized and secreted by the white adipose tissue (WAT). Leptin, acting on specific populations of neurons in the brain, including hypothalamic, midbrain, and brainstem neurons, plays a central role in weight control by suppressing food intake and increasing energy expenditure [111–113] and apparently it also plays an important role in reproduction. Mice that have leptin deficiency are infertile, but fertility can be restored by injections of recombinant leptin [114, 115]. Leptin and receptor transcripts were identified in the villous and extravillous trophoblast [116]. Interestingly, Lage et al. showed that a group of women who suffered spontaneous miscarriage showed leptin levels identical to women postpartum, but significantly reduced when compared with the control group and women in the first trimester of pregnancy, and significantly lower than nonpregnant control women. As these women were actually in the first trimester of pregnancy when the miscarriage occurred, higher levels of leptin should be expected [117]. The similar leptin values of post-partum and post-miscarriage groups suggests that leptin seems to be acting as an indicator that the pregnancy process has been stopped, either naturally at term or pathologically some time earlier. Larid et al. suggested that the significantly lower concentration of leptin in women who subsequently miscarried suggests that leptin may play a role in preventing miscarriage [118].

Annexin 5

As mentioned, among the leading candidates for the molecular basis of RPL are various inherited hypercoagulation disorders that promote thrombosis, collectively named "thrombophilias." Among these disorders are carriers of either factor V Leiden (FVL) mutation or the factor 2 (Prothrombin) G20210A (PTm) mutation that have proved by meta-analyses to be association with RPL [7].

Annexin-V is a member of a family of calcium-dependent phospholipid binding proteins [119]. It shows the essential tetrad structure and calcium-dependent phospholipid binding and is one of the few annexins that can be found extracellularly [120]. The annexin-V gene (ANXA5) is located in chromosome 4q27, and has several transcription options [121]. Annexin-V has been isolated from human placenta [122], blood vessels [123], and other sites as well. Annexin-V has anticoagulant activity in vitro, which is based on its high affinity for anionic phospholipids and its capacity to displace coagulation factors from the phospholipid surface [124] and/or its ability to downregulate the cell surface presentation of tissue factor [124].

It seems that Annexin-V forms an antithrombotic shield on the apical surface of placental syncytiotrophoblasts, and that it might be interrupted by antiphospholipid antibodies [125].

Annexin-V and aPL

A well-known major risk factor for RPL is the presence of circulating maternal antiphospholipid antibodies (aPL) [126]. APLA syndrome is marked by vascular thromboembolism or recurrent pregnancy losses, and by evidence for antibodies against anionic phospholipid–protein complexes in the plasma or serum of affected patients. The pathophysiologic pathways of this syndrome are not completely known [127].

Using atomic microscope, it was discovered that in the presence of aPL antibodies and cofactor, structures presumed to be aPL monoclonal antibody–antigen complexes, were associated with varying degrees of disruption to the Annexin-V structure, which is valuable for its anticoagulant activity [128].

Rand et al. [125] revealed that once trophoblasts and endothelial cells were exposed to antiphospholipid-antibody IgG, annexin-V levels were reduced. The antiphospholipid antibodies accelerated the coagulation of plasma on the trophoblasts and endothelial cells. The reduction of Annexin-V levels on vascular cells may be an important pathway in the aPL syndrome.

Annexin-V and RPL

Bogdanova et al. [129] analyzed 70 German RPL patients, all known to carry neither factor V Leiden nor a prothrombin mutation, and found that carriers of genetic variant, haplotype M2, in the ANXA5 gene promoter have two to four times higher risk for RPL compared to two different groups of noncarriers. Apparently M2 haplotype reduces the in vitro activity of the ANXA5 promoter to 37–42 % of the normal range.

Additionally, carrying the M2 haplotype of the ANAX5 gene was also found to be associated with delivering small-for-gestational age newborns [130].

Miyamura et al. [131] genotyped 243 Japanese women who suffered from RPL and 119 fertile control women for 4 ANXA5 gene promoter polymorphisms. Very similar to the M2 haplotype for Western women, one haplotype was found at a significantly greater frequency in RPL women than in the control group. Homozygotes of the SNP5 minor allele were more frequent in the RPL group ($p=0.02$), and this genotype conferred a sevenfold higher risk of RPL (OR = 7.76). These observations give rise to the thought that variations in the ANAX5 gene leading to Annexin-V structural change, or to its reduced expression, could be responsible for the immunological and hemostatic phenomena that, together, lead to fetal loss. Annexin-V is a potent anticoagulant that serves a thrombo-modulatory function in the placental circulation. One explanation might be that decreased expression of Annexin-V on the surface of the trophoblast might result in inefficient phospholipid shielding and hence in a potential enrichment of antigenic determinants, leading to aPL generation. Another explanation is that even in the absence of aPL, reduced expression of Annexin-V can cause a hypercoagulable state in the intervillous placental space [129]. Annexin-V might act as a genetic marker for RPL, taking us one step further in understanding and preventing RPL.

References

1. Christiansen OB, et al. Multifactorial etiology of recurrent miscarriage and its scientific and clinical implications. Gynecol Obstet Invest. 2008;66(4):257–67.
2. Stephenson M. Frequency of factors associated with habitual abortion in 197 couples. Fertil Steril. 1996;66(1):24–9.
3. Nielsen HS, Christiansen OB. Prognostic impact of anticardiolipin antibodies in women with recurrent miscarriage negative for the lupus anticoagulant. Hum Reprod. 2005;20(6):1720–8.
4. Creasy R. The cytogenetics of spontaneous abortion in humans. Early pregnancy loss. London: Springer; 1988. p. 293–304.
5. Bellver J, et al. Obesity and poor reproductive outcome: the potential role of the endometrium. Fertil Steril. 2007;88(2):446–51.
6. Homburg R. Pregnancy complications in PCOS. Best Pract Res Clin Endocrinol Metab. 2006;20(2):281–92.
7. Rey E, et al. Thrombophilic disorders and fetal loss: a meta-analysis. Lancet. 2003;361(9361):901–8.
8. Robertson L, et al. Thrombophilia in pregnancy: a systematic review. Br J Haematol. 2006;132(2):171–96.
9. Hattersley AT, McCarthy MI. What makes a good genetic association study? Lancet. 2005;366(9493):1315–23.
10. Hviid T, et al. Association between human leukocyte antigen-G genotype and success of in vitro fertilization and pregnancy outcome. Tissue Antigens. 2004;64(1):66–9.
11. Kruse C, et al. A study of HLA-DR and-DQ alleles in 588 patients and 562 controls confirms that HLA-DRB1* 03 is associated with recurrent miscarriage. Hum Reprod. 2004;19(5):1215–21.
12. Christiansen OB, et al. Association between HLA-DR1 and-DR3 antigens and unexplained repeated miscarriage. Hum Reprod Update. 1999;5(3):249–55.
13. Rull K, Nagirnaja L, Laan M. Genetics of recurrent miscarriage: challenges, current knowledge, future directions. Front Genet. 2012;3:34.
14. Topalidou M, et al. Low protein Z levels, but not the intron F G79A polymorphism, are associated with unexplained pregnancy loss. Thromb Res. 2009;124(1):24–7.

15. Iinuma Y, et al. Coagulation factor XII activity, but not an associated common genetic polymorphism (46C/T), is linked to recurrent miscarriage. Fertil Steril. 2002;77(2):353–6.

16. Cha J, Sun X, Dey SK. Mechanisms of implantation: strategies for successful pregnancy. Nat Med. 2012;18(12):1754–67.

17. Horcajadas J, Pellicer A, Simon C. Wide genomic analysis of human endometrial receptivity: new times, new opportunities. Hum Reprod Update. 2007;13(1):77–86.

18. Macklon NS, Geraedts JP, Fauser BC. Conception to ongoing pregnancy: the "black box" of early pregnancy loss. Hum Reprod Update. 2002;8(4):333–43.

19. Ledbetter DH. Chaos in the embryo. Nat Med. 2009;15(5):490–1.

20. Gellersen B, Brosens IA, Brosens JJ. Decidualization of the human endometrium: mechanisms, functions, and clinical perspectives. Semin Reprod Med. 2007;25(6):445–53.

21. Teklenburg G, et al. The molecular basis of recurrent pregnancy loss: impaired natural embryo selection. Mol Hum Reprod. 2010;16(12):886–95.

22. Teklenburg G, et al. Natural selection of human embryos: decidualizing endometrial stromal cells serve as sensors of embryo quality upon implantation. PLoS One. 2010;5(4):e10258.

23. Wilcox AJ, Baird DD, Weinberg CR. Time of implantation of the conceptus and loss of pregnancy. N Engl J Med. 1999;340(23):1796–9.

24. Serle E, et al. Endometrial differentiation in the peri-implantation phase of women with recurrent miscarriage: a morphological and immunohistochemical study. Fertil Steril. 1994;62(5):989–96.

25. Aplin J, Hey N, Li T. MUC1 as a cell surface and secretory component of endometrial epithelium: reduced levels in recurrent miscarriage. Am J Reprod Immunol. 1996;35(3):261–6.

26. Hey N, et al. MUC1 in secretory phase endometrium: expression in precisely dated biopsies and flushings from normal and recurrent miscarriage patients. Hum Reprod. 1995;10(10):2655–62.

27. Salker M, et al. Natural selection of human embryos: impaired decidualization of endometrium disables embryo-maternal interactions and causes recurrent pregnancy loss. PLoS One. 2010;5(4):e10287.

28. Weimar CH, et al. Endometrial stromal cells of women with recurrent miscarriage fail to discriminate between high-and low-quality human embryos. PLoS One. 2012;7(7):e41424.

29. Evers JL. Female subfertility. Lancet. 2002;360(9327):151–9.

30. Tietze C, Guttmacher AF, Rubin S. Time required for conception in 1727 planned pregnancies. Fertil Steril. 1950;1(4):338.

31. Brosens JJ, Gellersen B. Something new about early pregnancy: decidual biosensoring and natural embryo selection. Ultrasound Obstet Gynecol. 2010;36(1):1–5.

32. WHO. Model list of essential medicines. In: World Health Organization. World Health Organization; 2014.

33. Tyrrell DJ, Kilfeather S, Page CP. Therapeutic uses of heparin beyond its traditional role as an anticoagulant. Trends Pharmacol Sci. 1995;16(6):198–204.

34. Marcum J, et al. Anticoagulantly active heparin-like molecules from mast cell-deficient mice. Am J Physiol. 1986;250(5):H879–88.

35. Quaranta M, et al. The physiologic and therapeutic role of heparin in implantation and placentation. PeerJ. 2015;2:e691.

36. Staun-Ram E, et al. Expression and importance of matrix metalloproteinase 2 and 9 (MMP-2 and -9) in human trophoblast invasion. Reprod Biol Endocrinol. 2004;2:59.

37. Di Simone N, et al. Low-molecular-weight heparins induce decidual heparin-binding epidermal growth factor-like growth factor expression and promote survival of decidual cells undergoing apoptosis. Fertil Steril. 2012;97(1):169–77 e1.

38. D'Ippolito S, et al. Emerging nonanticoagulant role of low molecular weight heparins on extravillous trophoblast functions and on heparin binding-epidermal growth factor and cystein-rich angiogenic inducer 61 expression. Fertil Steril. 2012;98(4):1028–36 e1-2.

39. Hills FA, et al. Heparin prevents programmed cell death in human trophoblast. Mol Hum Reprod. 2006;12(4):237–43.

40. Jauniaux E, et al. Trophoblastic oxidative stress in relation to temporal and regional differences in maternal placental blood flow in normal and abnormal early pregnancies. Am J Pathol. 2003;162(1):115–25.

41. Wang X-F, et al. Low molecular weight heparin relieves experimental colitis in mice by downregulating IL-1β and inhibiting syndecan-1 shedding in the intestinal mucosa. PLoS One. 2013;8(7):e66397.

42. Black SC, et al. Cardioprotective effects of heparin or N-acetylheparin in an in vivo model of myocardial ischaemic and reperfusion injury. Cardiovasc Res. 1995;29(5):629–36.

43. Preuss JM, Page CP. Effect of heparin on antigen-induced airway responses and pulmonary leukocyte accumulation in neonatally immunized rabbits. Br J Pharmacol. 2000;129(8):1585–96.

44. Ahmed T, Garrigo J, Danta I. Preventing bronchoconstriction in exercise-induced asthma with inhaled heparin. N Engl J Med. 1993;329(2):90–5.

45. Evans R, et al. Treatment of corticosteroid-resistant ulcerative colitis with heparin – a report of 16 cases. Aliment Pharmacol Ther. 1997;11(6):1037–40.

46. Chande N, McDonald JW, MacDonald, JK. Unfractionated or low-molecular weight heparin for induction of remission in ulcerative colitis. Cochrane Database Syst Rev. 2008;2.

47. Brown RA, et al. Additional clinical benefit of enoxaparin in COPD patients receiving salmeterol and fluticasone propionate in combination. Pulm Pharmacol Ther. 2006;19(6):419–24.

48. Thornhill AR, ESHRE PGD Consortium, et al. Best practice guidelines for clinical preimplantation genetic diagnosis (PGD) and preimplantation genetic screening (PGS). Hum Reprod. 2005;20(1):35–48.

49. Brenner B, et al. Efficacy and safety of two doses of enoxaparin in women with thrombophilia and recurrent pregnancy loss: the LIVE-ENOX study. J Thromb Haemost. 2005;3(2):227–9.

50. Pasquier E, et al. Enoxaparin for prevention of unexplained recurrent miscarriage: a multicenter randomized double-blind placebo-controlled trial. Blood. 2015;125(14):2200–5.

51. Kaandorp SP, et al. Aspirin plus heparin or aspirin alone in women with recurrent miscarriage. N Engl J Med. 2010;362(17):1586–96.

52. Warning JC, McCracken SA, Morris JM. A balancing act: mechanisms by which the fetus avoids rejection by the maternal immune system. Reproduction. 2011;141(6):715–24.

53. Vacca P, et al. Origin, phenotype and function of human natural killer cells in pregnancy. Trends Immunol. 2011;32(11):517–23.

54. Raghupathy, Raj. Pregnancy: success and failure within the Th1/Th2/Th3 paradigm. Seminars in immunology. Vol. 13. No. 4. Academic Press, 2001.

55. Chaouat G. The Th1/Th2 paradigm: still important in pregnancy? Seminars in Immunopathol. Vol. 29. No. 2. New York: Springer-Verlag; 2007.

56. Costeas PA, et al. Th2/Th3 cytokine genotypes are associated with pregnancy loss. Hum Immunol. 2004;65(2):135–41.

57. Sones JL, et al. Role of decidual natural killer cells, interleukin-15, and interferon-γ in placental development and preeclampsia. Am J Physiol Regul Integr Comp Physiol. 2014;307(5):R490–2.

58. Fu B, et al. Natural killer cells promote immune tolerance by regulating inflammatory TH17 cells at the human maternal–fetal interface. Proc Natl Acad Sci. 2013;110(3):E231–40.

59. Jerzak M, Bischof P. Apoptosis in the first trimester human placenta: the role in maintaining immune privilege at the maternal-foetal interface and in the trophoblast remodelling. Eur J Obstet Gynecol Reprod Biol. 2002;100(2):138–42.

60. Brogin Moreli J, et al. Interleukin 10 and tumor necrosis factor-alpha in pregnancy: aspects of interest in clinical obstetrics. ISRN Obstet Gynecol. 2012;2012:230742.

61. Gormley M, et al. Maternal decidual macrophages inhibit NK cell killing of invasive cytotrophoblasts during human pregnancy. Biol Reprod. 2013;88(6):155.

62. Robertson SA. GM-CSF regulation of embryo development and pregnancy. Cytokine Growth Factor Rev. 2007;18(3):287–98.

63. Rahmati M, et al. Colony stimulating factors 1, 2, 3 and early pregnancy steps: from bench to bedside. J Reprod Immunol. 2015;109:1–6.

64. Orlando J, Coulam C. Is superfertility associated with recurrent pregnancy loss? Am J Reprod Immunol. 2014;72(6):549–54.

65. Aplin JD. The cell biological basis of human implantation. Best Pract Res Clin Obstet Gynaecol. 2000;14(5):757–64.

66. Weimar CH, et al. The motile and invasive capacity of human endometrial stromal cells: implications for normal and impaired reproductive function. Hum Reprod Update. 2013;19(5):542–57.

67. Bansal AS. Natural killer cells and their activation status in normal pregnancy. Int J Reprod Med. 2013;2013.

68. Hanna J, Mandelboim O. When killers become helpers. Trends Immunol. 2007;28(5):201–6.

69. Moffett-King A. Natural killer cells and pregnancy. Nat Rev Immunol. 2002;2(9):656–63.

70. El Costa H, et al. Critical and differential roles of NKp46-and NKp30-activating receptors expressed by uterine NK cells in early pregnancy. J Immunol. 2008;181(5):3009–17.

71. Hanna J, et al. Decidual NK cells regulate key developmental processes at the human fetal-maternal interface. Nat Med. 2006;12(9):1065–74.

72. Salker MS, et al. Disordered IL-33/ST2 activation in decidualizing stromal cells prolongs uterine receptivity in women with recurrent pregnancy loss. PLoS One. 2012;7(12):e52252.

73. Fock V, et al. Macrophage-derived IL-33 is a critical factor for placental growth. J Immunol. 2013;191(7):3734–43.

74. Hu W-T, et al. Decidual stromal cell-derived IL-33 contributes to Th2 bias and inhibits decidual NK cell cytotoxicity through NF-κB signaling in human early pregnancy. J Reprod Immunol. 2015;109:52–65.

75. Hu W-T, et al. IL-33 enhances proliferation and invasiveness of decidual stromal cells by up-regulation of CCL2/CCR2 via NF-κB and ERK1/2 signaling. Mol Hum Reprod. 2014;20(4):358–72.

76. Rosental B, et al. Proliferating cell nuclear antigen is a novel inhibitory ligand for the natural cytotoxicity receptor NKp44. J Immunol. 2011;187(11):5693–702.

77. Rosental B, et al. A novel mechanism for cancer cells to evade immune attack by NK cells: the interaction between NKp44 and proliferating cell nuclear antigen. Oncoimmunology. 2012;1(4):572–4.

78. Vacca P, et al. Regulatory role of NKp44, NKp46, DNAM-1 and NKG2D receptors in the interaction between NK cells and trophoblast cells. Evidence for divergent functional profiles of decidual versus peripheral NK cells. Int Immunol. 2008;20(11):1395–405.

79. Lash GE, Ernerudh J. Decidual cytokines and pregnancy complications: focus on spontaneous miscarriage. J Reprod Immunol. 2015;108:83–9.

80. Carp H. Cytokines in recurrent miscarriage. Lupus. 2004;13(9):630–4.

81. Fukui A, et al. Correlation between natural cytotoxicity receptors and intracellular cytokine expression of peripheral blood NK cells in women with recurrent pregnancy losses and implantation failures. Am J Reprod Immunol. 2009;62(6):371–80.

82. Shemesh A, et al. First trimester pregnancy loss and the expression of alternatively spliced NKp30 isoforms in maternal blood and placental tissue. Front Immunol. 2015;6:189.

83. Barber EM, Pollard JW. The uterine NK cell population requires IL-15 but these cells are not required for pregnancy nor the resolution of a Listeria monocytogenes infection. J Immunol. 2003;171(1):37–46.

84. Murphy SP, et al. Uterine NK cells mediate inflammation-induced fetal demise in IL-10-null mice. J Immunol. 2005;175(6):4084–90.

85. Sharma S. Natural killer cells and regulatory T cells in early pregnancy loss. Int J Dev Biol. 2014;58:219.

86. Berman J, Girardi G, Salmon JE. TNF-α is a critical effector and a target for therapy in antiphospholipid antibody-induced pregnancy loss. J Immunol. 2005;174(1):485–90.

87. Weinblatt ME, et al. Adalimumab, a fully human anti–tumor necrosis factor α monoclonal antibody, for the treatment of rheumatoid arthritis in patients taking concomitant methotrexate: the ARMADA trial. Arthritis Rheum. 2003;48(1):35–45.

88. Moreland LW, et al. Etanercept therapy in rheumatoid arthritis: a randomized, controlled trial. Ann Intern Med. 1999;130(6):478–86.

89. Winger EE, Reed JL. Treatment with tumor necrosis factor inhibitors and intravenous immunoglobulin improves live birth rates in women with recurrent spontaneous abortion. Am J Reprod Immunol. 2008;60(1):8–16.

90. Winger EE, et al. Treatment with adalimumab (Humira®) and intravenous immunoglobulin improves pregnancy rates in women undergoing IVF*. Am J Reprod Immunol. 2009;61(2):113–20.

91. Würfel W. Treatment with granulocyte colony-stimulating factor in patients with repetitive implantation failures and/or recurrent spontaneous abortions. J Reprod Immunol. 2015;108:123–35.

92. Scarpellini F, Sbracia M. Use of granulocyte colony-stimulating factor for the treatment of unexplained recurrent miscarriage: a randomised controlled trial. Hum Reprod. 2009;24(11):2703–8.

93. Santjohanser C, et al. Granulocyte-colony stimulating factor as treatment option in patients with recurrent miscarriage. Arch Immunol Ther Exp (Warsz). 2013;61(2):159–64.

94. Alijotas-Reig J, Garrido-Gimenez C. Current concepts and new trends in the diagnosis and management of recurrent miscarriage. Obstet Gynecol Surv. 2013;68(6):445–66.

95. Patil R, et al. Elevated procoagulant endothelial and tissue factor expressing microparticles in women with recurrent pregnancy loss. PLoS One. 2013;8(11):e81407.

96. Distler JH, et al. Microparticles as regulators of inflammation: novel players of cellular crosstalk in the rheumatic diseases. Arthritis Rheum. 2005;52(11):3337–48.

97. Zahra S, et al. Microparticles, malignancy and thrombosis. Br J Haematol. 2011;152(6):688–700.

98. Bretelle F, et al. Circulating microparticles: a marker of procoagulant state in normal pregnancy and pregnancy complicated by preeclampsia or intrauterine growth restriction. Thromb Haemost. 2003;89(3):486–92.

99. Alijotas-Reig J, Palacio-Garcia C, Vilardell-Tarres M. Circulating microparticles, lupus anticoagulant and recurrent miscarriages. Eur J Obstet Gynecol Reprod Biol. 2009;145(1):22–6.

100. González-Quintero VH, et al. Elevated plasma endothelial microparticles: preeclampsia versus gestational hypertension. Am J Obstet Gynecol. 2004;191(4):1418–24.

101. Alijotas-Reig J, et al. Circulating cell-derived microparticles in women with pregnancy loss. Am J Reprod Immunol. 2011;66(3):199–208.

102. Kaptan K, et al. Platelet-derived microparticle levels in women with recurrent spontaneous abortion. Int J Gynecol Obstet. 2008;102(3):271–4.

103. Van der Post JA, et al. The functions of microparticles in pre-eclampsia. Seminars in Thrombosis and Hemostasis. Vol. 37. No. 2. 2011.

104. Jeschke U, et al. Stimulation trials of trophoblast cells in vitro using PP14. Z Geburtshilfe Neonatol. 1995;200(5):199–201.

105. Toth B, et al. Glycodelin protein and mRNA is downregulated in human first trimester abortion and partially upregulated in mole pregnancy. J Histochem Cytochem. 2008;56(5):477–85.

106. Salim R, et al. A comparative study of glycodelin concentrations in uterine flushings in women with subseptate uteri, history of unexplained recurrent miscarriage and healthy controls. Eur J Obstet Gynecol Reprod Biol. 2007;133(1):76–80.

107. Jeschke U, et al. Glycodelin and amniotic fluid transferrin as inhibitors of E-selectin-mediated cell adhesion. Histochem Cell Biol. 2003;119(5):345–54.

108. Carp H. Recurrent miscarriage and hCG supplementation: a review and metaanalysis. Gynecol Endocrinol. 2010;26(10):712–6.

109. Lin J, et al. Lymphocytes from pregnant women express human chorionic gonadotropin/luteinizing hormone receptor gene. Mol Cell Endocrinol. 1995;111(1):R13–7.

110. Schumacher A, et al. Human chorionic gonadotropin attracts regulatory T cells into the fetal-maternal interface during early human pregnancy. J Immunol. 2009;182(9):5488–97.

111. Maffei M, et al. Leptin levels in human and rodent: measurement of plasma leptin and ob RNA in obese and weight-reduced subjects. Nat Med. 1995;1:1155–61.

112. Myers MG, et al. Obesity and leptin resistance: distinguishing cause from effect. Trends Endocrinol Metab. 2010;21(11):643–51.

113. Panariello F, et al. The role of leptin in antipsychotic-induced weight gain: genetic and non-genetic factors. J Obes. 2012;2012:572848.

114. Chehab FF, Lim ME, Lu R. Correction of the sterility defect in homozygous obese female mice by treatment with the human recombinant leptin. Nat Genet. 1996;12(3):318–20.

115. Cunningham MJ, Clifton DK, Steiner RA. Leptin's actions on the reproductive axis: perspectives and mechanisms. Biol Reprod. 1999;60(2):216–22.

116. Henson MC, Swan KF, O'Neil JS. Expression of placental leptin and leptin receptor transcripts in early pregnancy and at term. Obstet Gynecol. 1998;92(6):1020–8.

117. Lage M, et al. Serum leptin levels in women through-out pregnancy and the postpartum period and in women suffering spontaneous abortion. Clin Endocrinol (Oxf). 1999;50(2):211–6.

118. Laird S, et al. Leptin and leptin-binding activity in women with recurrent miscarriage: correlation with pregnancy outcome. Hum Reprod. 2001;16(9):2008–13.

119. Cookson BT, et al. Organization of the human annexin V (ANX5) gene. Genomics. 1994;20(3):463–7.

120. Gerke V, Creutz CE, Moss SE. Annexins: linking Ca2+ signalling to membrane dynamics. Nat Rev Mol Cell Biol. 2005;6(6):449–61.

121. CARCEDO M, et al. Functional analysis of the human annexin A5 gene promoter: a downstream DNA element and an upstream long terminal repeat regulate transcription. Biochem J. 2001;356:571–9.

122. Reutelingsperger CP, et al. Purification and charac-terization of a novel protein from bovine aorta that inhibits coagulation. Eur J Biochem. 1988;173(1):171–8.

123. Creutz CE. The annexins and exocytosis. Science. 1992;258(5084):924–31.

124. Ravassa S, et al. Annexin A5 down-regulates surface expression of tissue factor a novel mechanism of regulating the membrane receptor repertoir. J Biol Chem. 2005;280(7):6028–35.

125. Rand JH, et al. Pregnancy loss in the antiphospholipid-antibody syndrome – a possible thrombogenic mechanism. N Engl J Med. 1997;337(3):154–60.

126. Empson M, et al. Recurrent pregnancy loss with antiphospholipid antibody: a systematic review of therapeutic trials. Obstet Gynecol. 2002;99(1):135–44.

127. Rand JH. Antiphospholipid antibody-mediated dis-ruption of the annexin-V antithrombotic shield: a thrombogenic mechanism for the antiphospholipid syndrome. J Autoimmun. 2000;15(2):107–11.

128. Rand JH, et al. Human monoclonal antiphospholipid antibodies disrupt the annexin A5 anticoagulant crystal shield on phospholipid bilayers: evidence from atomic force microscopy and functional assay. Am J Pathol. 2003;163(3):1193–200.

129. Bogdanova N, et al. A common haplotype of the annexin A5 (ANXA5) gene promoter is associated with recurrent pregnancy loss. Hum Mol Genet. 2007;16(5):573–8.

130. Tiscia G, et al. Haplotype M2 in the annexin A5 (ANXA5) gene and the occurrence of obstetric com-plications. Thromb Haemost. 2009;102(2):309–13.

131. Miyamura H, et al. Polymorphisms in the annexin A5 gene promoter in Japanese women with recurrent pregnancy loss. Mol Hum Reprod. 2011;17(7):447–52.

132. Diamond MS, et al. Heparin is an adhesive ligand for the leukocyte integrin Mac-1 (CD11b/CD1). J Cell Biol. 1995;130(6):1473–82.

133. Koenig A, et al. Differential interactions of heparin and heparan sulfate glycosaminoglycans with the selectins. Implications for the use of unfractionated and low molecular weight heparins as therapeutic agents. J Clin Invest. 1998;101(4):877.

134. Skinner MP, et al. GMP-140 binding to neutrophils is inhibited by sulfated glycans. J Biol Chem. 1991;266(9):5371–4.

135. Revelle BM, Scott D, Beck PJ. Single amino acid residues in the E-and P-selectin epidermal growth factor domains can determine carbohydrate binding specificity. J Biol Chem. 1996;271(27):16160–70.

136. Ley K, Cerrito M, Arfors K-E. Sulfated polysaccha-rides inhibit leukocyte rolling in rabbit mesentery venules. Am J Physiol. 1991;260(5):H1667–73.

137. Tyrrell DJ, et al. Heparin in inflammation: potential therapeutic applications beyond anticoagulation. Adv Pharmacol. 1999;46:151–208.

138. Petitou M, et al. Synthesis of thrombin-inhibiting heparin mimetics without side effects. Nature. 1999;398(6726):417–22.

139. Tabeur C, et al. Oligosaccharides corresponding to the regular sequence of heparin: chemical synthesis and interaction with FGF-2. Bioorg Med Chem. 1999;7(9):2003–12.

140. Lundin L, et al. Selectively desulfated heparin inhibits fibroblast growth factor-induced mitogenicity and angiogenesis. J Biol Chem. 2000;275(32):24653–60.

141. Fath MA, et al. Interaction of secretory leukocyte protease inhibitor with heparin inhibits proteases involved in asthma. J Biol Chem. 1998;273(22):13563–9.

142. Darien BJ, et al. Low molecular weight heparin pre-vents the pulmonary hemodynamic and pathomor-phologic effects of endotoxin in a porcine acute lung injury model. Shock. 1998;9(4):274–81.

143. Li L-F, et al. Unfractionated heparin and enoxaparin reduce high-stretch ventilation augmented lung injury: a prospective, controlled animal experiment. Crit Care. 2009;13(4):R108.

144. Kennedy T. Use of heparin to inhibit interleukin-8. International patent application, WO94/18989, 1994.

145. Gaffney A, Gaffney P. Rheumatoid arthritis and hep-arin. Rheumatology. 1996;35(8):808–9.

146. Lilly JD, Parsons CL. Bladder surface glycosamino-glycans is a human epithelial permeability barrier. Surg Gynecol Obstet. 1990;171(6):493–6.

147. Parsons CL. Epithelial coating techniques in the treatment of interstitial cystitis. Urology. 1997;49(5):100–4.

Index

A

Acquired thrombophilias, 70, 71. *See also* Inherited thrombophilias
Acquired uterine structural malformations
  intrauterine adhesions, 104, 105
  myomas, 102, 103
  uterine polyps, 104
Activated partial thromboplastin time (aPTT), 156
Advanced maternal age (AMA), 5, 10, 13, 60, 61
Alcohol
  behavioural effects, 137
  growth restriction, 137
  neurological effects, 137
  pregnancy failure, 137
  recurrent miscarriage, 138
AMA. *See* Advanced maternal age (AMA)
Annexin A5, 161
Annexin-V and aPL, 197, 198
Annexin-V and RPL
  ANAX5 gene, 198
  fetal loss, 198
  prothrombin mutation, 198
  SNP5 minor allele, 198
Antinuclear antibody (ANA), 76, 157
Antiphospholipid antibodies (aPLs), 13, 67, 156, 157, 197, 198
Antiphospholipid syndrome (APS)
  aCL, 156
  acquired thrombophilia, 12
  ANA, 157
  aPLs, aPTT and RVVT, 156
  assays, 156, 157
  β2GPI, 156
  cutoff value, 156
  diagnosis, 155
  gestation, 157
  incidence, 156
  inherited thrombophilia and antinuclear antibodies, 157
  LA, 156
  live birth rate, 157
  murine model, 196
  phospholipid-binding plasma proteins, 157
  RPL, 156

APS. *See* Antiphospholipid syndrome (APS)
Autoantibodies
  ANA, 76
  autoimmune diseases, 76, 83
  cytokines, 76, 77
  MBL, 77
  NK cells, 77–79
  T regulatory (Treg), 79

B

Basic evaluation tests, 145
β2glycoprotein I (β2GPI), 156, 157
Bicornuate uterus, 10, 97, 98, 101, 102
Biomarkers
  microRNAs, 57
  couples/placenta, 186
  DNA-based tests, 83
  genetics, 186
  polymorphisms, 186
  RPL, 75

C

Caffeine
  environmental factors, 13
  foetal cell growth, 135–136
  pregnancy, 136
  teratogenic effect, 135
  toxicity, 135
Cardiovascular and respiratory disease, 134
Chromosomal micro array (CMA), 56, 59, 60
Cigarette smoking
  death syndrome, 137
  nicotine, 137
  toxic components, 136
CMA. *See* Chromosomal micro array (CMA)
Cognitive Behavior Therapy (CBT), 171–173
Congenital uterine anomaly
  bicornuate/septate uterus, 158
  chromosomal karyotype rates, 158
  classification, 98
  defect/cavity ratio, 158
  3D ultrasound, 92

© Springer International Publishing Switzerland 2016
A. Bashiri et al. (eds.), *Recurrent Pregnancy Loss*, DOI 10.1007/978-3-319-27452-2_5